The Mechanical Vibration: Therapeutic Effects and Applications

Edited by:

Raoul Saggini

Physical and Rehabilitation Medicine, Department of Medical
Oral and Biotechnological Sciences Director of the School of Specialty
in Physical and Rehabilitation Medicine, "Gabriele d'Annunzio" University,
Chieti-Pescara, Italy
National Coordinator of Schools of Specialty in Physical and
Rehabilitation Medicine

General:

1. Any dispute or claim arising out of or in connection with this License Agreement or the Work (including non-contractual disputes or claims) will be governed by and construed in accordance with the laws of the U.A.E. as applied in the Emirate of Dubai. Each party agrees that the courts of the Emirate of Dubai shall have exclusive jurisdiction to settle any dispute or claim arising out of or in connection with this License Agreement or the Work (including non-contractual disputes or claims).
2. Your rights under this License Agreement will automatically terminate without notice and without the need for a court order if at any point you breach any terms of this License Agreement. In no event will any delay or failure by Bentham Science Publishers in enforcing your compliance with this License Agreement constitute a waiver of any of its rights.
3. You acknowledge that you have read this License Agreement, and agree to be bound by its terms and conditions. To the extent that any other terms and conditions presented on any website of Bentham Science Publishers conflict with, or are inconsistent with, the terms and conditions set out in this License Agreement, you acknowledge that the terms and conditions set out in this License Agreement shall prevail.

Bentham Science Publishers Ltd.
Executive Suite Y - 2
PO Box 7917, Saif Zone
Sharjah, U.A.E.
Email: subscriptions@benthamscience.org

**BENTHAM
SCIENCE**

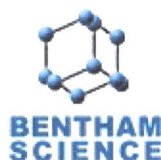

CONTENTS

FOREWORD

Vibrations. Good vibes. Bad vibes. Too much of vibes. Not enough of them. When I first heard of vibrations, I was in my teens, and it was all about the good vibes coming from great music bands. After that, as an orthopaedic trainee, I was taught that vibrations were bad: helicopter pilots and truck drivers were exposed to exactly the kind of vibrations which induced asynchronous contractions of the back muscles, and had direct deleterious effects on the vertebral discs. The result includes low back pain and osteoarthritis of the lumbar spine. Following this, somebody had the great idea to test vibrations in clinical practice. Lo and behold, some science was injected into vibration science, and it was found that if too much is not too good (actually, it is pretty bad), a measured amount of the right kind of vibration can bring good. Prof. Saggini has been on the forefront of this "good vibes movement".

Prof. Saggini is a thoughtful, skilled clinician, armed with foresight and rigour. He started observing and experimenting, and has been able to produce much of the present day scientific evidence on this fascinating topic. "Mechanical vibration: therapeutic effects and applications" show, as Prof. Saggini would say, that "nothing rests". Indeed, we are moving all the time, and vibration is at the centre of our life.

Progressing from the basic sciences of vibration, the scene is set for clinical applications, in a variety of forms. The truth, however, is that: this edition of "Mechanical vibration: therapeutic effects and applications", provides the beginning, and, through the strict scientific work that Prof. Saggini will continue to perform, more truth will come out of it.

Enjoy!

Nicola Maffulli
School of Medicine Surgery and Dentistry, University of Salerno
Italy

PREFACE

Current evidence shows that the entire Universe vibrates; gravitational waves may be regarded as ripples in the curvature of space-time propagating in an oscillatory fashion and travelling outward from the source.

Any given complex body is capable of vibrating in several different ways, each one being characterized by its own frequency.

The inorganic matter is made up of atoms that are in a constant state of motion; depending on the atomic speed, inorganic matter will exist in a solid, liquid, or gaseous state. By the same token, the human body is made up of atoms in continuous vibration, the latter being necessary for the homeostatic maintenance of the organism.

Several essential cellular processes, including cytoskeleton activity, enzymatic reactions, chromosome packaging and replication, nucleic acids transcription and translation, and protein folding and unfolding, generate forces resulting in intracellular movement. For instance, protein polar oscillation during cell division and cytoskeleton assembly greatly contribute to such intracellular dynamics by generating polarizing ionic currents and charge-induced nanoscale movements. The net effect of these events is the vibration of the entire cell and its components.

It is currently thought that the transduction of intracellular movements allows the cell to emit vibration waves carrying information about intracellular metabolic status. The latter mirrors the energy internal to the cell, being the proportional to intensity and frequency of the ensuing vibrations.

Mechanotransduction analysis assesses the causal relationship between mechanical forces, intracellular signaling, and subsequent changes in cell behavior. Indeed, mechanical forces seem to play a crucial role in several aspects of living tissues, including organization, growth, maturation, and normal functioning.

Physical signals are known to travel faster than signaling through chemical mediators, the latter being limited by dependence on diffusion. Accordingly, physical signals appear to represent a more effective way of cell signaling whenever a rapid response is required.

The human body is constantly subjected to vibrations deriving from the surrounding environment, including sources such as industrial machinery as well as common means of transport (terrestrial, nautical, and aerial). Overall, such vibrations may be viewed as different forms of the same primitive mechanical oscillation – *i.e.*, endless "variations on the theme" acting at both the macroscopic and the microscopic level. Any vibration or oscillation will induce a tuning response by the cell through changes in signal transduction, resulting in potentially healthy (therapeutic) or adverse effects. Indeed, to quote Paracelsus, «*Omnia venenum sunt: nec sine veneno quicquam existit. Dosis sola facit, ut venenum non fit*».

In sum, it appears indisputable that nothing rests: everything surrounding the human body vibrates at an exclusive frequency, and so does the human body. Accordingly, it seems crucial to develop a deeper understanding of the physical parameters of vibration (amplitude, frequency, direction of the stimulation, and duration of the exposure), as well as to gain better knowledge regarding ways to modulate vibrations in order to improve body homeostasis by means of:

• relief of pain and pathological inflammation, both acute and chronic;
• bone and soft tissues regeneration, and musculoskeletal functional improvement;
• amelioration of common neurological diseases, including motor impairment.

My hope in writing this book is to clarify further the medical role of vibrations in improving human health.

Raoul Saggini
Physical and Rehabilitation Medicine
Department of Medical Oral and Biotechnological Sciences
School of Specialty in Physical and Rehabilitation Medicine
"Gabriele d'Annunzio" University, Chieti-Pescara
Italy

ACKNOWLEDGEMENTS

My sincere thanks to all co-authors, Nicola Maffulli for the Foreword, my wife Susanna Morici Saggini whose constant encouragement and sustain my life.

The excellent staff of Bentham Science Publishers.

ABOUT THE EDITOR

Professor Raoul Saggini was born in 1953 in Florence, where he graduated in Medicine and Surgery in 1979. Later he specialized in Orthopedics and Traumatology, Physical and Rehabilitation Medicine, Sports Medicine, always obtaining the highest grades and honors.

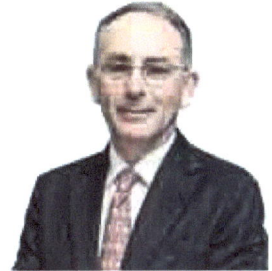

At the University of Florence, Institute of Orthopedic Clinic, he performed activities initially as intern (1979-'81) and later as an Assistant Professor. In this period he carried out scientific activities taking care of foot surgery, orthopedic aspects of some genetic diseases and knee arthroscopic diagnostics. In 1986-'90, at the Institute of Orthopedic Clinic of the University of Florence, and in collaboration with the Institute of Orthopedic Clinic of the Catholic University of the Sacred Heart in Rome, he carried out scientific activities concerning the field of biomechanics of the human body movement and study of gait analysis.

Since 1991, he has continued the academic research and teaching at the "Gabriele d'Annunzio" University of Chieti-Pescara, Italy. Today in the same University he is Full Professor, President of the degree course in Physiotherapy, and the Director of the School of Specialty in Physical and Rehabilitation Medicine.

He is also a permanent member of the National Commission for the Degree Courses in Physiotherapy, and National Coordinator of Schools of Specialty in Physical and Rehabilitation Medicine, as well as Coordinator of the Rehabilitation in Sport sector of the Italian Society of Physical and Rehabilitation Medicine (SIMFER), and former President of the Italian Society of Shock Wave Therapy (SITOD).

The current research activity ranges from posture and applied body dynamics, treatment of acute and chronic overload diseases of foot and trunk and musculoskeletal pain syndromes, to rehabilitation approaches during cancer treatment and therapeutic aspects of major neurological disabilities. Furthermore, in the field of research on advanced physical therapies and applications on human body to create an increase in homeostasis during the pathological state.

List of Contributors

Andrea Saggini Dermatology Specialist Anatomic Pathology, Department of Biomedicine and Prevention, University of Rome Tor Vergata, Rome, Italy

Elisabetta Giuliani International Commission for Electromagnetic Safety (ICEMS), Venice, Italy

Emilio Ancona School of Specialty in Physical and Rehabilitation Medicine, "Gabriele d'Annunzio" University, Chieti-Pescara, Italy

Enrico Corsetti Research and Development Unit Director, "Salvator Mundi International Hospital", Rome, Italy

Livio Giuliani International Commission for Electromagnetic Safety (ICEMS), Venice, Italy Istituto per la Medicina Molecolare "Giuliano Preparata" SCE, Rome-Copenhagen Manuela Lucarelli International Commission for Electromagnetic Safety (ICEMS), Venice, Italy Istituto Nazionale per l'Assicurazione contro gli Infortuni sul Lavoro e le malattie professionali (INAIL), Rome-Copenhagen, Italy

Maria Cristina D'Agostino Head of Shock Waves Therapy and Research Centre, Humanitas Research Hospital, Adjunct Professor, "Humanitas" University, Rozzano, Italy

Michele Casciani Chief Executive Officer, "Salvator Mundi International Hospital", Rome, Italy

Manuela Lucarelli International Commission for Electromagnetic Safety (ICEMS), Venice, Italy Istituto Nazionale per l'Assicurazione contro gli Infortuni sul Lavoro e le malattie professionali (INAIL), Rome, Italy

Raoul Saggini Physical and Rehabilitation Medicine, Department of Medical Oral and Biotechnological Sciences, Director of the School of Specialty in Physical and Rehabilitation Medicine, "Gabriele d'Annunzio" University , Chieti-Pescara, Italy National Coordinator of Schools of Specialty in Physical and Rehabilitation Medicine,

Rosa Grazia Bellomo Physical and Rehabilitation Medicine, Department of Medical Oral and Biotechnological Sciences, "Gabriele d'Annunzio" University, Chieti-Pescara, Italy

Simona Maria Carmignano School of Specialty in Physical and Rehabilitation Medicine , "Gabriele d'Annunzio" University, Chieti-Pescara, Italy

The Mechanical Vibration: Therapeutic Effects and Applications

2

The Mechanical Vibration: Therapeutic Effects and Applications

Editor: Raoul Saggini

eISBN (Online): 978-1-68108-508-1

ISBN (Print): 978-1-68108-509-8

© 2017, Bentham eBooks imprint.

Published by Bentham Science Publishers – Sharjah, UAE. All Rights Reserved.

First published in 2017.

CHAPTER 1

The Study of Vibrations: Mathematical Modelling and Classifications

Enrico Corsetti[*] and **Michele Casciani**

"Salvator Mundi International Hospital", Rome Italy

Abstract: The matter is made up of particles, firmly assembled, as in the solids, or rarefied, as in the gases. When a force acts on a particle it moves determining different physical phenomena depending on the different characteristics of that particle and the surrounding ones.-This model represents the action of a blast or a mechanical pulse, just one hit and the system can manage the supplied energy by damping and distributing it.

Each system has a specific behavior, mainly depending on the frequency of the stressing force; if the system has a frequency of resonance whose value is close to the frequency of the stressing force, energy is stored in the system, movements of the particles become larger and, at the end of the energy supply, the system continues to oscillate, giving back the stored energy, implying that the longer the oscillation the lower is the damping.

The vibration of a physical system can propagate the movement through a vibrational wave, generated by the application of external forces generating internal stress, strain and reaction, a *disturbance* that travels through a medium from one place to another like a wave. When the vibration is forced by a mechanical system, the stimulus can be applied in order to generate a different kind of vibration. In order to generate a vibration, it is necessary to apply an external force: however, the response of a mechanical system to an external force can vary not only depending on the nature of the stimulus, but also according to the composition of the system itself. The mathematical model of a vibration system may take the form of acoustic waves.

Keywords: Mathematical modelling, Matter, Vibrations, Ways of propagation.

Matter is made up of particles, tightly assembled, as in the solid, or rarefied, as in the gases. When a force acts on a particle, it moves it, but the other particles of the whole system try to limit its movement, propagating its momentum in the same

[*] **Corresponding authors Enrico Corsetti:** Research and Development Unit Director "Salvator Mundi International Hospital", Rome Italy; Tel: +39 06 588961; Fax: +39 06 58896 023; E-mail: e.corsetti@salvatormundi.it

Raoul Saggini (Ed.)

direction of the acting force (transmission), distributing its momentum among the other particles (absorption), degrading its phase and propagation direction (diffraction) or bouncing it back (reflection) [1] (Fig. **1**).

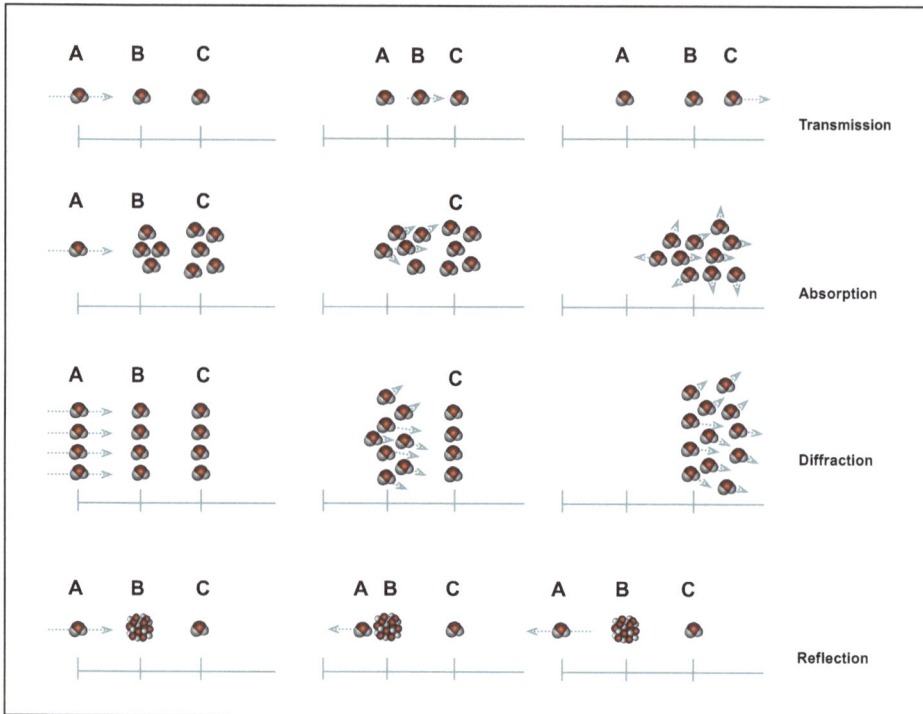

Fig. (1). Energy distribution of the whole system when a force acts on a particle.

This model is the action of a gust of wind or mechanical impulse, one shot and the system can handle the energy provided by damping and distribution.

If the force is applied for a duration longer than the time of strain it decays and if it is, eventually, variable in time, the system can react and store part of the supplied energy, starting a vibrational movement/strain variable in time. From an energy perspective, in a time longer than decay time, the supplied energy is equal to the distributed energy.

Each system has a specific behavior, mainly depending on the frequency of the stressing force (harmonic oscillation); if the resonance frequency of the system has a value which is near to the frequency of the stressing force, energy is stored in the system. So the movements of the particles become larger and, as the energy supply stops, the system continues to oscillate, and releases the energy previously stored, implying that the longer the oscillation is the lower the damping.

Matter transmits variable applied oscillating forces, through propagating waves, and it is able to store part of the supplied energy as static waves: the latter are good for resonators in order to reach a sharp frequency, a larger and steady amplitude, a phase variation, but are not good when the medium has to transfer energy, *i.e.* when the medium is a feeder.

In the latter case, resonances must be avoided either by increasing the propagation resistance (absorption related to damping) or keeping the transmitted signals away from resonance situations.

A mechanical vibration is a periodic back-and-forth motion of the particles of an elastic body or medium (*i.e.* with a mass and volume). The phenomenon occurs when the physical system is displaced from its equilibrium condition and responds to the stimulation with an internal motion that tends to restore equilibrium.

This general assumption has to be completed with the consideration that the medium has an elastic behaviour; this means that the particles in the solid can periodically and symmetrically oscillate around their position of a small Δx ($\Delta x = x_f - x_i$, where x_f is the final position and x_i is the initial position). The possible change in the solid position and shape generates a reaction force which is able to restore the original configuration.

Whereas the elastic behaviour releases all the energy stored by the body deformation, plastic behaviour keeps part of the deformation/strain permanently and releases only part of the supplied energy.

In physical systems, only small forces/strains/displacements can be considered as elastic.

The vibration of a physical system can propagate the movement through a vibrational wave, which is generated by the application of external forces generating internal stress, strain and reaction, a disturbance that travels through a medium from one place to another like a wave.

Vibrations can be divided into two main categories: free and forced. Free vibrations occur when the system is transiently disturbed by an external force (such as an impulse) and then allowed to move without restraint. A classic example is the mass-spring system. In the equilibrium position, the system has minimum energy and the mass is at rest. If an impulsive force is applied to the mass, the system will respond with a periodic vibration around the initial position, and in case of a damped system, the mass will tend to return to the equilibrium position of minimum potential energy with smaller and smaller displacements.

Mechanical waves transport energy as they travel through the medium, but they do not carry any matter along with them.

Forced vibrations occur if a system is continuously driven by an external force. Considering the above example, if the force applied to the mass is a function of time, the resulting oscillation of the system will be dependant by this force and by the geometrical characteristics of the mass-spring system. The forced signal can be generated by some kind of sources, such as acoustic wave generators, laser generators and mechanical vibrators.

An acoustic wave is a particular kind of vibration that propagates through a longitudinal wave, that consists of a sequence of pressure pulses or elastic displacements of the medium where the wave propagates (as exposed below).

Sound waves need to travel through a medium such as a solid, liquid, or gas. In gases and liquids, the wave is transmitted through a sequence of compressions (dense fluid) and rarefactions (less dense fluid) The sound waves move through each of these mediums by vibrating the molecules in the matter. The molecules in solids are packed very tightly. Liquids are not packed as tightly as solids, gases are very loosely packed. The spacing of the molecules enables sound to travel much faster through a solid than a gas. Sound travels about four times faster and farther in water than it does in air (Fig. **2**).

The frequency of an acoustic wave is the number of times the wave reaches its maximum in a second. Frequency is measured in Hertz; a snapshot of a travelling wave would show many crests and troughs; the distance between two crests is the wavelength.

Audible sounds are within the range of 20 – 20.000 Hertz, about 10 octaves: sounds below 20 Hertz are called infrasound, (air resonance, earthquake, beat), sounds above 20.000 Hertz are called ultrasounds (Figs. **3, 4**).

Ultrasounds with very high frequency (f > 3 MHz) are used in diagnostic imaging, as they generate echo images of reflected waves; high density structures (bones) generate neat and sharp echoes, while soft tissues generate low or no echoes.

The pressure wave has an elastic behaviour while the pressure variation is little compared to the medium pressure.

If there is a variation in the pressure, which is comparable to medium pressure, then the medium cannot be considered as elastic. At sea level (0.1 MPa) a wave of

10 Pa amplitude acts like a wave, whereas a 1 MPa amplitude blast creates asymmetric pulses made of steep high pressure peaks and long vacuum intervals (Fig. **5**).

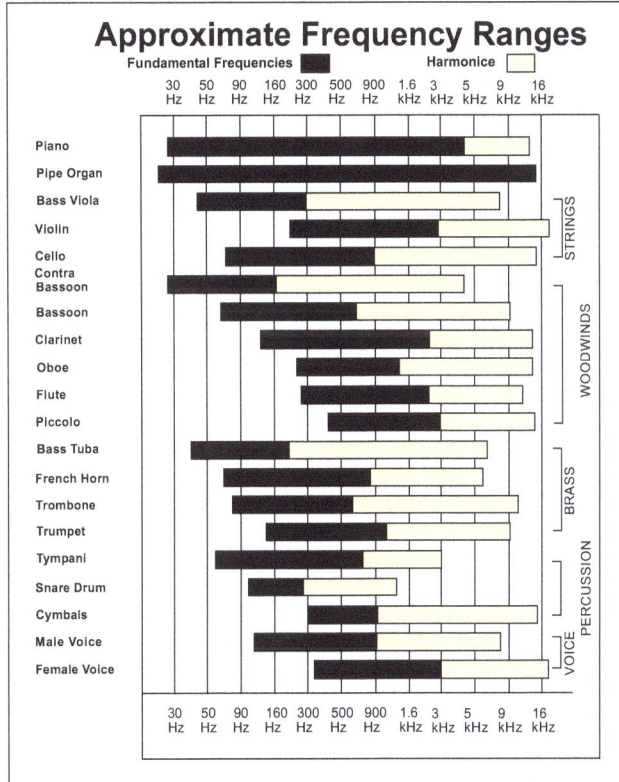

Fig. (2). Frequency range of musical instruments. From: http://www.dak.com.

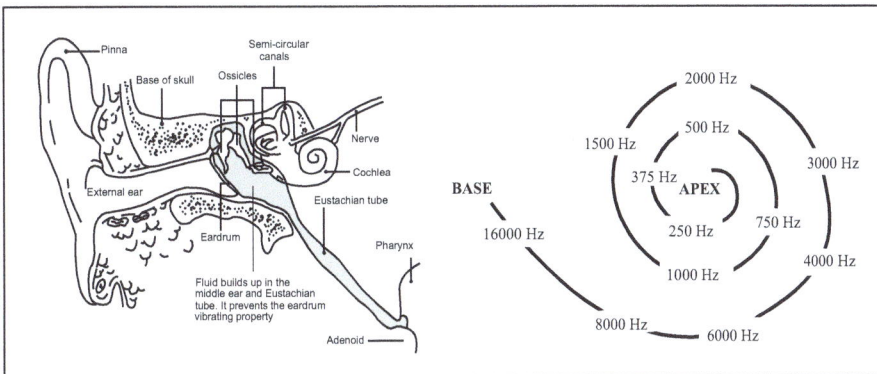

Fig. (3). Audible sound frequencies. From: http://patient.info/health/perforated-eardrum.

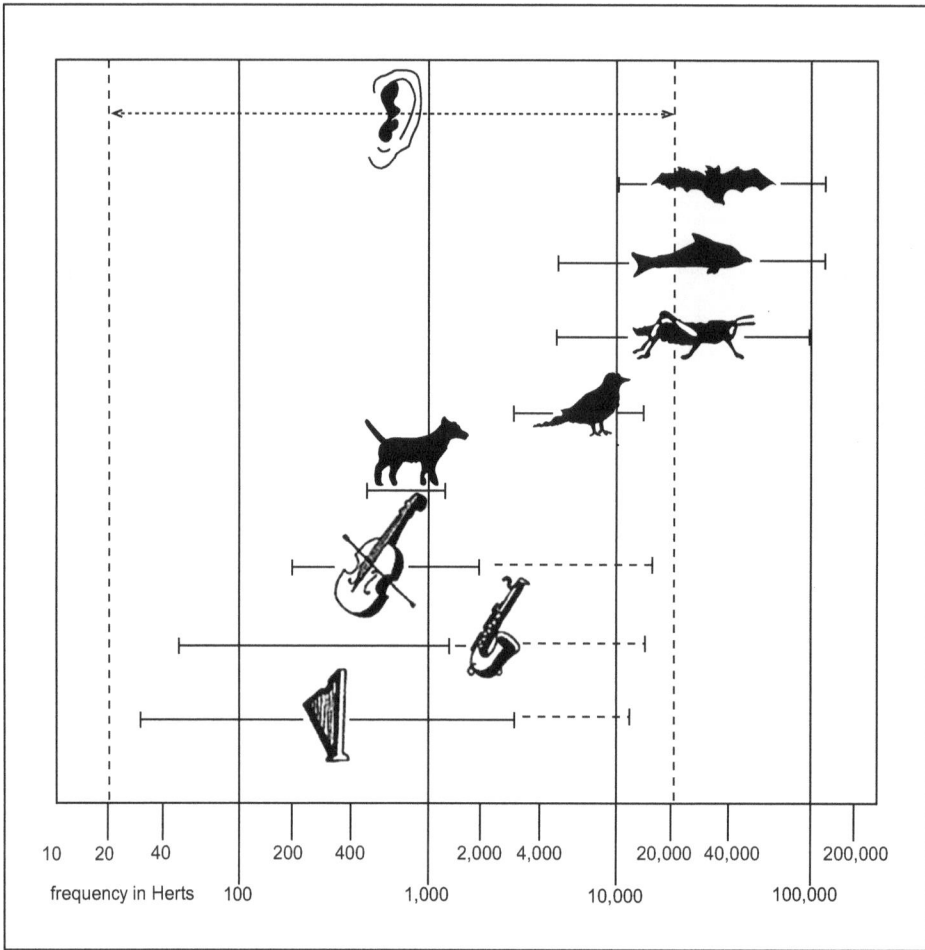

Fig. (4). Frequency vibration range. From: http://www.everydayhearing.com/hearing-loss/what-is-my-hearing-range.

Whereas the minimum rarefaction value is 0, the upper limit of compression is very high; blasts and shock waves create vacuum bubbles in liquids (cavitation), which are able to generate queer conditions in medium interfaces.

The term "laser" is an acronym for "light amplification by stimulated emission of radiation". Lasers work as a result of resonant effects. The output of a laser is a coherent electromagnetic field, a coherent beam of electromagnetic energy: all the waves have the same frequency and phase.

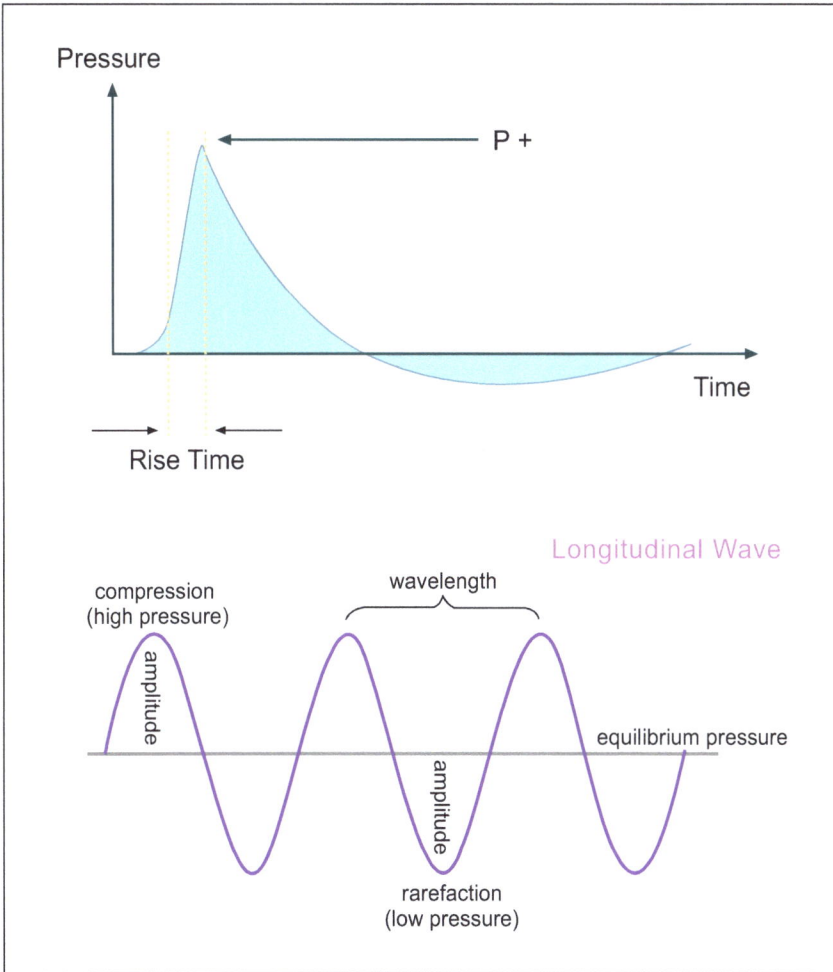

Fig. (5).   Shockwave and acoustic wave. From: http://www.electrotherapy.org/modality/shockwave-therapies; http://dev.physicslab.org/.

In a basic laser, a chamber called cavity, is designed to internally reflect infrared (IR), visible-light, or ultraviolet (UV) waves so that they reinforce each other. The cavity can contain gases, liquids, or solids. The choice of cavity material determines the wavelength of the output. At each end of the cavity, there is a mirror. One mirror is totally reflective and it impedes allowing none of the energy to pass through; the other mirror is partially reflective, allowing approximately 5 percent of the energy to pass through. Electromagnetic energy is pumped into the cavity from an external source. As a result of pumping, an electromagnetic field appears inside the laser cavity at the natural (resonant) frequency of the atoms of the material that fills the cavity. The waves reflect back and forth between the mirrors. The length of the cavity is such that the reflected and re-reflected wave fronts reinforce each other in the phase at natural frequency of the cavity substance creating a standing wave. Electromagnetic waves at this resonant frequency emerge from the end of the cavity that has the partially-reflective mirror. The output may appear as a continuous beam, or as a series of brief, intense pulses that can heat the medium, generating pressure waves, *i.e.* vibrations [2].

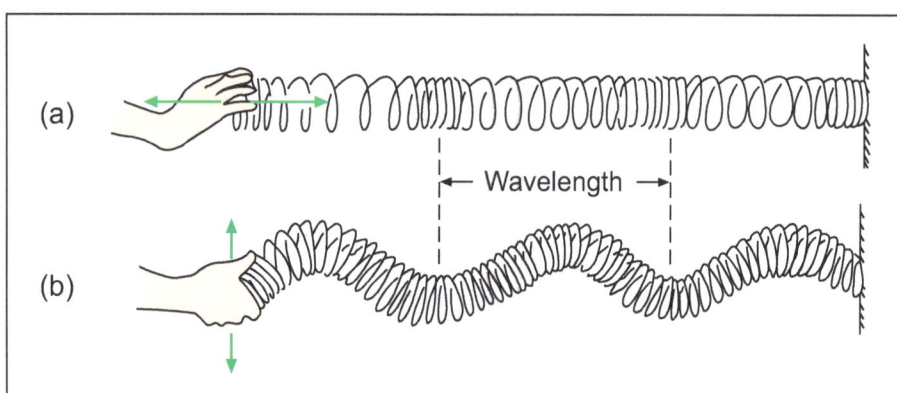

Fig. (6). Longitudinal (**a**) and transverse (**b**) forced system. From: http://www.danielcelton.com.

When the vibration is forced by a mechanical system, the stimulus can be applied in order to generate different kinds of vibrations. In a mass-spring system, if a force is impressed parallel to the direction of the movement (single degree of freedom), it will generate a longitudinal wave (pressure wave, like in gases), with movements along the abscissa axis; a force perpendicular to the movement will generate a transversal wave, with movements along the ordinate axis. The combination of the two kinds of waves described above, generates a superficial wave.

Among the forced systems, we should focus on systems driven by forces that are periodic functions. This kind of applied forces leads to the important phenomenon of resonance. Resonance occurs when the frequency of the periodic force applied in the system approaches the natural (free) frequency of vibration of the medium (like the laser optical cavity). The resulted energy in the vibrating system, determines an increase in the amplitude (Figs. **6, 7**).

The stored increase in the amplitude of resulting signal can be limited by the presence of a damper, but the response can be very great. Indeed, soldiers marching across a bridge can set up resonant vibrations sufficient to destroy the bridge structure. A similar folklore exists about opera singers shattering wine glasses.

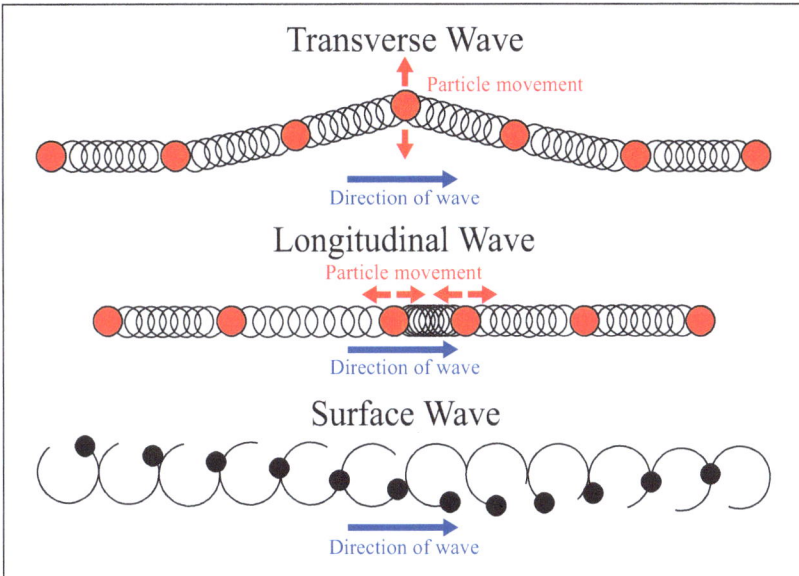

Fig. (7). Particles movement in mechanic waves. From: http://www.acs.psu.edu/ drussell/ Demos/ waves/wavemotion.html.

Let us focus on the resonance principle, approaching with the mass-spring taken as an example (with mechanical force applied to the system) (Fig. **8**).

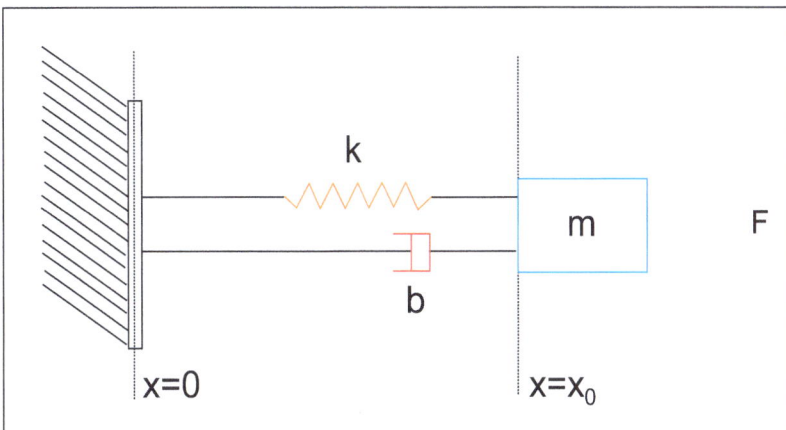

Fig. (8). Mass-spring system. Modified from: http://www.mdpi.com.

In this simple example, a mass is connected to a wall through a spring and a damper. Let $x(t)$ denotes the displacement, as a function of time of the mass relative to its equilibrium position (x_0). The general equation of the displacement $x(t)$ is as follows:

$$mx'' + bx' + kx = F \qquad (1)$$

Where, m is the mass, b is the damping constant, k is the spring constant and the dependency of x and F by time is omitted.

Consider the case of undamped, free vibration ($b = 0$ and $F = 0$):

$$mx'' + kx = 0 \qquad (2)$$

The characteristic equation is:

$$my^2 + k = 0 \qquad (3)$$

And the solutions are:

$$y = \pm \sqrt{\frac{k}{m}} i \qquad (4)$$

The general solution for $x(t)$ is,

$$x(t) = c_1 \cos(w_0 t) + c_2 \sin(w_0 t) \qquad (5)$$

that can be expressed as:

$$x(t) = R \cos(w_0 t + \varphi) \qquad (6)$$

Where, $w_0 = \sqrt{k/m}$ is the natural pulsation (*i.e.* $2\pi f$ with f frequency of the system).

The vibrating movement has a frequency which is equal to the number of oscillations in a second, and that can be composed of a single frequency or by several components. The vibration signals are usually created by many frequencies which appear simultaneously, so it can be very difficult to determine instantly how many vibrating components there are in the signal by only analysing the time domain profile.

The energy derived by various oscillations can be measured by Fourier analysis in the frequency spectrum. The Fourier transform allows us to deal with non-periodic functions.

The plane wave decomposition in the individual frequency components is called frequency analysis, with the graphical representation of different energy contributions in frequency.

Now consider the case of forced vibration, that is to say the same system as before with an applied force:

$$mx'' + kx = F \tag{7}$$

If we apply a sinusoidal force with a frequency equal to the natural frequency of the system, we will be able to observe the resonance phenomenon:

$$F(t) = F_0 \cos(w_0 t) \tag{8}$$

$$x(t) = R \cos(w_0 t + \varphi) + \frac{F_0}{2mw_0} t\sin(w_0 t) \tag{9}$$

The first term in the solution is considered as described previously, while the third term is a sinusoidal wave whose amplitude increases proportionally with the elapsed time. This phenomenon is called *resonance* (Fig. **9**).

The first term in the solution is as seen previously, while the third term is a sinusoidal wave whose amplitude increases proportionally with elapsed time. This phenomenon is called *resonance* (Fig. **9**).

As said, in order to generate a vibration, it is necessary to apply an external force: the response of a mechanical system to an external force can change not only depending on the nature of the stimulus, but also on the composition of the system itself. Starting from this consideration, the vibrational waves can be classified using multiple approaches, for example, based on the linearity of the system, the degrees of freedom of the system's mathematical model, or considering the kind of vibration observed.

In the latter case, the mechanical vibrations are usually classified into 5 categories: shear (or transverse), longitudinal (or compression), torsional, bending and surface waves.

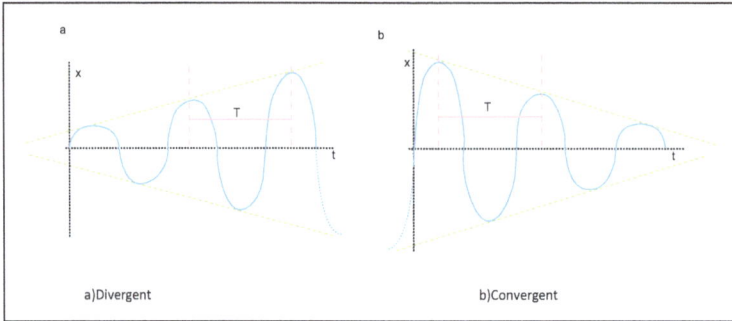

Fig. (9). Response to a resonant signal.

Solid systems can carry (propagate) all kinds of waves, while fluid systems can propagate longitudinal (compression) waves only. Instead, at the boundary of fluid, there is a specific condition: *i.e.* the sea surface can carry transversal (surface) waves whose energy can vary not only with the wave's eight (amplitude), but also with the wavelength: high and short waves carry more energy than the small and long waves [3] (Fig. **10**).

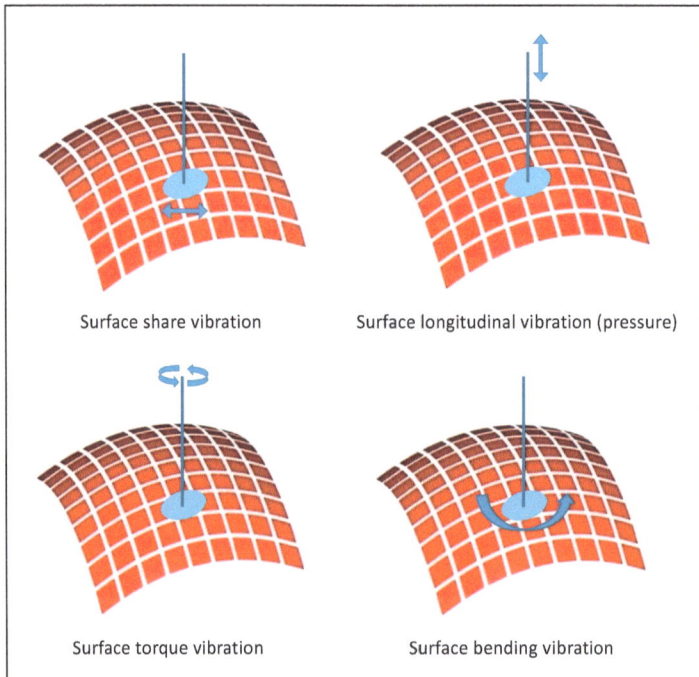

Fig. (10). Classification of mechanical vibrations.

In a transversal vibration, the motion of the particles in the medium is perpendicular to the direction of the wave. In this kind of wave, the particles do not move along with the wave, they simply oscillate around their individual equilibrium position as the wave passes by. The up-and-down position of the particles determines the amplitude of the wave, while the distance from a peak to another peak is called wavelength. The simplest transverse wave has a waveform which is easy to imagine, since the movement with crests and troughs generates a sine wave that propagates in the surrounding space.

Whereas the snapshot of a transversal wave is a sine function plot, the movement of a particle of the medium propagating the wave is a mass-spring straight oscillation perpendicular to the direction of propagation.

A longitudinal wave in an elastic solid makes the particles oscillate along the direction of the propagation, and the motion of the oscillating medium is parallel to the motion of the wave itself.

A longitudinal wave changes the local density of the medium, that is; its pressure: a longitudinal wave begins with a compression, that is, the point of maximum density on the medium of the wave. The opposite of the compression is the rarefaction, the point of minimum density on the wave medium. Compressions and rarefactions are observed alternate along the length of the medium, and the wavelength is the measurement of the distance between compressions, or between rarefactions. In a longitudinal wave, compressions and rarefactions slide from one end to the other, in the same direction that the wave travels.

The pressure change generates a secondary pressure wave which is transversal to the direction of propagation of the wave, according to the medium Poisson's ratio, and creates the geometric effect of the wave propagation: for example, a sphere for a sound in free air, wavy circles on water surfaces.

A torsional wave is a motion in which the vibrations in the medium are periodic rotational motions around the direction of propagation.

A surface wave is an example of waves that involves a combination of both longitudinal and transverse movements. A surface wave is observed in the sea water motion and, like a wave travels through the waver, the particles travel in clockwise circles. The radius of the circles decreases which is inversely proportional to the depth of the water.

In deep water, when the water depth is bigger than both the wavelength and the wave amplitude, surface waves can be considered just as transversal wave with up and down particle motion.

The mathematical model of a vibration system may take the form of acoustic waves [4]. In order to write the equations, it is necessary to use the equation of continuity, Newton's law and the gas law. The definitions that will be used to describe the model are the following:

$\xi(x,t)$ particle displacement

ρ_0 equilibrium density

$\delta(x,t)$ relative change in density

p_0 equilibrium pressure

$\frac{\partial \xi(x,t)}{\partial t}$ particle velocity

$\rho(x,t)$ density

$\rho(x,t) = \rho_0(1 + \delta(x,t))$

$p(x,t)$ change in pressure

Equation Of Continuity: Assuming that the wave propagates in the air, we consider a small portion of the medium, modelled as a cylinder of surface and length (Fig. **11**).

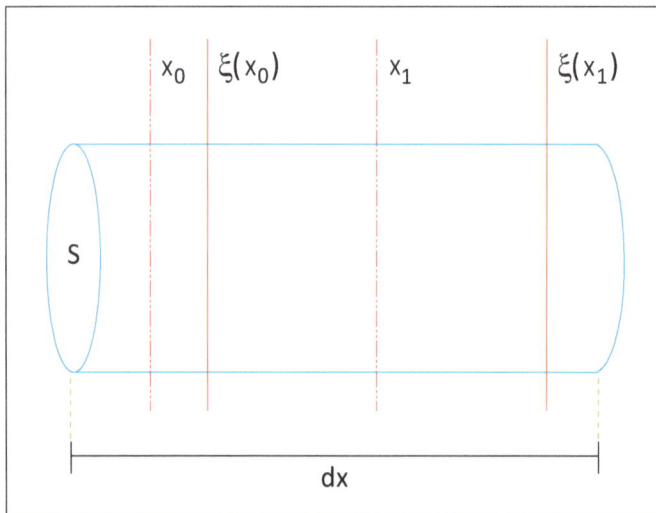

Fig. (11). Geometry of a small cylinder of air.

According to the hypothesis, dx is so small that any variable changes linearly in the cylinder, and the mass is conserved in the cylinder dx. So the equation for mass conservation can be written as (V_0 is the volume without displacement):

$$\rho_0 S dx = \rho_0 V_0 \tag{10}$$

$$V_0 = S dx \tag{11}$$

As assumed before, all variables are linear in the cylinder, so we can express the particle displacement (Taylor series) as:

$$\xi(dx) = \xi(0) + \frac{\partial \xi}{\partial x} dx \tag{12}$$

$$\frac{\partial \xi}{\partial x} dx = \xi(dx) - \xi(0) \tag{13}$$

So we can express the volume with the displacement as:

$$V = S(dx + \xi(dx) - \xi(0)) \tag{14}$$

$$V = S\left(dx + \frac{\partial \xi}{\partial x} dx\right) \tag{15}$$

Because of the mass conservation, the displaced mass equals the mass without displacement as shown below:

$$\rho(x,t) S dx \left(1 + \frac{\partial \xi}{\partial x}\right) = \rho_0 S dx \tag{16}$$

$$\rho_0 [1 + \delta(x,t)] S dx \left(1 + \frac{\partial \xi}{\partial x}\right) = \rho_0 S dx \tag{17}$$

$$\rho_0 S dx \left[1 + \delta(x,t) + \frac{\partial \xi}{\partial x} + \frac{\partial \xi}{\partial x} \delta(x,t)\right] = \rho_0 S dx \tag{18}$$

The last term of the left side in (18) can be omitted, so the final form of the continuity equation is:

$$\delta(x, t) + \frac{\partial \xi}{\partial x} = 0 \tag{19}$$

Perfect gas law: In order to write the gas law, we have to assume that there is no energy transfer in the cylinder due to propagation, so the system is considered adiabatic.

$$dQ = \frac{\partial Q}{\partial V} dV + \frac{\partial Q}{\partial P} dP \tag{20}$$

$$Q = CT \tag{21}$$

$$dQ = T \left(\frac{C_p}{V_0} dV + \frac{C_v}{P_0} dP \right) \tag{22}$$

We can express dV using the volume formula with particle displacement using (15):

$$V = V_0 + dV = S dx + S \frac{\partial \xi}{\partial x} dx \tag{23}$$

$$dV = S \frac{\partial \xi}{\partial x} dx \tag{24}$$

We can as well express dP as the pressure equation:

$$dP = p(x, t) \tag{25}$$

We can now write (22) using (24) and (25) and considering that in the adiabatic process, $dQ = 0$:

$$\frac{C_p}{V_0} S dx \frac{\partial \xi}{\partial x} = -\frac{C_v}{P_0} p(x, t) \tag{26}$$

$$p(x, t) = -\frac{P_0}{C_v} \frac{C_p}{V_0} S dx \frac{\partial \xi}{\partial x} \tag{27}$$

$$V_0 = Sdx; \quad \text{(a)}$$

$$\frac{c_p}{c_v} = \gamma_c \quad \text{(b)}$$

(28)

$$p(x,t) = -P_0\gamma_c \frac{\partial \xi}{\partial x}$$

(29)

Using (19) in (29), we can derive the final form of the gas law:

$$p(x,t) = P_0\gamma_c\delta(x,t)$$

(30)

Newton's law: Consider the cylinder with surface S and length dx. We can model the forces that act on the cylinder at the opposite sides (Fig. **12**):

$$F_{x=0} = [P_0 + p(x)]S$$

(31)

$$F_{x=dx} = \left[P_0 + p(x) + \frac{\partial p}{\partial x}dx\right]S$$

(32)

$$F = F_{x=dx} - F_{x=0}$$

(33)

$$F = \frac{\partial p}{\partial x}Sdx$$

(34)

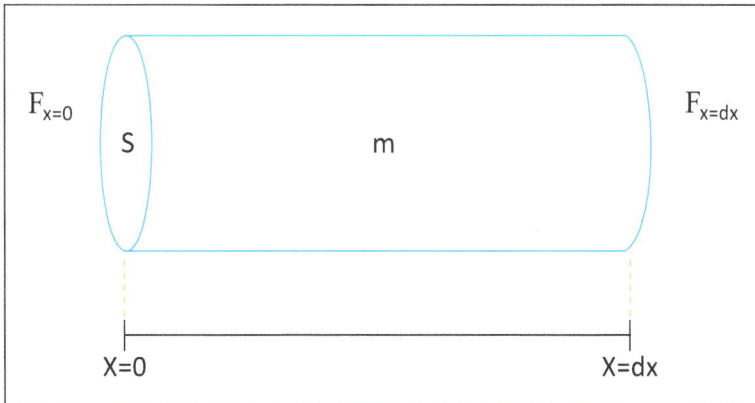

Fig. (12). Geometry of the force acting on a cylinder.

The force in (34) accelerates the air which creates a counter-force:

$$-ma = -\rho_0 S dx \frac{\partial^2 \xi}{\partial t^2}$$

$$\frac{\partial p}{\partial x} S dx = -\rho_0 S dx \frac{\partial^2 \xi}{\partial t^2}$$

(35)

$$-\frac{\partial p}{\partial x} = \rho_0 \frac{\partial^2 \xi}{\partial t^2}$$

(36)

Eq. (36) is the Euler equation.

Wave equation: Finally, we can write the wave equation, initiating from (29) and deriving each member as follows:

$$-\frac{\partial p}{\partial x} = P_0 \gamma_c \frac{\partial^2 \xi}{\partial x^2}$$

(37)

Using (37) in (36):

$$P_0 \gamma_c \frac{\partial^2 \xi}{\partial x^2} = \rho_0 \frac{\partial^2 \xi}{\partial t^2}$$

$$\frac{\partial^2 \xi}{\partial x^2} = \frac{\rho_0}{P_0 \gamma_c} \frac{\partial^2 \xi}{\partial t^2}$$

(38)

By defining the speed of sound c as:

$$c = \sqrt{\frac{P_0 \gamma_c}{\rho_0}},$$

(39)

we can finally write the wave equation for displacement $\xi(x, t)$:

$$\frac{\partial^2 \xi}{\partial x^2} = \frac{1}{c^2} \frac{\partial^2 \xi}{\partial t^2}$$

(40)

To express the wave equation for the pressure, we have to derive each member in equation (36) as follows:

$$\frac{\partial^2 p}{\partial x^2} = -\rho_0 \frac{\partial^2}{\partial t^2}\left(\frac{\partial \xi(x,t)}{\partial x}\right) \tag{41}$$

And using (19) and then (30):

$$\frac{\partial^2 p}{\partial x^2} = \rho_0 \frac{\partial^2 \delta(x,t)}{\partial t^2} \tag{42}$$

$$\frac{\partial^2 p}{\partial x^2} = \frac{1}{c^2}\frac{\partial^2 p}{\partial t^2} \tag{43}$$

Speed of waves: A possible solution for the wave equation (40) is as follows:

$$\xi(x,t) = \xi_0 \sin(kx + wt) \tag{44}$$

Where ξ_0 is the maximum displacement of the particles or the amplitude of oscillation, $w = 2\pi f = \frac{2\pi}{T}$ is the natural frequency, $k = \frac{2\pi}{\lambda}$ is the wave number, and λ is the wavelength.

Deriving (44) and applying the results in (40):

$$\frac{\partial^2 \xi}{\partial x^2} = -\xi_0 k^2 \sin(kx + wt)$$

$$\frac{\partial^2 \xi}{\partial t^2} = -\xi_0 w^2 \sin(kx + wt) \tag{45}$$

$$-\xi_0 k^2 \sin(kx + wt) = -\frac{1}{c^2}\xi_0 w^2 \sin(kx + wt)$$

$$c^2 = \frac{w^2}{k^2} = \frac{P_0 \gamma_c}{\rho_0}$$

This is a fairly profound result. It tells us that the plane wave solution for particle displacement is a good solution, defining the speed of the wave (speed of sound) not arbitrary, but dependant on the gas variables. At room temperature and sea surface pressure, this results in the nominal speed of sound in the air of 345 m/s.

If instead of the equation of gas we used the bulk liquid equation, we would have found a similar result:

$$c^2 = \frac{w^2}{k^2} = \frac{B}{\rho} \tag{46}$$

This is the bulk module. When the bulk module and density of water are used, a nominal value for the speed of sound (longitudinal waves) in water is 1500 m/s.

In the human body, soft tissues respond to vibration/sound like a soft container full of water, but the stiff structures of the body reflect, diffract or refract the longitudinal (pressure) waves that propagate in it, allowing the use of reflected waves for ultrasound imaging.

Table **1** summarizes the speed of wave in different mediums.

Table 1. Speed of sound in different mediums.

	Air	Water	Steel
Bulk modulus	$1.4(1.01 \times 10^5)Pa$	$2.2 \times 10^9 Pa$	$2.5 \times 10^{11} Pa$
Density	$1.21 \, kg/m^3$	$1000 \, kg/m^3$	$10^4 \, kg/m^3$
Speed	$343 \, m/s$	$1500 \, m/s$	$5000 \, m/s$

Energy of waves: The energy carried by the wave can be modelled considering the main kind of waves: the longitudinal and the transverse ones. If we consider one dimensional longitudinal or transverse waves propagating in an elastic medium, the energy can be expressed in terms of kinetics energy. The total mechanical energy of an infinitesimal mass element *dm* in the elastic medium is:

$$dE = \frac{1}{2}\omega^2 \xi_0^2 dm \tag{47}$$

Where, we should consider that the mass can be related to the density of the medium in the space *dx*:

$$dm = \mu dx \tag{48}$$

So, the final expression for the energy is:

$$E_l = \frac{1}{2}\mu\omega^2\xi_0{}^2 \tag{49}$$

Wave energy defines how much energy the wave can carry, but another important information is how deep in the body the wave can travel before absorption, *i.e.* in a long way, the wave can interact more deeply in the molecules of body [5] (Fig. **13**).

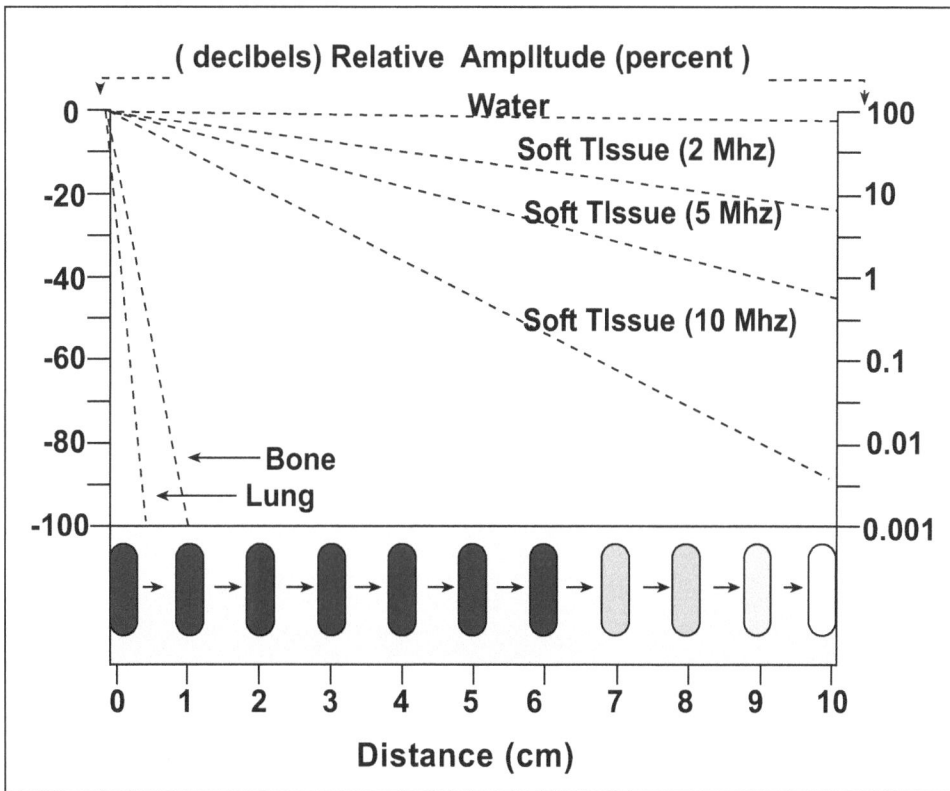

Fig. (13). Mechanic vibration penetration in body tissues. From: http://caputino-bme.blogspot.it/.

The higher the frequency, the better is the image resolution and smaller is the depth of penetration in the tissues.

CONFLICT OF INTEREST

The author (editor) declares no conflict of interest, financial or otherwise.

ACKNOWLEDGEMENTS

Declared none.

REFERENCES

[1]   Auld BA. Acoustic fields and waves in solid. Рипол Классик 1974.

[2]   Ristic V. Principles of acoustic devices. John Wiley & Sons: Australia 1983.

[3]   Royer D, Dieulesaint E. Elastic waves. In: Solids I, Ed. Free and Guided Propagation. Springer Science & Business Media 1999.

[4]   Cronk EW, Heald MA. Physics of Waves. Courier Corporation 1969.

[5]   Tucker JW. Microwave ultrasonics in solid state physics. North-Holland Pub. Co. 1973.

CHAPTER 2

The Applied Mechanical Vibration as Whole-body and Focal Vibration

Raoul Saggini[1,*] and **Emilio Ancona**[2]

[1] *Physical and Rehabilitation Medicine, Department of Medical Oral and Biotechnological Sciences, Director of the School of Specialty in Physical and Rehabilitation Medicine, "Gabriele d'Annunzio" University, Chieti-Pescara, Italy; National Coordinator of Schools of Specialty in Physical and Rehabilitation Medicine*

[2] *School of Specialty in Physical and Rehabilitation Medicine, "Gabriele d'Annunzio" University, Chieti-Pescara, Italy*

Abstract: The mechanical vibration is the simplest and purest form of vibratory energy application in physical and rehabilitation medicine. After the first observations of the effects of vibrations, the scientific research has been directed to the identification of the molecular mechanisms that mediate signal trans-duction at the tissue level. Although these mechanisms are still not fully understood, and despite the adverse effects observed in subjects improperly exposed to vibratory sources for various reasons, during the last century, the mode of application of mechanical vibration has gradually evolved from whole-body to focal and mechano-acoustic forms, as much as the field of application has gradually expanded spreading from the initial skeletal and muscle applications to the current motor impairment conditions associated with the most common neurological diseases.

Keywords: Amplitude, Focal vibration, Frequency, Mechanical vibration, Mechano-acoustic vibration, Mechanoreceptors, Mechanostat theory, Muscle spindle, Musculoskeletal system, Neurorehabilitation, Resonance, Somatosensory cortex, Tensegrity, Tonic vibration reflex, Tuning response, Whole-body vibration.

INTRODUCTION

The musculoskeletal system is a complex biological machine designed for movement and locomotion. This system is structured in such a way to respond

* **Corresponding authors Raoul Saggini:** Physical and Rehabilitation Medicine, Department of Medical Oral and Biotechnological Sciences, Director of the School of Specialty in Physical and Rehabilitation Medicine, "Gabriele d'Annunzio" University, Chieti-Pescara, Italy; Tel: 03908713555306; Fax: 03909713553224; E-mail: raoul.saggini@unich.it

with modifications both in metabolism and in structure to the functional needs of the organism and to the stresses transmitted from the environment, according to the principle of the so-called "Wolff's law", for which «form follows function» [1].

To describe the conditions that allow the maintenance of the system, a theory of the stimulus of everyday stress was formulated, which describes the intensity of a mechanical stress in terms of stimulation of daily stress. According to this theory, if a stimulus stressful for the system is greater than a threshold stimulus, the homeostatic balance will be positive (and oriented towards anabolism), while if the stimulus is lower than the threshold stimulus, the homeostatic balance will be negative (and oriented towards catabolism). When daily loads to be supported are drastically reduced (as occurs in disuse for palsy or immobilization, chronic degenerative diseases, or in case of reduced gravity), it results in degradation of the protein structure that forms the contractile component of the muscle and changes in microarchitecture of the bone, with reduced muscle tone and bone mass.

A type of mechanical stress is represented by vibratory stimulation. From a purely mechanical point of view, vibration is the mechanical oscillation of some measure or mobile body around an equilibrium point; the oscillation being the motion that it makes to return to the starting position. In a mechanical model constituted by a body of mass m, bound to a spring whose elastic constant is denoted by k, and put into oscillation, the mass m moves with regularity with respect to the reference position. In addition, the movement may reproduce self-identically to regular time intervals, having a so-called "periodic character" (Fig. **1**).

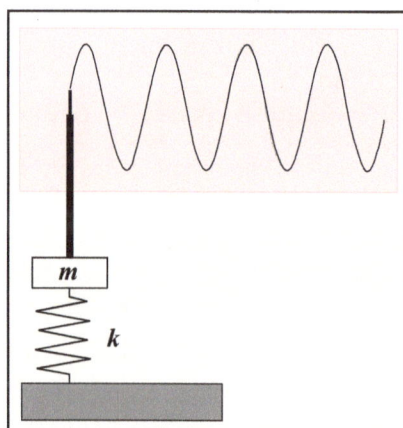

Fig. (1). In a system consisting of a mass constrained to a spring and placed in oscillation it will produce a smooth movement of a periodic nature.

The simplest periodic function is the *simple* or *natural harmonic motion*, whose trend in function of time is represented by a *sinusoid* or *sinewave* with constant amplitude and period. In a periodic oscillation, *amplitude* or *magnitude* is the maximum extent of the motion (peak-to-peak displacement of the wave, measured in millimeters), whereas *period* is the duration of time between two consecutive passages of the mobile body at the equilibrium point (a cycle) and is the reciprocal of *frequency*, that is the number of cycles per unit of time; thus, period and frequency are related through the following relationship:

$$f = 1 / T$$

Where f is the frequency (expressed in Hertz, Hz), and T is the period (usually measured in seconds). Frequency has also an inverse relationship to the *wavelength*, that is the spatial period of the wave (usually determined by considering the distance between two consecutive crests, troughs, or zero crossings):

$$f = v / \lambda$$

Where f is the frequency, v is the propagation velocity, and λ (lambda) is the wavelength (Fig. **2**).

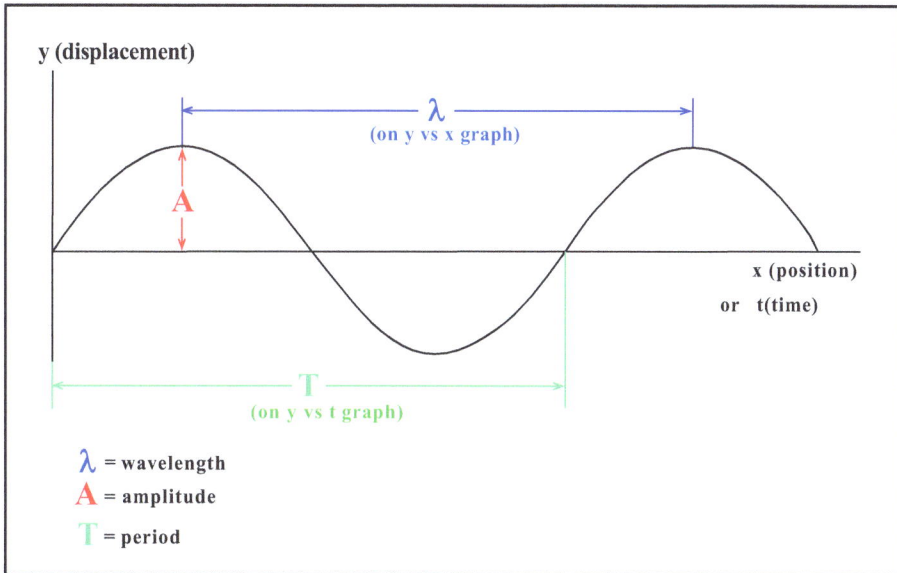

Fig. (2). Basic characteristics of the sinusoid or sinewave.

ANATOMICAL DISTRIBUTION OF MECHANORECEPTORS

The vibratory perception constitutes a type of mechanical sensitivity, and hence involves receptors structures sensitive to mechanical pressure or distortion, i.e., the mechanoreceptors [2]. Mechanoreceptors are found in various types of tissues, as skin, muscles, tendons, ligaments, articular capsules, periosteum, blood vessels.

Mechanoreceptors In Skin

In the skin, there are four principal types of mechanoreceptors (all innervated by myelinated Aβ fibers), categorized by morphology, perceived sensation, receptive field size, and rate of adaptation [3, 4] (Fig. **3**).

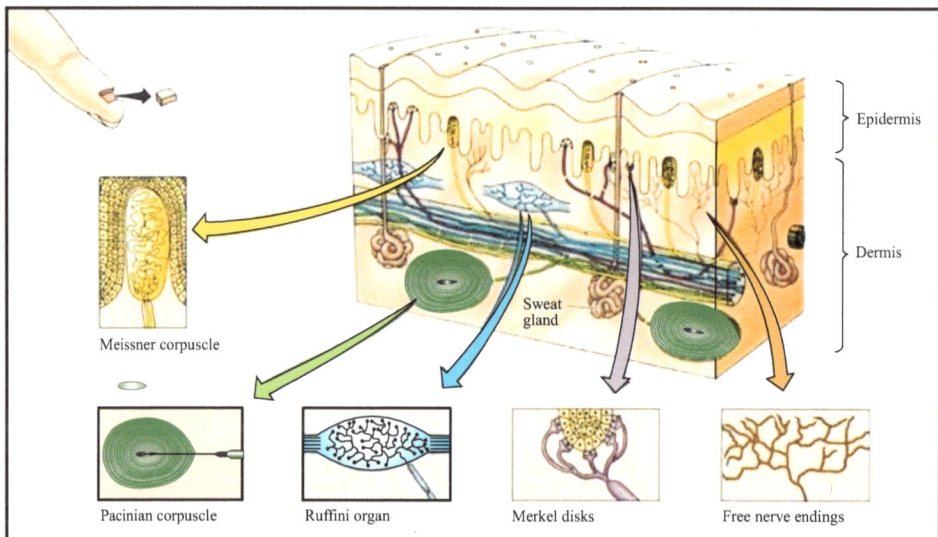

Fig. (3). Schematic representation of cutaneous mechanoreceptors. From: Purves D, Augustine GJ, Fitzpatrick D, Hall WC, LaMantia AS, McNamara JO, Williams SM, Eds. Neuroscience. 3rd ed. Sunderland (MA): Sinauer Associates 2004; 8: p. 193.

Tactile corpuscles (Meissner corpuscles) consist of flattened supportive cells arranged as horizontal lamellae surrounded by a connective tissue capsule and located in the papillary ridges of the dermis, have the highest sensitivity (lowest threshold) and respond to light touch. Bulbous corpuscles (Ruffini endings), located in the dermis, consist of nerve terminals interspersed in collagen fibrils longitudinally passing through a thin and spindle-shaped capsule and linking the corpuscle up to the dermal collagen at its poles, thus providing the mechanical connection to the fibrous tissues of the dermis and detecting tension deep in the skin and fascia and change of joint angle. Merkel discs consist of expanded extremities of branches of myelinated axons enclosed into specialized epithelial cells (Merkel cells), are placed at the tip of the intermediate epidermal ridges and have sustained response to pressure. Lamellar corpuscles (Pacinian corpuscles), located in the deeper layers of the skin, consist of a single unmyelinated afferent neuron wrapped in 20-60 concentric lamellae constituted by flat epithelial cells, fibroblasts and fibrous connective tissue (mainly types II and IV collagen network) separated by gelatinous material (more than 92% of which is water); the lamellae filter mechanical deformations thus responding to gross pressure changes and especially rapid vibrations [5 - 7] (Fig. **4**).

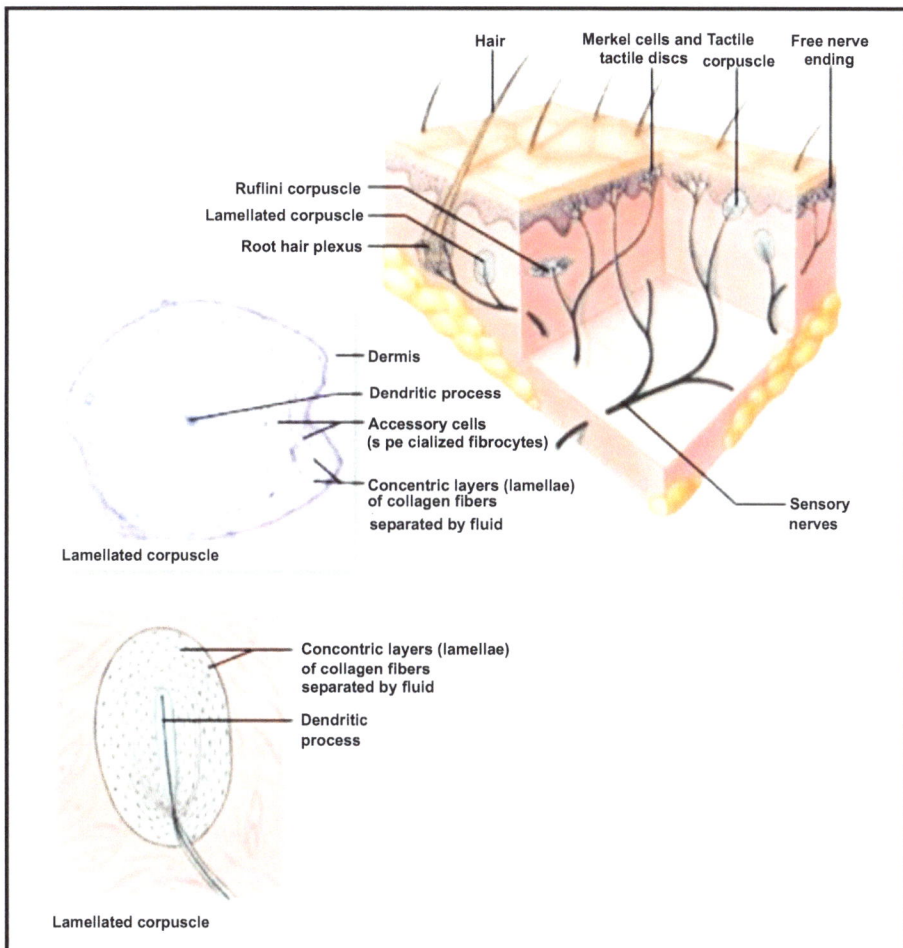

Fig. (4). Light microscopy and schematic representation of a Pacinian corpuscle. Copyright© 2012 Pearson Education, Inc.

Vibration of frequency between 20-40 Hz are detected by Meissner corpuscles [8], stimuli of frequency above 60 Hz are detected by Pacinian corpuscles, which have the highest sensitivity (1 mm) at a frequency of 250-300 Hz, thus representing the vibration receptors for excellence [9]. Any deformation in the Pacinian corpuscle causes bending or stretching of the afferent neuron, thus opening pressure-sensitive sodium ion channels in the axon membrane and hence generating action potentials (Fig. **5**); this happens only when the skin is rapidly distorted but not when pressure is continuous, because of the mechanical filtering of the stimulus in the lamellar structure that envelop the nerve ending and because the latter does not carry on indefinitely depolarization. Ultimately, the stimulation perceived by the Pacinian corpuscle is the velocity of deformation and the information transmitted to the central nervous system is the frequency of stimulus rather than the pressure of the exerted load [10, 11].

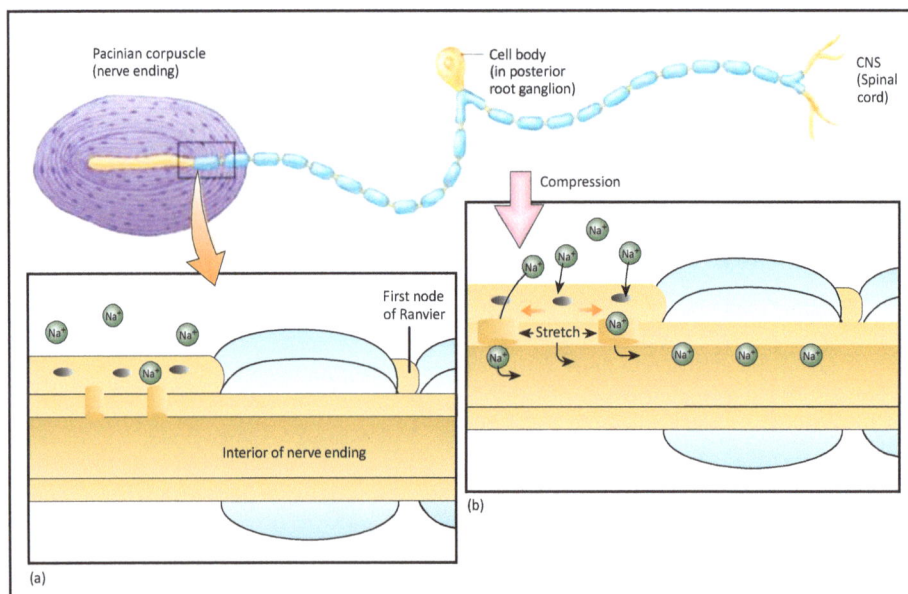

Fig. (5). A Pacinian corpuscle consists of a neuron wrapped in layers of connective tissue, with a myelinated nerve ending (axon) **(a)** A tactile (pressure or vibration) stimulus causes the neuron within the connective tissue to deform, opening the Na^+ channels and allowing the ion to enter the cell **(b)**. This produces initially a depolarizing generator potential and then an action potential. From: Rhoades R, Pflanzer RG. Human Physiology. 4th ed. Pacific Grove: Brooks/Cole 2003.

The receptive field of a receptor is defined as the cutaneous area in which a stimulus triggers the firing of the corresponding afferent neuron; thus, if the skin is stimulated in two points in the same receptive field, the spatial difference is not perceived (Fig. **6**).

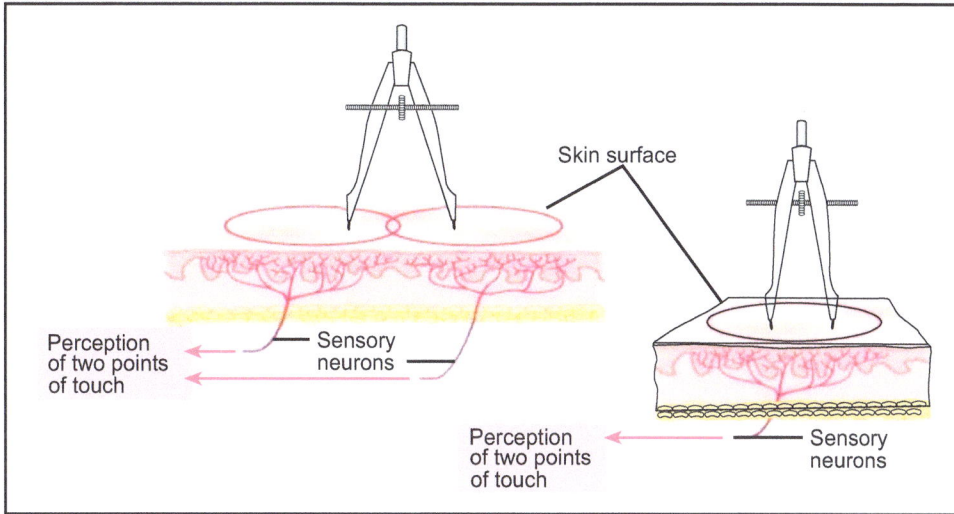

Fig. (6). Receptive field in tactile perception.

Depending on the properties of their receptive fields, two different types of mechanoreceptor have been distinguished: the type I has a small and well defined field, whereas the type II has a wider field with obscure border. The receptive field of type I mechanoreceptors contains several zones of maximal sensitivity within a sharply demarcated area of high and relatively uniform sensitivity; the receptive field of type II mechanoreceptors consists of a single zone of maximal sensitivity and a wide surrounding area where the sensitivity fades out gradually [4]. Since the receptive field size increases with the depth of receptor in the skin, Pacinian corpuscles that are the deepest ones have the largest receptive field (Fig. **7**).

Depending upon the nature of their response to a prolonged step indentation of the skin, cutaneous mechanoreceptors have been further classified into two major categories: 56% are fast-adapting (FA, also called rapidly adapting or RA) and respond with a burst of impulses only at the onset and removal of the stimulus, *i.e..* when the stimulus is moving; the remaining 44% are slow-adapting (SA) and respond with a prolonged discharge [12 - 14] (Fig. **8**).

The FA I mechanoreceptors are mostly sensitive to the rate of skin indentation, whereas the FA II mechanoreceptors are highly sensitive to acceleration and higher derivatives; overall, the fast-adapting mechanoreceptors, particularly the FAII, respond not only when the indentation is increasing, but also when the stimulus is retracted. The SA I mechanoreceptors show a high dynamic sensitivity and often a quite irregular sustained discharge, having an excellent sensitivity to edge outlines of objects indenting the skin, the SA II mechanoreceptors on the other hand have a less pronounced dynamic sensitivity and a very regular sustained discharge; overall, the slow-adapting mechanoreceptors exhibit a sustained discharge during constant skin indentation in addition to their discharge during increasing skin indentation, and often show a spontaneous discharge in the absence of tactile stimulation [4].

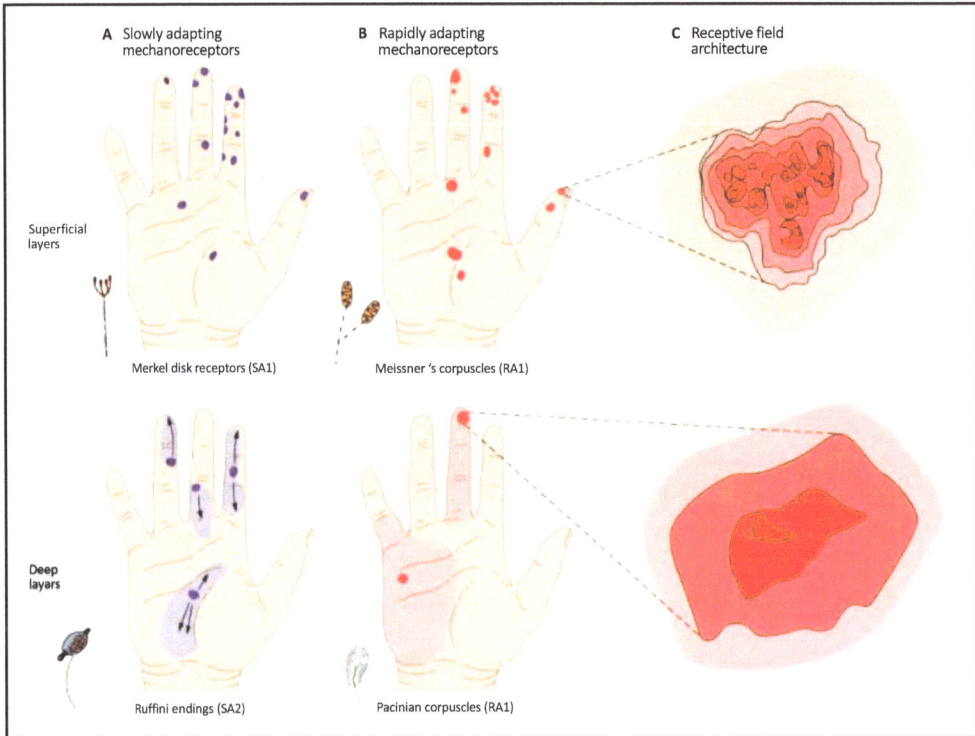

Fig. (7). Receptive field size of cutaneous mechanoreceptors as measured with von Frey hairs. Redrawn from: Johansson RS, Vallbo ÅB. Tactile sensory coding in the glabrous skin of the human hand. Trends neurosci 1983; 6: 27-32.

Since there are no radical differences in receptive field properties between units in the various regions of the glabrous skin, a critical factor for the resolution is the density of afferent units. Indeed, the distribution of cutaneous mechanoreceptors is not homogeneous on body surface, their density being higher in certain regions (*e.g.*, on fingertips) than in others (*e.g.*, on forearm).

In the hand, the density is characterized by a pronounced regional variation, increasing in the proximo-distal direction, with a slight increase from the palm (relative density: 1.0) to the main part of the finger (relative density: 1.6) and an abrupt increase from the main part of the finger to the fingertip (relative density: 4.2), which is the preferred site for tactual exploration. Whilst the differences in overall density are essentially explained by the type I units, the type II units are almost evenly distributed over the whole glabrous skin area. The spatial distribution of densities of the type I units, as much as their receptive field properties, is coherent with their role in tactile spatial discrimination; at the same time, the findings that the type II units have a low density, which is also relatively uniform from the wrist to the finger, and that they are widely distributed in deep fibrous structures (*i.e.,* joint capsule, interosseous membranes and tendon sheets), corroborates the conclusion that their main role in tactile sensibility does not lie as much as in detailed spatial discrimination but rather in proprioception and kinesthesia [15] (Fig. **9**).

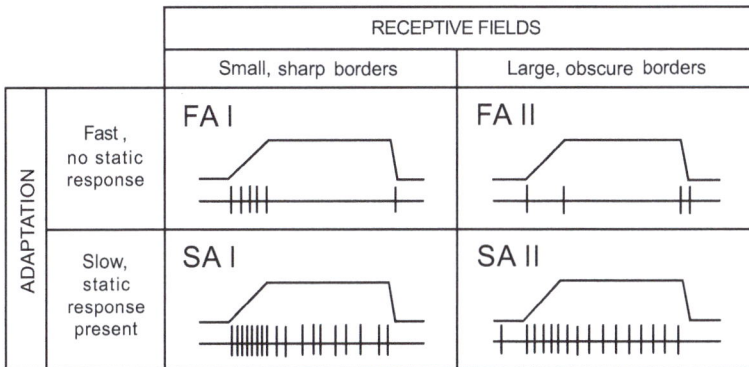

Fig. (8). Rate of adaptation of cutaneous mechanoreceptors. Graphs show the impulse discharge (lower trace) to perpendicular slope indentation of the skin (upper trace) for each mechanoreceptor type. FA, fast adaptation; SA, slow adaptation. From: Johansson RS, Vallbo ÅB. Tactile sensory coding in the glabrous skin of the human hand. Trends neurosci 1983; 6: 27-32.

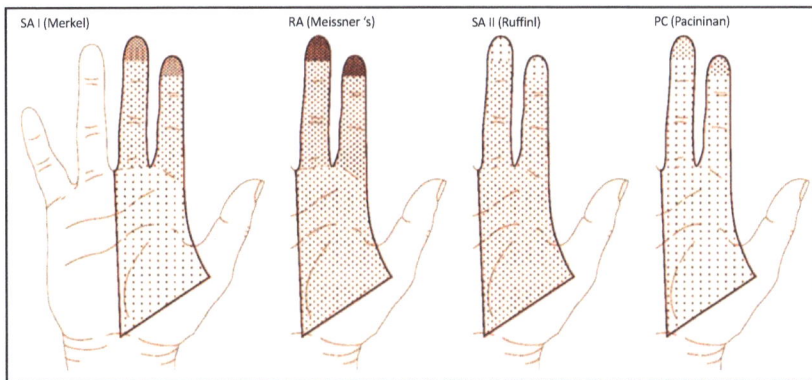

Fig. (9). Distribution density of cutaneous mechanoreceptors in the palm. From: Vallbo AB, Johansson RS. The tactile sensory innervation of the glabrous skin of the human hand. In: Gordon G, Ed. Active Touch, the Mechanism of Recognition of Objects by Manipulation. Oxford: Pergamon Press Ltd 1978; pp. 29-54.

In the palm there are about seventeen thousand mechanoreceptive units [15]; the density of distribution is so high as to lead to the overlapping of single receptive fields, up to a two-point discrimination (that is the minimum distance at which two points of touch can be perceived as separate) of 2 mm in fingertips (Fig. **10**).

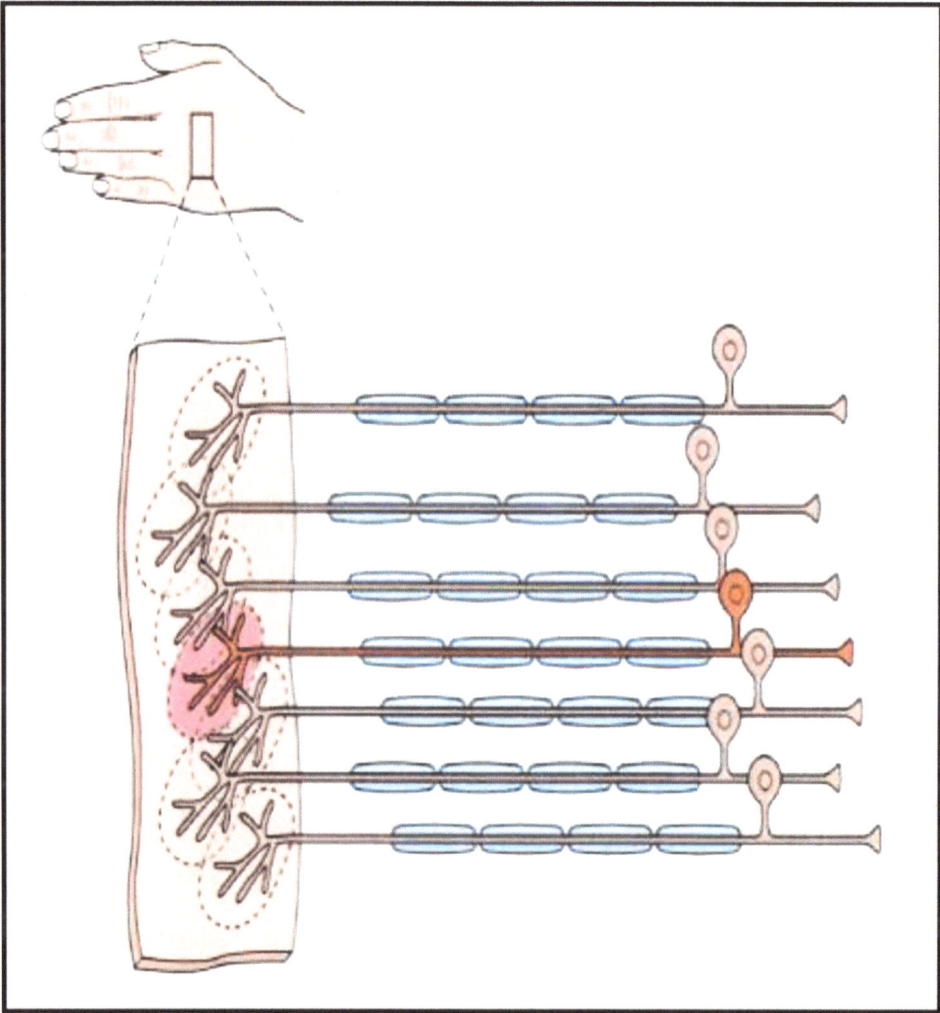

Fig. (10). Overlapping of receptive fields in the hand.

Together, the receptive field size and the distribution density of cutaneous mechanoreceptors determine the spatial resolution with which stimuli are perceived, and the spatial resolution is not uniform in different areas of body surface, as illustrated in Fig. (**11**).

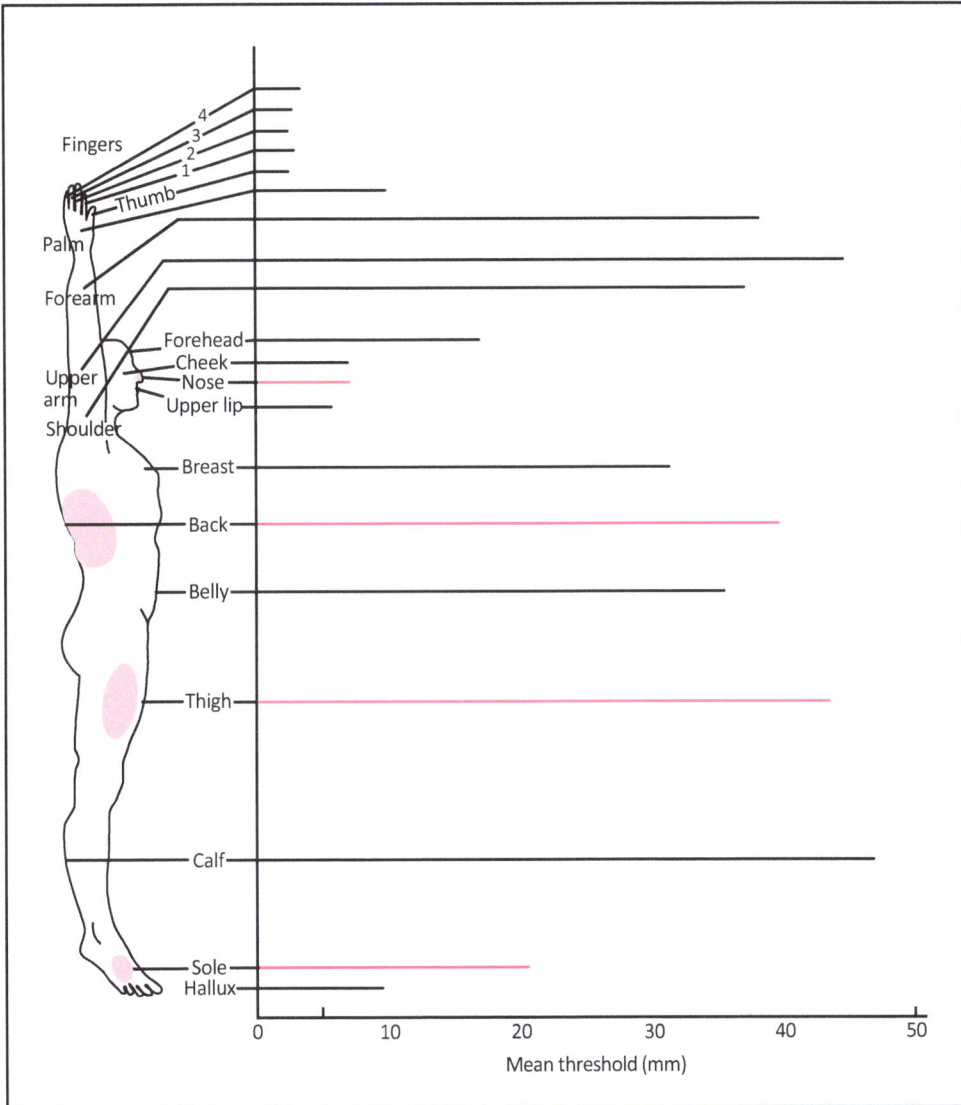

Fig. (11). Spatial resolution (as the distance in mm where the two points can be felt as separate) in different areas of body surface. From: Weinstein S. Intensive and Extensive Aspects of Tactile Sensitivity as a Function of Body Part, Sex, and Laterality. In: Kenshalo DR, Ed. The Skin Senses. Springfield (IL): Charles C. Thomas 1968; pp. 195-222.

In the foot, cutaneous mechanoreceptors act differently from those of the palm: firstly, a large percentage (70%) are fast-adapting and randomly distributed throughout the plantar surface of the foot (without accumulation in the toes);

secondly, they have larger (three times greater) receptive fields predominantly gathered on the plantar surface of the metatarsal-tarsal region of the sole and elevated activation thresholds compared to the palm [16] (Fig. **12**).

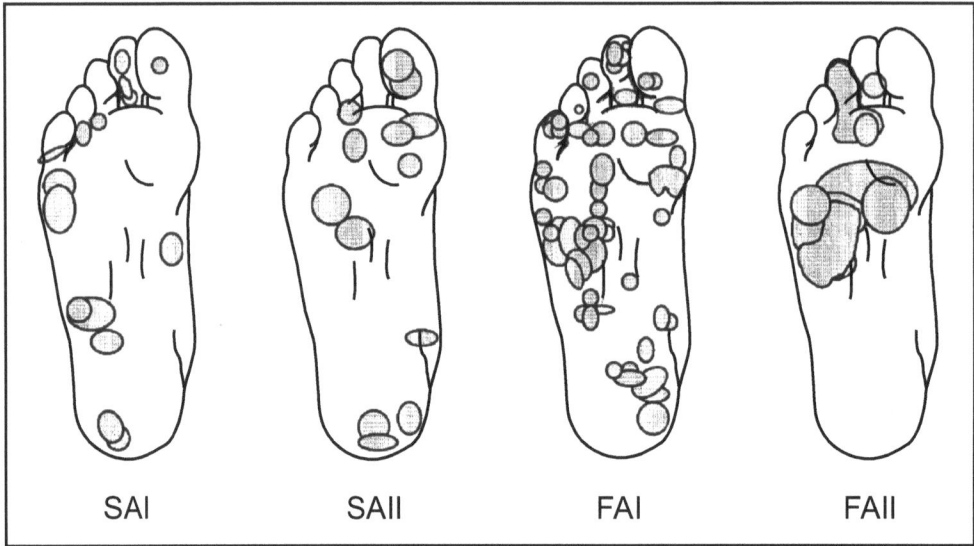

Fig. (12). The receptive field for each receptor type in the foot sole. The receptive field has been outlined with a monofilament 4-5 times greater than the initial threshold value. From: Kennedy PM, Inglis JT. Distribution and behaviour of glabrous cutaneous receptors in the human foot sole. J Physiol. 2002; 538(Pt 3): 995-1002.

Lastly, whereas they show no background discharge activity with the foot in an unloaded position and in absence of intentionally applied stimulation, they are sensitive to contact pressures [17] and to modifications in the distribution of pressure, conditioning spatially oriented whole-body tilts whose direction depends on the foot areas stimulated and is always opposite to vibration-simulated pressure increase [18, 19] (Fig. **13**).

For details, see: Kavounoudias A, Roll R, Roll JP. The plantar sole is a 'dynamometric map' for human balance control. Neuroreport 1998; 9(14): 3247-52.

Therefore, *somatosensory input from the foot has been recognized as an important source of sensory information in controlling standing balance and movement control* [20, 21] – as well as visual [22, 23], vestibular [24 - 27] or muscular [28, 29] systems – making the sole a "dynamometric map" equipped with numerous sensors able to spatially code every pressure applied against the sole (Table **1**).

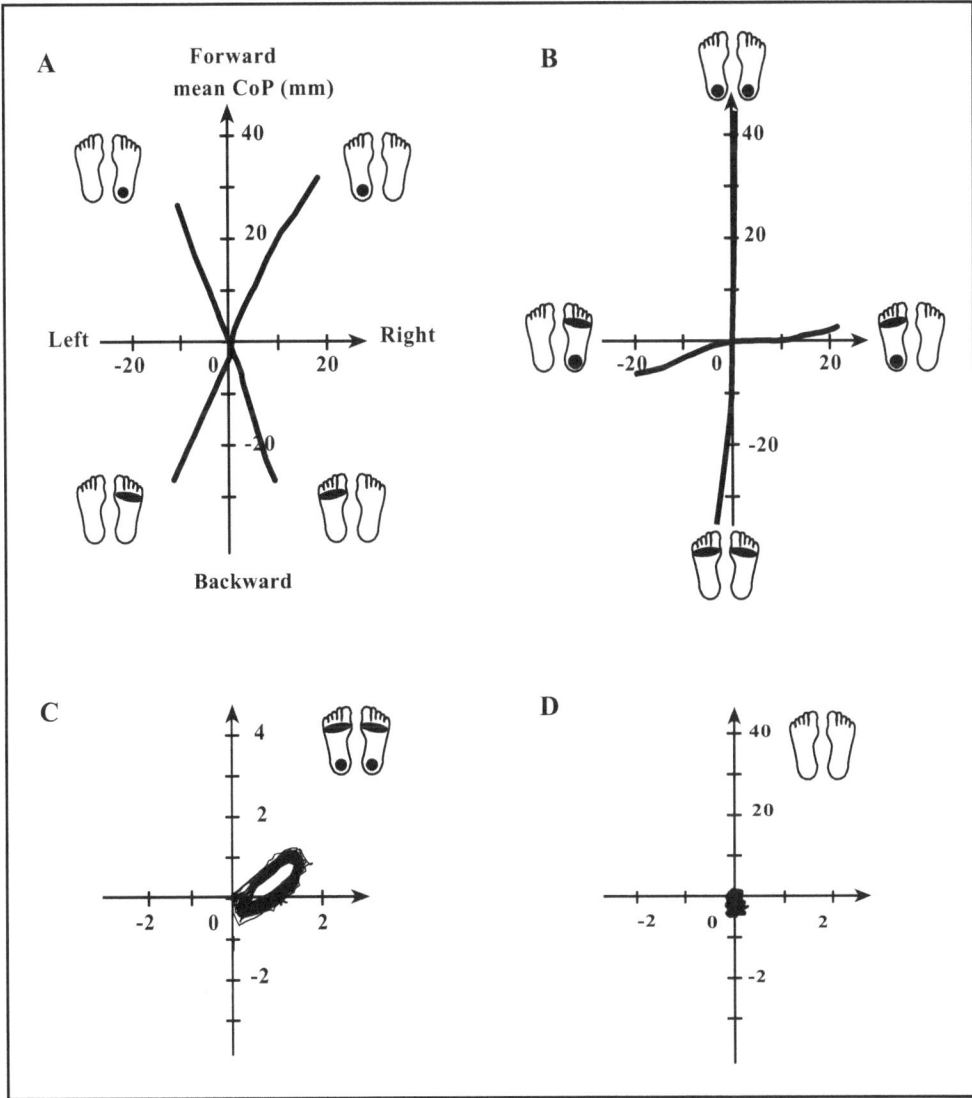

Fig. (13). Mean oriented postural responses induced by applying vibratory stimulation (100 Hz, 0.2-0.5 mm) to the anterior and posterior areas of the soles. Traces are the mean trajectories (mm) of the Center of Pressure (CoP) during the first 3 seconds of recording. The pictograms indicate the vibration sites. Because the subjects' displacements were very small under both control and four vibration conditions, a larger scale was used in C and D.

The processing of the cutaneous messages from the sole together with the other sensory messages allow the central nervous system to constantly acquire information about body position and trigger adequate responses to reduce the gap between the body position and the equilibrium position [18, 19]. Data supporting the role of plantar cutaneous messages in postural control have been obtained through two different experimental approaches. A first method consists of temporarily eliminating the exteroceptive and/or proprioceptive inputs by cooling [17, 30 - 38] or anesthetizing [39, 40] the sole, or applying an ischemic block of afferent fibers: in all cases, the suppression of these inputs increased the postural instability [20, 41 - 43]. The second approach consists of changing the characteristics of the supporting surface on which the subject is standing [39, 44, 45].

Table 1. Profiles of cutaneous mechanoreceptors in the foot sole.

Profiles of cutaneous mechanoreceptors in the foot sole						
Type	Number	Per cent of total	Median threshold (mN)	Range (mN)	Receptive field size (mm²)	
					Median	Range
SAI	15	14.4	35.6	4–744	70.9	11.8–277.5
SAII	16	15.4	115.3	36–2800	127.4	44.0–296.2
FAI	59	56.7	11.8	0.7–282	38.0	5.8–333.6
FAII	14	13.5	4.0	0.5–2800	284.2	41.7–1248.0
Total	104	100	—	—	—	—

The total number of units for each subpopulation, the threshold levels as estimated with calibrated nylon monofilaments, and the receptive field properties were calculated.

From: Kennedy PM, Inglis JT. Distribution and behaviour of glabrous cutaneous receptors in the human foot sole. J Physiol 2002; 538(Pt 3): 995-1002.

Mechanoreceptors In Muscle

Mechanoreceptors in muscle tissue are corpuscles 10-12 mm long and 1-2 mm in diameter called *muscle spindles*, highly specialized sensory structures that are able to determine position of the muscle and to detect amount and rate of change in length of the muscle, hence conveying information to the central nervous system via sensory neurons. Placed in the interfascicular connective tissue within the belly of a skeletal muscle and arranged with their longitudinal axis in parallel to the extrafusal muscle fibers, spindles are composed of 3-12 *intrafusal muscle fibers*: the central nuclear bag fibers, with nuclei concentrated in bags, and the smaller nuclear chain fibers, with nuclei aligned in a chain [46, 47]. In their central non-contractile parts intrafusal muscle fibers are coiled by two types of sensory nerve endings: primary (Ia) afferent and secondary (II) afferent fibers (Fig. **14**). The first ones are larger and faster and because of their rapid adaptation they stop firing when muscle stops changing length, constantly monitoring the velocity of muscle stretching; on the contrary, the second ones are non-adapting and continue firing when movement has ceased, constantly informing on instantaneous length or position of still muscle [48, 49].

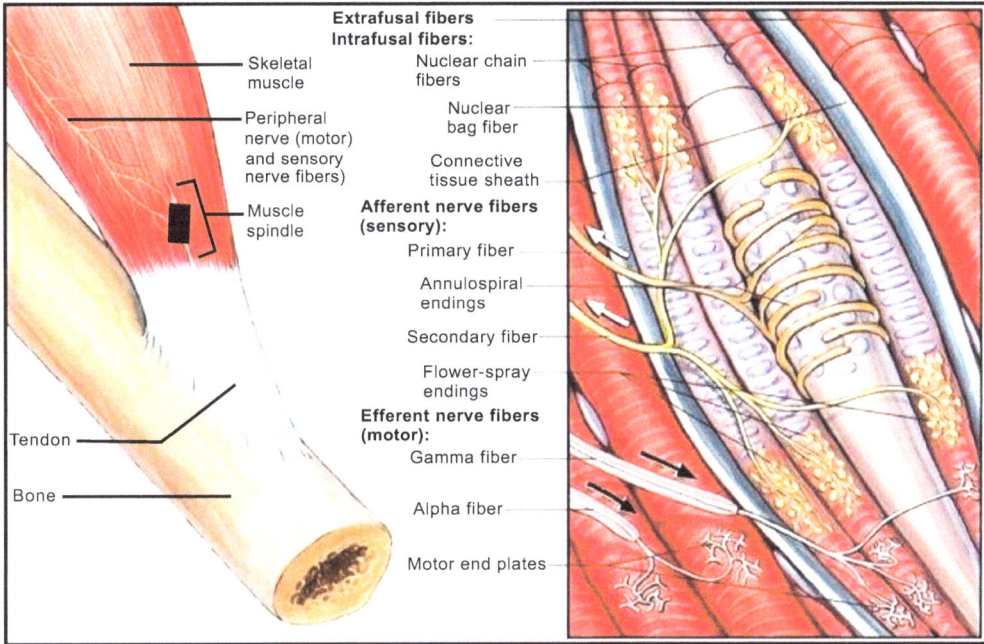

Fig. (14). Detailed representation of a muscle spindle.

In the dorsal horn of the spinal cord, the Ia afferent fiber of the muscle spindle bifurcates. One branch make synapse directly on alpha motoneurons that innervate the same (homonymous) muscle; in this way, activation of the Ia afferent induces a monosynaptic activation of the alpha motoneuron, which in turn generates the muscle contraction, and as a result the stretch of the muscle is quickly counteracted (stretch or myotatic reflex) (Fig. **15a**). The other branch innervates the Ia inhibitory interneuron, which in turn innervates the alpha motoneuron that synapses onto the opposing (antagonist) muscle; because the interneuron is inhibitory, it prevents the firing of the opposing alpha motoneuron, thus reducing the contraction of the opposing muscle (reciprocal inhibition in the stretch reflex) (Fig. **15b**).

It has been demonstrated that mechanical vibration on a single muscle is able to activate Ia and II afferent nerve fibers of the muscle spindle [50], and hence the alpha motoneurons: this elicits the so-called "Tonic Vibration Reflex" (TVR)

[51 - 53], consisting in the sustained contraction of the vibrated muscle and simultaneous relaxation of its prime antagonist [54 - 60].

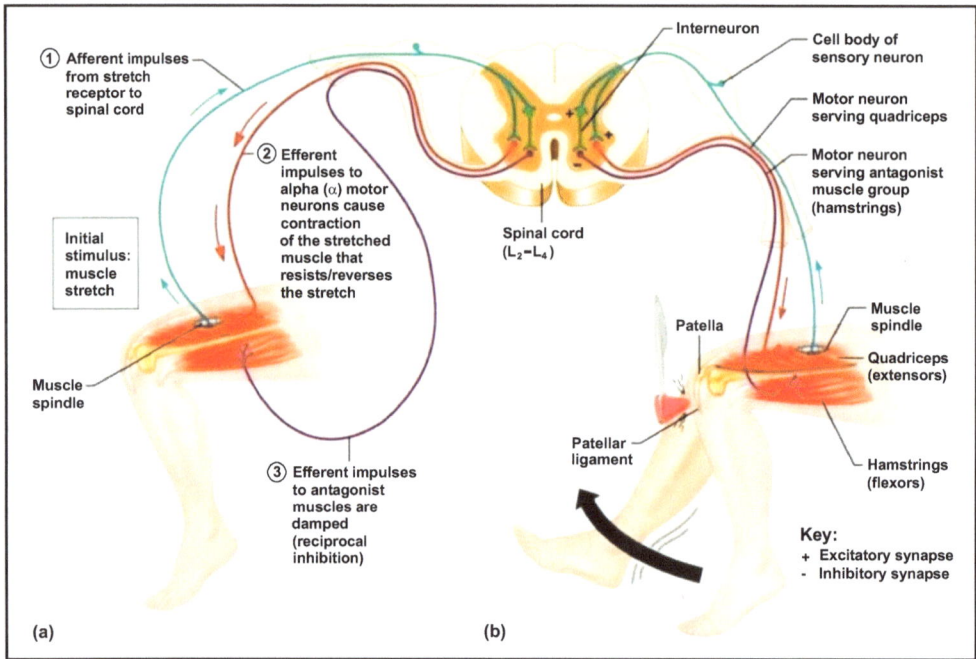

Fig. (15). Physiology of spinal reflexes. Copyright© 2006 Pearson Education, Inc., publishing as Benjamin Cummings.

VIBRATIONS, RESONANCE AND TUNING RESPONSE: THE TENSEGRITY MODEL

In daily life, the body interacts with the external environment and experiences externally applied forces. During walking, a train of vibratory waves is generated and transmitted along the body upon impact of the foot to the ground; these vibrations (with frequency typically between 10-20 Hz) are transmitted through the foot, leg, and spine [61 - 63], thus making walking the most widespread mechanical stress adequate to maintain muscles and bones within a range of functionality.

Overall, during most recreational or occupational activities, vibrations within the tissues of the body can be induced from the collision of either a part of the body or sporting or working equipment in contact with the body against an object (as occurs when the heel strikes the ground during each running stride [64] or the hand or a racket hits a ball); after every impact the tissues continue to vibrate as a free oscillation, that is vibrating at their natural frequency, with the amplitude of these vibrations decaying because of damping within the tissues. In the event of less irregular forms of vibration (as may occur during bike riding or driving) the continuously oscillating input force leads the soft tissue vibrations to attuning to the same frequency as the input force, but at a greater amplitude if the natural frequency of the tissues is close to that of the input force (resonance) [65].

Table 2. Summarizes the major classes of somatic sensory receptors.

The Major Classes of Somatic Sensory Receptors

Receptor type	Anatomical characteristics	Associated axons[a] (and diameters)	Axonal conduction velocities	Location	Function	Rate of adaptation	Threshold of activation
Free nerve endings	Minimally specialized nerve endings	C, Aδ	2–20 m/s	All skin	Pain, temperature, crude touch	Slow	High
Meissner's corpuscles	Encapsulated; between dermal papillae	Aβ 6–12 μm		Principally glabrous skin	Touch, pressure (dynamic)	Rapid	Low
Pacinian corpuscles	Encapsulated; onionlike covering	Aβ 6–12 μm		Subcutaneous tissue, interosseous membranes, viscera	Deep pressure, vibration (dynamic)	Rapid	Low
Merkel's disks	Encapsulated; associated with peptide-releasing cells	Aβ		All skin, hair follicles	Touch, pressure (static)	Slow	Low
Ruffini's corpuscles	Encapsulated; oriented along stretch lines	Aβ 6–12 μm		All skin	Stretching of skin	Slow	Low
Muscle spindles	Highly specialized (see Figure 8.5 and Chapter 15)	Ia and II		Muscles	Muscle length	Both slow and rapid	Low
Golgi tendon organs	Highly specialized (see Chapter 15)	Ib		Tendons	Muscle tension	Slow	Low
Joint receptors	Minimally specialized	—		Joints	Joint position	Rapid	Low

[a]In the 1920s and 1930s, there was a virtual cottage industry classifying axons according to their conduction velocity. Three main categories were discerned, called A, B, and C. A comprises the largest and fastest axons, C the smallest and slowest. Mechanoreceptor axons generally fall into category A. The A group is further broken down into subgroups designated α (the fastest), β, and δ (the slowest). To make matters even more confusing, muscle afferent axons are usually classified into four additional groups—I (the fastest), II, III, and IV (the slowest)—with subgroups designated by lowercase roman letters!

From: Purves D, Augustine GJ, Fitzpatrick D, Hall WC, LaMantia AS, McNamara JO, Williams SM, Eds. Neuroscience. 3rd ed. Sunderland (MA): Sinauer Associates 2004; 8: p. 190.

The natural frequency of a vibrating system depends on its mass and stiffness. The latter is based on the skeletal muscle tone, which in turn is modulated by the interaction between the actin and myosin myofilaments [66], and so increases in muscle activity can increase the tissue stiffness (and therefore the tissue natural frequency). Indeed, studies have shown that increments in the natural frequency of whole muscle groups match with the joint torques developed by the muscle and typically range between 10-50 Hz for the lower extremity muscles (zero to maximal activity [67]). Conversely, muscles can also damp externally applied vibrations, and indeed vibration energy is more absorbed by activated muscle [62, 68] than by muscles in rigor [69], suggesting that the actomyosin bundles play an important role in the vibration damping process. Wakeling and Nigg determined the natural frequencies for the tissues for each posture by measuring the vibration response to a complex vibration covering a range of frequencies (10-65 Hz, amplitude 5 mm) and therefore described changes in resonance that occurred with altered limb posture and muscle activity; they found that most vibration damping occurred at the resonant frequencies of the tissues, match with the highest levels of muscle activity. Since the responses of the lower extremities to continuous vibrations or sequences of single, impact-like input were similar, they suggests that *the body has a strategy of "tuning" its muscle activity to minimize the vibrations that pass through the soft tissue regardless of the features of the input force, in an attempt to tolerate more vibration energy and reduce potential harmful effects* [64, 70].

Actually, the effect of the input force amplitude on the tuning response has not yet been determined, nor is it known if there is a minimum amplitude below which the tissue reaction is not triggered. Conversely, at high force amplitudes, the tissue maximum damping will not be as effective at scattering the vibration energy, so we do not yet know which is the most effective range of vibration amplitudes that can be applied safely in order to evoke a significant tuning response. Indeed, it has been shown that improper vibratorious exposure may have deleterious effects on the soft tissues, including muscle fatigue [71], reduction in muscle contraction force [72] and motor unit firing rate [73], delay in nerve conduction velocity, and weakened perception [74]. More specifically, for vibratory stimulation frequency greater than 75 Hz, and acceleration greater than 1 g (where 1 g is the acceleration due to the Earth's gravitational field or 9.81 m/s^2), several adverse effects are reported in literature, including low back pain, circulatory disorders such as Raynaud's syndrome, nervous alterations, disorders of perception, dizziness [75 - 77]; however, the evidence of a dose-response association is feeble and the causal link remains to be clarified. Moreover, most of the adverse effects of vibrations are related to prolonged exposure to occupational reasons [78 - 80]. Hence, precise regulation exists at least in occupational medicine, expressly for some categories of individuals are subject to different types of vibration for occupational reasons: use of jackhammer and other utensil, drive of heavy vehicles, and much more [81]. On the other hand, vibration therapy – at least using the whole-body technique – also has various contraindications, as shown in Table **3**.

Nevertheless, *according to the muscle tuning theory, the muscular response to externally applied forces is related not only to the interaction between the amplitude and frequency of the vibration input but also to the muscle tone (state of relaxation or contraction), intercurrent length variation (shortening or elongation movement), combined effect of all the muscles interlinked with a same joint as much as the position of the body* [82, 83]. In human body, pre-stress (pre-

Table 3. Contraindications to whole-body vibration.

Contraindications to whole-body vibration
• Kidney or bladder stones
• Arrhythmia
• Pregnancy
• Epilepsy
• Seizures
• Cancer
• Pacemaker
• Untreated orthostatic hypotension
• Recent implants (joint/corneal/cochlear, etc)
• Recent surgery
• Recently placed intrauterine devices or pins
• Acute thrombosis or hernia
• Acute rheumatoid arthritis
• Serious cardiovascular disease
• Severe diabetes
• Migraines

From: Kasturi GC, Adler RA. Osteoporosis: nonpharmacologic management. PM R 2011; 3(6): 562-72.

existing) tension is provided by a matrix of connective tissue, whereas the counterbalancing compression is provided by the bones and fluids. Since tension is continuous and compression is discontinuous, such that continuous pull is balanced by oppositely discontinuous pushing forces, according to a model inspired by R. Buckminster Fuller's structural principle of «tensegrity» (portmanteau of "tensional integrity") – which describes «a structural-relationship principle in which structural shape is guaranteed by the finitely closed, comprehensively continuous, tensional behaviors of the system and not by the discontinuous and exclusively local compressional member behaviors» [84] – *the human body can be seen as a tensegrity structure which distributes stresses to establish a force balance and stabilize itself against shape distortion* [85] (Fig. **16**).

Hence, pre-stress plays an important role in determining the mechanics of the musculoskeletal system [86]. As engineers have developed reinforced concrete beams with pretensioned steel bars as "pre-stress" structures, similarly muscles, tendons and ligaments are endowed with tensile properties that allow them to put

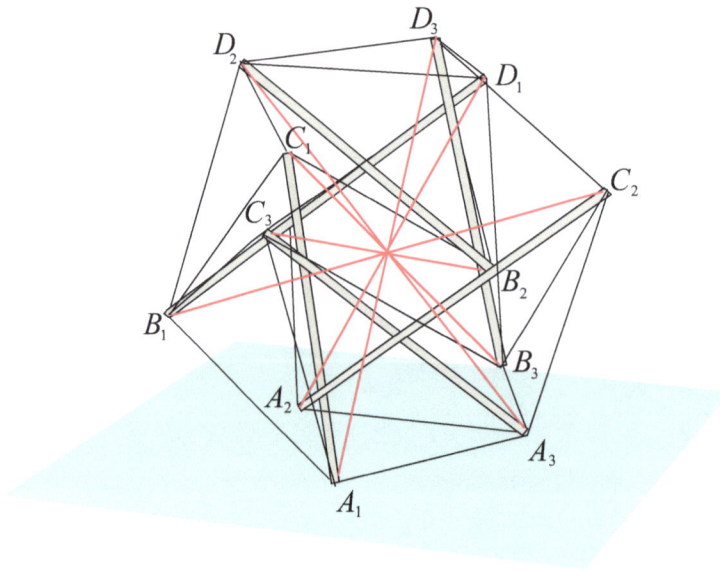

Fig. (16). A tensegrity structure with cytoskeletal filaments network used to generate the computational tensegrity model. Black lines represent microfilaments, red lines represent intermediate filaments, the thick gray beams represent microtubules, the black triangles (A1, A2, and A3) indicate the anchoring points to the substrate (blue). From: Sultan C, Stamenović D, Ingber DE. A computational tensegrity model predicts dynamic rheological behaviors in living cells. Ann Biomed Eng 2004; 32(4): 520-30.

together the bones articulated at any joint, stabilizing body in any posture: in this way, even when the bones diverge from each other, the joint does not dislocate. Moreover – since the structure of each joint is assembled by a number of muscles, tendons and ligaments – a critical role in defining the joint potential strength, power, speed, and range of motion is played by the number and position of these tensile elements (*i.e.*, the architectural arrangement): indeed, where tendons and ligaments loosen, it results in joint instability, increased wear on the articular cartilage, pain, and loss of function [87] (Fig. **17**).

The variety of structural components that constitute the musculoskeletal system possess a broad spectrum of mechanical properties without using many types of materials. This is possible because of a hierarchical organization of tissues in several length scales, so that the smaller building elements themselves show specialized architecture [88, 89]. The existence of discrete networks within bones, cartilage, tendons, ligaments and muscles maximizes their structural efficiency (*e.g.*, strength/mass ratio) as much as stress damping, since the same stress will be distributed to and resist by many smaller elements rather than a single continuum [85]. Even on the smallest size scale (the molecular level), architectural organization contributes significantly to the mechanical strength of biologic tissue, as explained beyond. In the bone, the mineral component containing hydroxyapatite crystals accounts for the compressive stiffness, while the collagen fibrils augment the tensile strength [88] (Fig. **18**).

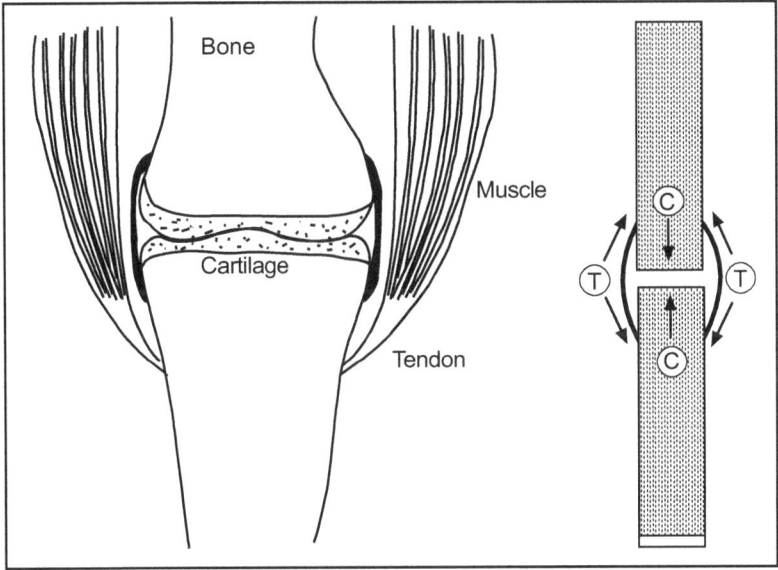

Fig. (17). Schematic diagram of a generic articular joint (left) and grossly simplified corresponding internal stresses in bone, cartilage, and ligaments (right). External forces acting on the joint are indicated as compressive (C) or tensile (T). From: Chen CS, Ingber DE. Tensegrity and mechanoregulation: from skeleton to cytoskeleton. Osteoarthritis Cartilage 1999; 7(1): 81-94.

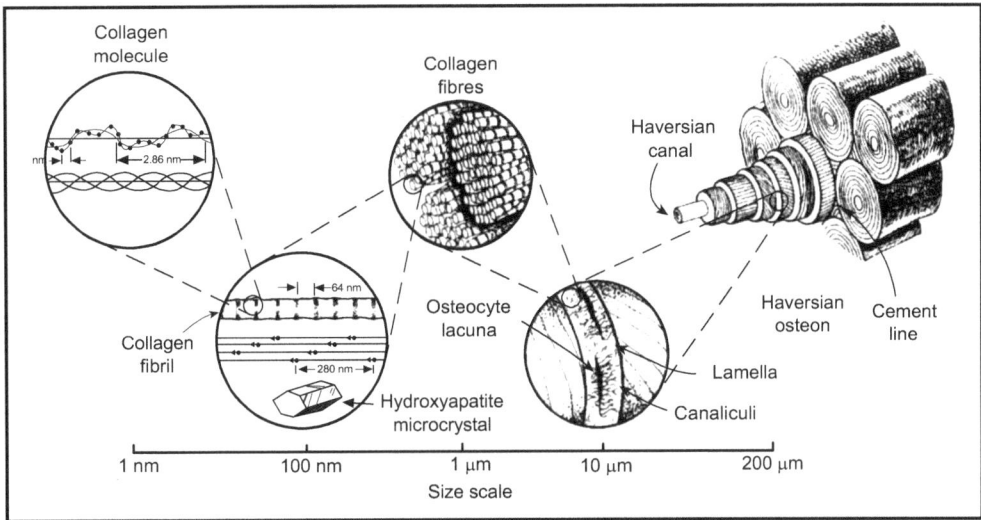

Fig. (18). Hierarchical structure of the human compact bone. From: Lakes R. Materials with structural hierarchy. Nature 1993; 361: 511-5.

The action of stress in bone is influenced by the shape of the bone itself, its loading conditions, and the strain exerted by the surrounding muscles and tendons; contractile fibroblasts also conceivably pre-stress the collagen network during the process of tissue development and remodeling, before the surrounding extracellular matrix mineralizes (Fig. **19**).

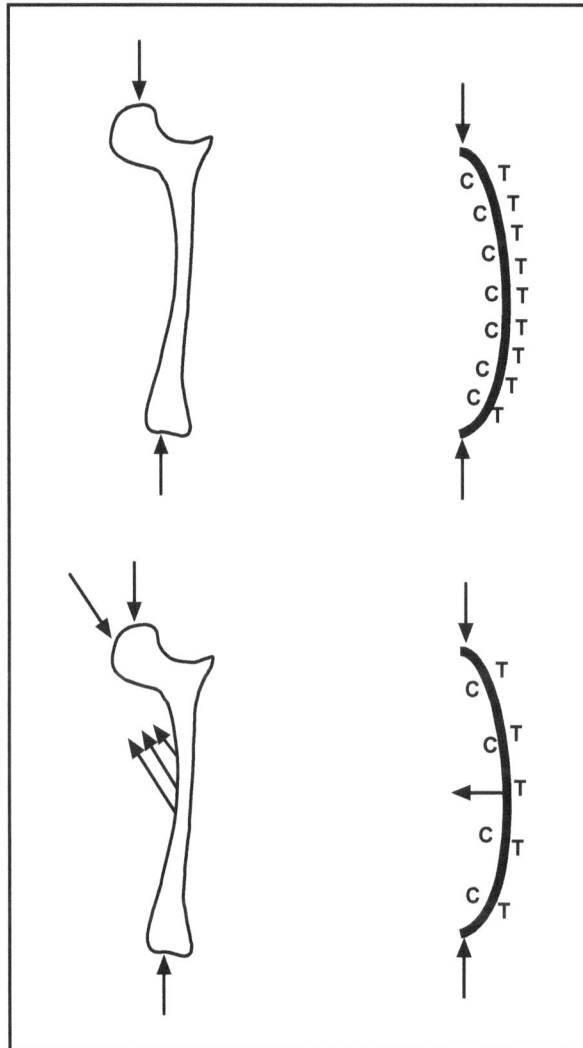

Fig. (19). The loading of the femur in upright position and its modulation by the muscular tension. External forces acting on the bone are indicated as compressive (C) or tensile (T). For details, see: Chen CS, Ingber DE. Tensegrity and mechanoregulation: from skeleton to cytoskeleton. Osteoarthritis Cartilage 1999; 7(1): 81-94.

Pre-stress also plays an important role in determining the mechanics of cartilage and soft tissues [86]. In cartilage and ligaments, the collagen network is pre-stressed and stretched by the osmotic force of hydration of embedded proteoglycan molecules [89 - 93] (Fig. **20**); the cellular elements themselves may bear some mechanical loads.

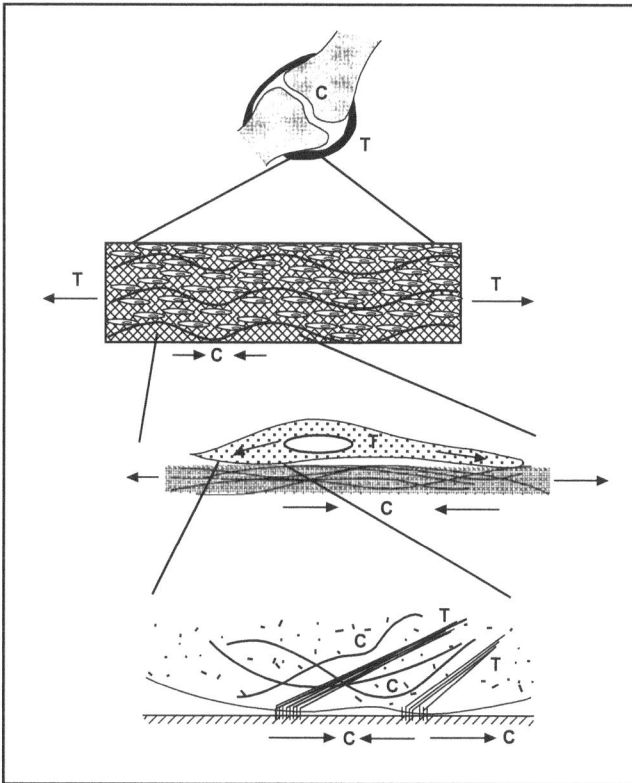

Fig. (20). Hierarchical tensegrity structure of a ligament from an articular joint. External forces acting on the ligament are indicated as compressive (C) or tensile (T). For details, see: Chen CS, Ingber DE. Tensegrity and mechanoregulation: from skeleton to cytoskeleton. Osteoarthritis Cartilage 1999; 7(1): 81-94.

Besides small amounts of proteoglycans (depending on the site and the mechanical loading conditions), glycoproteins (including tenascin-C and fibronectin), elastic fibers (including elastin and microfibrillar proteins), water and cells (mainly fibroblasts, but also endothelial and synovial cells and chondrocytes) [94], tendon is primarily made up of collagen molecules (almost entirely type I collagen, followed by types III and V and traces of other collagens, probably reflecting differences in mechanical properties [95]) self-assembled into cross-striated fibrils and arranged in a hierarchical structure composed of fibrils, fiber bundles, fascicles and tendon unit aligned with its long axis [96] (Fig. **21**).

The end-to-end crosslinks between collagen molecules within fibrils are responsible for the elastic response of tendon, whose magnitude is directly related to the collagen fibril length (more than the fibril diameter) and therefore the number of collagen molecules that are cross-linked end-to-end in series [97, 98].

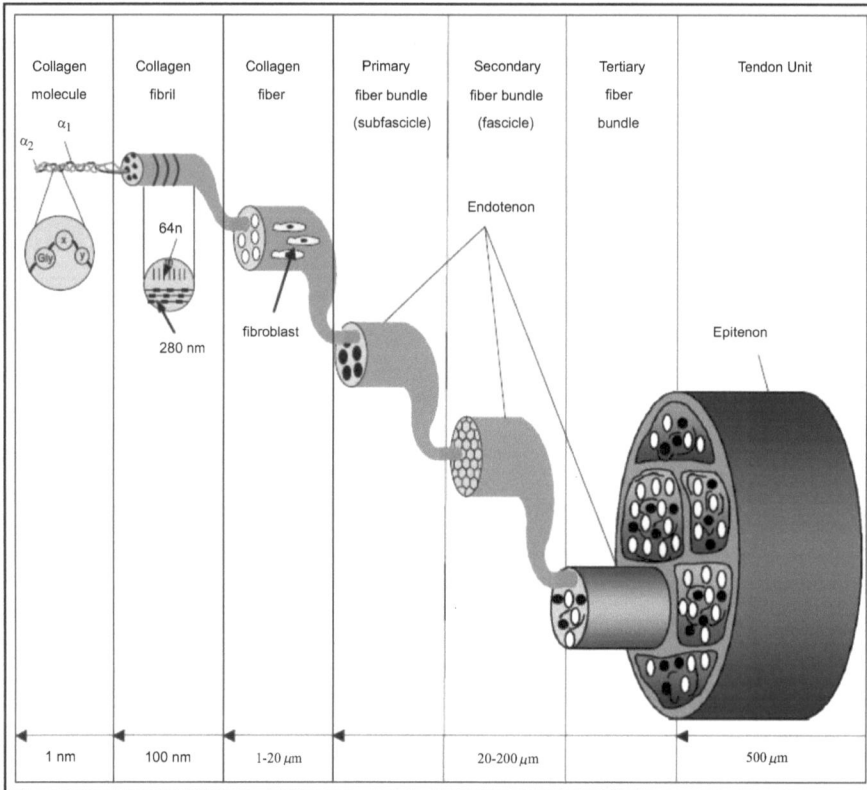

Fig. (21). Schematic representation of the hierarchical structure of the tendon. Modified from: Silver FH, Freeman JW, Seehra GP. Collagen self-assembly and the development of tendon mechanical properties. J Biomech 2003; 36(10): 1529-53.

Hence, according to the tensegrity model, mechanical forces – applied to either the whole body (*e.g.*, gravity) or a part of the body (*e.g.*, stretching or compression) – are transmitted across structural elements that results physically interconnected, inducing a response that depends on the level of pre-stress tension and, more importantly, is orchestrated at a cellular and molecular level [99 - 102]. This occurs because cells express on their surface specific transmembrane receptors (such as integrins) able to recognize and respond to mechanical stimuli, transmitting them from the extracellular matrix to the cytoskeletal filament network (Fig. **22**). The integrin-transmitted mechanical deformation ("outside-in signaling") triggers perturbations in kinetic or thermodynamic parameters (molecular motion, dissociation and association constants) and modifications in cytoskeletal scaffold organization (conformational changes in actin bundle assembly and microtubule polymerization) [103 - 106] (Fig. **23**) and affects different cellular functions through activation of membrane ion channels (direct chemical response), signal-transducing molecules in cooperation with growth factor receptors (with release of chemical second messengers such as kinases), interference on binding interaction between cytoskeletal filaments and various organelles (with proteic synthesis and secretion), or even changes in nuclear matrix structure (with induction of the expression of specific genes). This retroactively allows to regulate force transmission across the cell surface by altering ability of integrins to anchor to the cytoskeleton or by modulating exposure of their extracellular binding sites ("inside-out signaling") (Fig. **22**). In this way, the balance between inward and outward forces results to be critical for control of cell shape, migration, growth, proliferation, differentiation, and eventually survival or death [107].

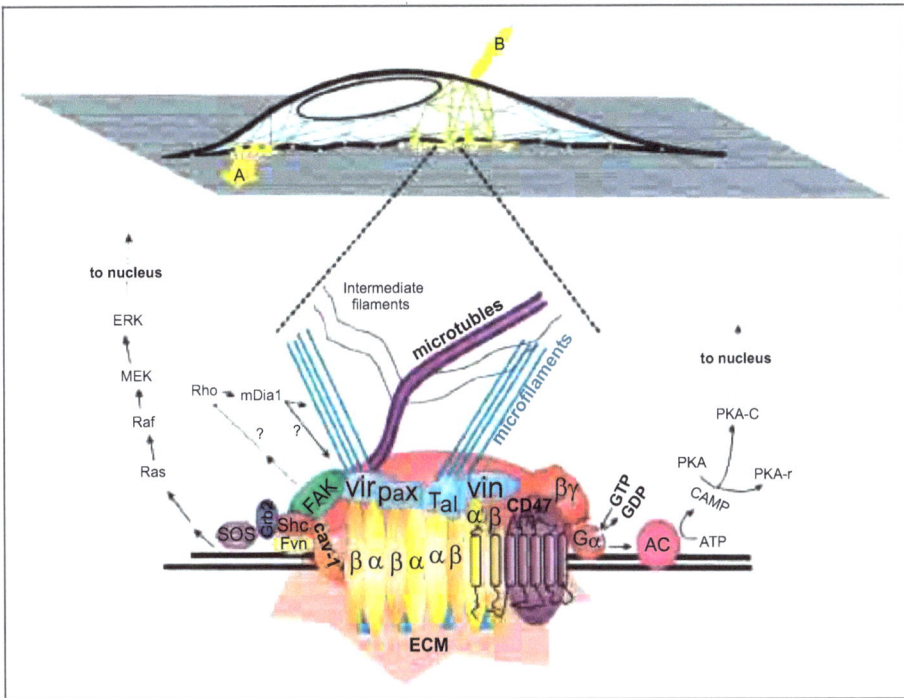

Fig. (22). Schematic representation of the transmission of mechanical stimuli from the basement membrane (A) or the extracellular matrix (B) to the cytoskeletal scaffold, through clustering of dimeric (α,β) integrin receptors and induced recruitment of focal adhesion proteins (such as Vinculin [Vin], Paxillin [Pax], Talin [Tal]), and examples of signaling cascade.

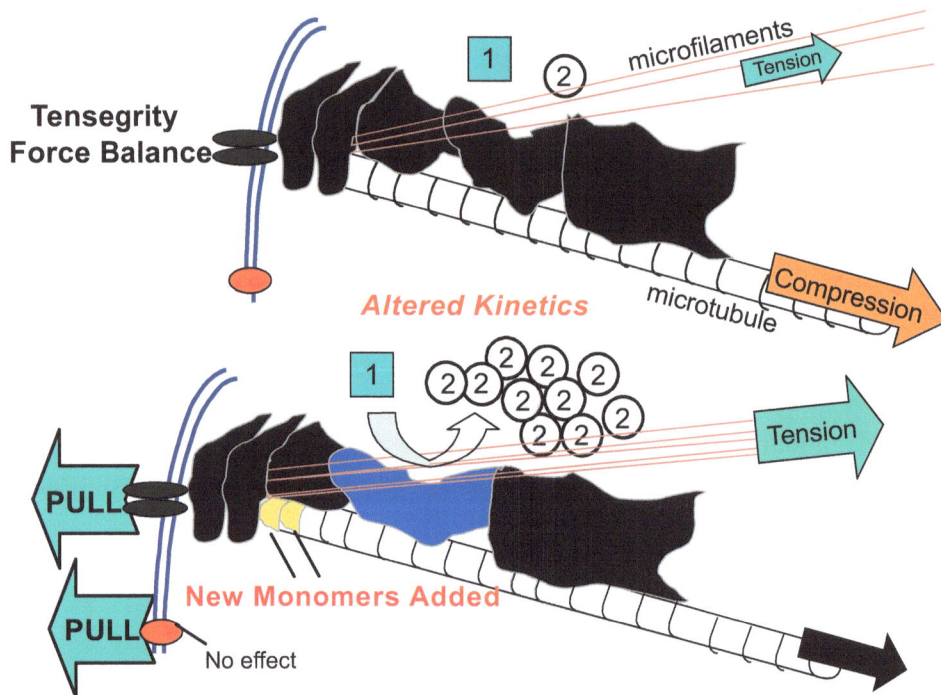

Fig. (23). Contribution of cellular tensegrity to mechanochemical transduction through perturbations in kinetic or thermodynamic parameters and modifications in cytoskeletal scaffold organization. For details, see: Ingber DE. Tensegrity II. How structural networks influence cellular information processing networks. J Cell Sci 2003; 116(Pt 8): 1397-408.

In conclusion, it is clear that tensegrity provides a mechanism of conversion of mechanical stress into cellular responses through a variety of molecular pathways, and, in wider terms, a mechanistic basis to explain how application of physical therapies might condition and influence cell and tissue physiology [108 - 110].

VIBRATION AND THE MUSCULOSKELETAL SYSTEM: THE MECHANOSTAT THEORY

Within the so-outlined tensegrity model, it has been proposed that vibrations could be used as a rehabilitation and a training aid.

In 1880s, the French neurologist Jean-Martin Charcot, observing that patients suffering from Parkinson's disease experienced a reduction in their rest tremor and a better sleep after a train carriage ride or after horseback riding, fashioned a vibratory chair (*fauteuil trépidant*) that simulated the rhythmic shaking of a carriage and where he replicated the experience seating patient for 30-minute daily sessions [111]. His student and junior colleague Georges Gilles de la

Tourette extended these observations and fashioned a helmet that vibrated the head on the premise that the brain responded directly to the pulsations, reporting efficacy in «neurasthenic invalids» and migraine [112] (Fig. 24).

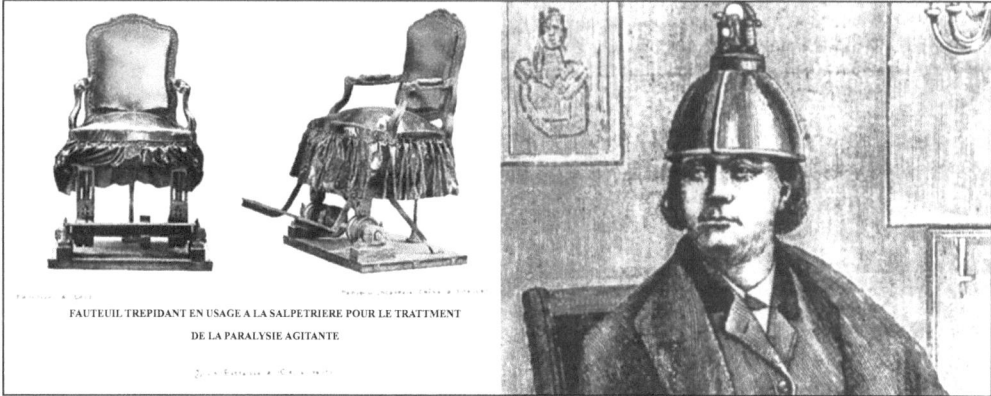

FAUTEUIL TREPIDANT EN USAGE A LA SALPETRIERE POUR LE TRATTMENT DE LA PARALYSIE AGITANTE

Fig. (24). Charcot observed that patients with Parkinson's disease experienced a reduction in their rest tremor after taking a train carriage ride or after horseback riding, so he developed a therapeutic vibratory chair that simulated the rhythmic shaking of a carriage (left). His student Gilles de la Tourette later developed a vibratory helmet to shake the head and brain (right). From: Goetz CG. The history of Parkinson's disease: early clinical descriptions and neurological therapies. Cold Spring Harb Perspect Med 2011; 1(1): a008862.

Although after Charcot's death vibratory therapy was not widely pursued, his ideas were developed further by different therapists and vibratory appliances reemerged in 21st century medicine: since between 1890 and 1910, G. Taylor and JH. Kellogg in USA, and G. Zander in Sweden adapted Charcot's protocols producing different kinds of vibration therapy for arms and back. The first application of whole-body vibration (WBV) technique dates back to 1949, when Whedon *et al.* reported the positive effects achieved through the application of vibrations generated by an oscillating bed on metabolic and physiological alterations of bedridden in plaster cast patients [113]. In this direction, in experiments conducted on animal models, the vibratory stimulation at high frequency seemed to be able to greatly stimulate osteogenesis [114 - 117], whereas studies in human indicate that it improves bone mineral density, muscle strength and proprioception, especially in people with osteoporosis or those with motor impairment from neuromuscular diseases of various etiologies [83, 118 - 124]. The effect of vibration exercises on bone tissue directly through micro deformation of tissue matrix and cells (particularly osteocytes and bone lining cells seem to be located in the bone to act as the sensors of local strains [125]) [126 - 136], through mechanocoupling of shear stresses transmitted by the intramedullary pressure [137 - 140], and/or through mechanotransduction of electric fields (called "streaming potentials" [138, 141 - 147]) generated in endocanalicular and intra-lacunar fluid flow [148 - 153], and probably for this seems to be greater at trabecular level [138, 154 - 157] (Fig. **25**).

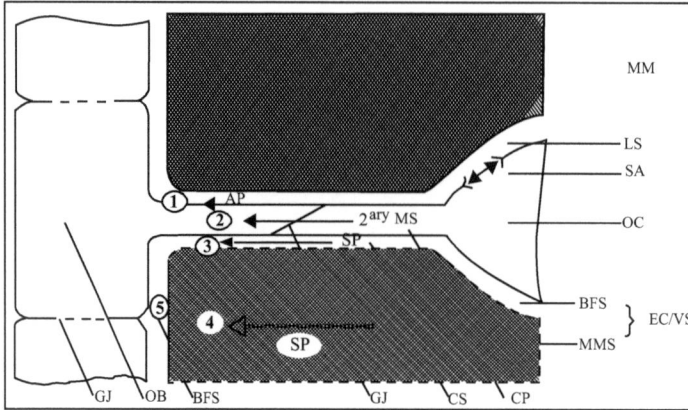

Fig. (25). Schematic representation of several possible pathways for the transmission of mechanosensory information in an osseous, connected cellular network. The following notations are employed to label features in the diagram: (MM) mineralized matrix, (MMS) mineralized matrix fluid space, (SA) stretch-activated ion channel in osteocytic plasma membrane, (Oc) osteocyte, (Ob) osteoblast, (BFS) bone fluid space, (CS) canalicular space, (LS) lacunar space, (CP) cell process, (GJ) gap junction, (EC/VS) extra-cellular extravascular bone fluid space, (SP) streaming potential, (AP) action potential, (2^{ary} MS) secondary messengers. The fluid in the bone fluid space (BFS) is equal to the sum of the lacunar space (LS) and the canalicular space (CS), (BFS) = (LS) + (CS). Together the bone fluid space (BFS) and the mineralized matrix fluid space (MMS) form the extra-cellular, extravascular bone fluid space (EC/VS), (EC/VS) = (BFS) + (MMS) = (MMS) + (LS) + (CS). The bone tissue is assumed to be mechanically strained unevenly so that the right side sustains a greater strain than the left side. The external surface of the bone is to the left of the diagram. One periosteal osteoblast (Ob) is depicted as interconnected by gap junctions (GJ) to adjacent osteoblasts and similarly to one osteocytic cell (canalicular) process (CP). Three possible transductive mechanisms and related pathways are depicted: along the cell membrane [with the propagation of an action potential along the cell plasma membranes (1), and the gap junction acting as an electrical synapse]; intracellular [with the passage of one or more secondary messengers (2)]; extracellular [streaming potentials (SP) would be generated in the deformed mineralized matrix (MM)]. Under the conditions depicted, (+) charges would flow (4) towards the less strained bone surface on the left. It is possible that additional streaming potentials (3) may also be generated within the bone fluid space (BFS) in both the osteocytic lacunar (LS) and canalicular spaces (CS). These mechanisms and pathways are not mutually exclusive. Whatever the pathway and mechanism, an appropriate signal must reach the genomic apparatus to regulate the functional responses of the osteoblast (Ob). With the extracellular transmission of streaming potentials (SP), (3) and/or (4), the effective electrical events must occur in the bone fluid space (BFS), (5), intervening between the plasma membrane of the osteoblast (Ob) and the external surface of the mineralized matrix (MM). Activation of the stretch-activated ion channel (SA) in the plasma membrane of the cell bodies and/or cell processes of the osteocyte (Oc) could invoke both the action potential (AP) of (1) and the secondary messengers (2^{ary} MS) of (2). From: Cowin SC, Moss-Salentijn L, Moss ML. Candidates for the mechanosensory system in bone. J Biomech Eng 1991; 113(2): 191-7.

Regardless of the actual mechanisms, and *consistently with the Wolff's law and the theory of everyday stress stimulus, to describe the mechanical conditions that allow the maintenance of bone mass Harold M. Frost put forth the hypothesis of a "mechanostat", which describes windows of mechanical usage that should be considered physiological or not*, each separated by a minimum effective strain (MES): when local mechanical signals do not reach the lower limit of the physiological MES, bone tissue will be resorbed (until the local strains are increased); on the other hand, when local mechanical signals exceed the upper limit of the physiological MES, bone will undergo increasing modeling (until a fracture) [158 - 173] (Fig. **26**).

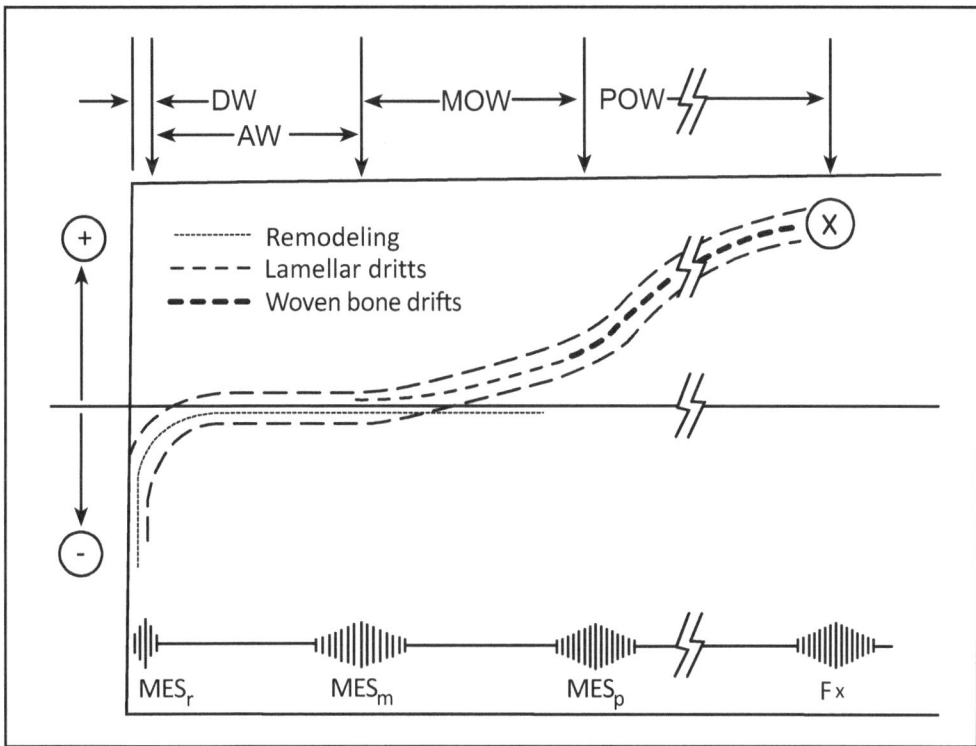

Fig. (26). Combined modeling and remodeling effects on load-bearing bone strength. DW, disuse window; AW, adapted window; MOW, mild overload window; POW, pathological overload window; MESr, remodeling minimum effective strain; MESm, modeling minimum effective strain; MESp, pathologic minimum effective strain; Fx, fracture strain.
For details, see: Frost HM. Strain and other mechanical influences on bone strength and maintenance. Curr Opin Orthop 1997; 8: 60-70.

According to the mechanostat theory, the effect of mechanical strains on bone depends upon the amplitude and duration of the applied load. Lower amplitude loads applied for longer duration has the same anabolic effect as loads with short duration and high amplitude [174 - 180] (Fig. **27**). For instance, Rubin and Lanyon demonstrated that an applied strain of 2,050 microstrain (1 micro strain equals 1 micrometer of deformation per meter of length) applied for 4 cycles per day produced the same maintaining effect on bone mass in immobilized limbs as an applied strain of 1,000 micro strain applied for 100 cycles per day [181, 182]. Therefore, it is supposed that the bone responds to the cyclic muscular contraction and relaxation induced by the TVR generated by the stimulation of mono- and polysynaptic neuronal pathways [183].

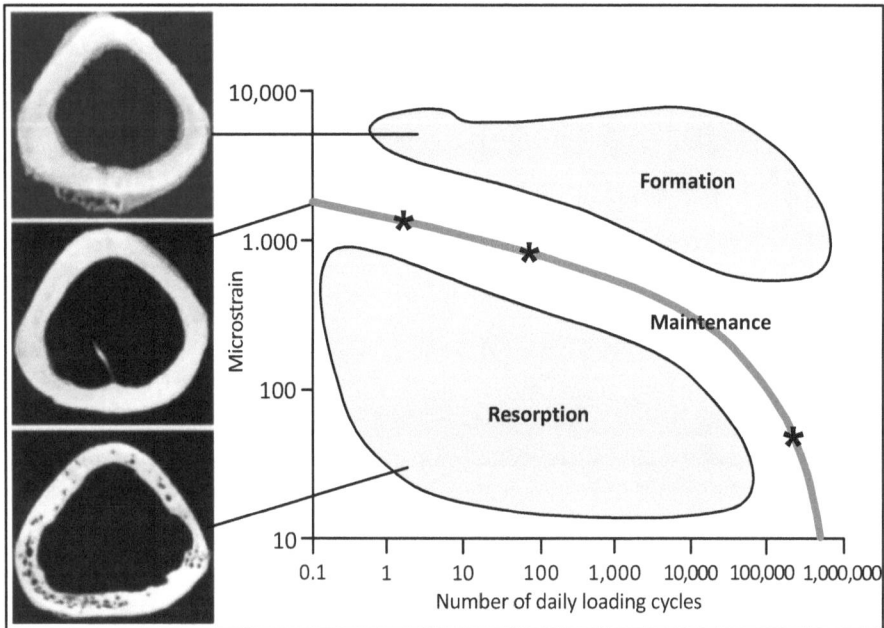

Fig. (27). Interrelationship between loading cycles and bone adaptation. Redrawn from: Qin YX, Rubin CT, McLeod KJ. Nonlinear dependence of loading intensity and cycle number in the maintenance of bone mass and morphology. J Ortop Res 1998; 16: 482-9.

Besides the amplitude and duration, critical factors for the response of the skeletal system to vibration therapy are the direction (vertical or lateral) and frequency of the vibration and the position of the body on the platform [154, 156, 184].

With regard to the position of the body on the platform, it is known that a person standing on a platform requires muscle activation from the lower limbs in order to dampen the vibrations coming up from the vibrating plate. Wakeling *et al.* observed that standing with the heel in contact with the vibration platform resulted in uncomfortable and unsustainable vibrations traveling through the body; however, the long vibration loads could be sustained by subjects standing on their forefeet with the heels raised 1 cm above the ground. To mimic the knee posture at heel strike during running, the same authors used a slightly flexed knee, resulting in muscle activities of 20-193% of those found at heel strike during running [70]. Using transcutaneous pins placed in the spinous process of L4 and the greater trochanter of the femur, Rubin *et al.* were able to demonstrate decreased transmissibility of vibration with varying postures in six subjects standing on an oscillating platform which provided sinusoidal loading at discrete frequencies from 15 to 35 Hz, and accelerations ranging up to 1 g. With the subjects standing erect, transmissibility at the hip exceeded 100% for loading frequencies less than 20 Hz, indicating a resonance; at frequencies more than 25 Hz, transmissibility decreased to approximately 80% at the hip and spine; in relaxed stance, transmissibility decreased to 60%; with 20-degree knee flexion, transmissibility was reduced even further to approximately 30%; a phase-lag reached as high as 70 degrees in the hip and spine signals [185].

The currently marketed devices that deliver vibration to the whole body use two different types of vibrating plates: in one type, the plate oscillates uniformly up and down with only a vertical translation; in the other type, the plate oscillates with reciprocal vertical displacements on the left and right side of a fulcrum (Fig. **28**).

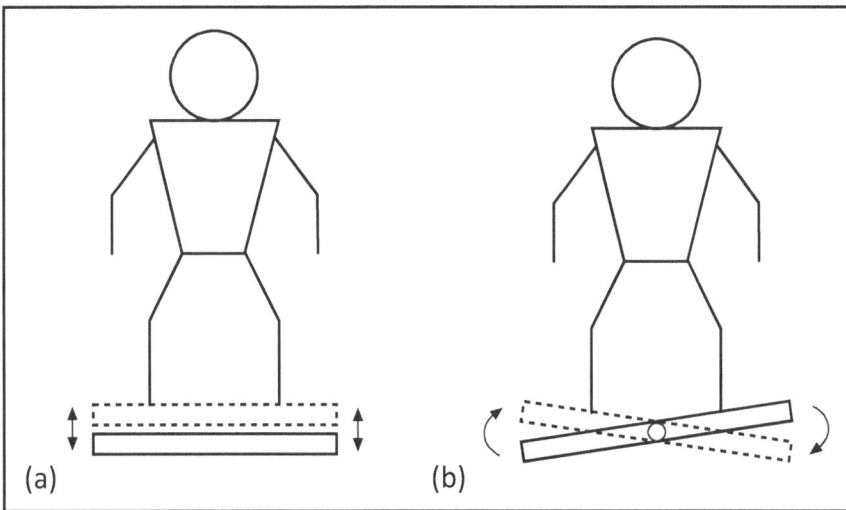

Fig. (28).   Designs of currently marketed whole body vibrating plates. Platform displacements are exaggerated for demonstrative purposes. Modified from: Cardinale M, Wakeling J. Whole body vibration exercise: are vibrations good for you? Br J Sports Med 2005; 39(9): 585-9.

Performing a series of static and dynamic unloaded squatting using two different directions of vibration, vertical and rotational, and removing large vibration-induced artefacts from recorded electromyographic data, Abercromby *et al.* found that the average responses of the tibialis anterior were significantly greater during vertical than rotational vibration while responses of the vastus lateralis and gastrocnemius (leg extensor muscles) were significantly greater during rotational than vertical vibration [186]. As regards the risk of adverse health effects, in another study the same authors concluded that it may be lower on a short duration (< 10 minutes) exposures to rotational than vertical vibration and at half-squats (knee flexion angle between 26-30°) rather than full-squats or upright stance [187].

Currently available WBV exercise devices deliver vibrations at a range of frequencies from 15 to 60 Hz and displacements from <1 mm to 10 mm; the acceleration delivered can reach 15 g. Considering the numerous combinations of amplitudes and frequencies possible with current technology, it is clear that there are several WBV protocols that could be used on humans [65]. Studies with the most significant results utilizes frequencies between 25-45 Hz and accelerations of 0.3 g [188 - 198]; are recommended, furthermore, cycles of short duration (2-20 minutes), interlaced with variable-duration periods of rest [199], and the assumption of an upright posture with hips and knees in modest flexion, to ensure better transmissibility of the forces at the hip and spine [184]. Owing to the differences in WBV protocols used in the different studies, it is difficult to compare studies and standardize the application of the WBV training (WBVT) interventions on the skeletal and muscular systems.

The reaffirmed transient and long-term enhancement of the muscle mechanical behavior (increase in sectional area and reduction in adipose tissue inside the muscle itself, increase in contractile velocity, force and power, improvement in vertical jumping ability, isometric lower-limb extension strength, and dynamic or static body balance) is strongly suggestive for a neurogenic adaptation that may occur in response to the vibration treatment [65, 122, 188, 192 - 195, 200 - 207].

VIBRATION AND THE CENTRAL NERVOUS SYSTEM: APPLICATIONS IN NEUROREHABILITATION

Prolonged observations seem to demonstrate that the vibration-induced muscle mechanical activation could lead to a modulation of the spinal reflex excitability [208] *via* short spindle-Moto neuron connections [209]. In general, it is controversial whether in addition to reflex (involuntary) muscle work there is a mechanism of central (voluntary) control [72, 210 - 213]. It has been demonstrated that low amplitude muscle vibration (80 Hz, 0.5 mm, duration 1.5 s) increases the amplitude of motor evoked potentials produced by transcranial magnetic stimulation in the vibrated muscle compared to that evoked at rest, whereas the opposite occurs in non-vibrated muscles, and that vibratory stimulation can produce differential changes in the excitability of populations of cortical inhibitory neurons that project to different output zones of the motor cortex [214 - 216], probably because the input from muscle spindles is important in shaping the excitability of intracortical GABAergic circuits [217 - 221].

Furthermore, *vibration appears to be much more specific than cutaneous electrical stimulation*, having opposite rather than graded effects on the vibrated and non-vibrated muscle. The reason is not completely clear: it may be that vibration is a more natural input than electrical stimulation of nerves, since it activates muscle spindles and thus elicits the TVR, whereas electrical nerve stimulation activates afferent fibres directly; alternatively, it may be that the muscle spindle input activated by vibration has a more specific action on cortical circuits than cutaneous input activated by electrical nerve stimulation. The latter explanation is consistent with the different (segregated) distribution of cutaneous and proprioceptive afferents to areas of the somatosensory cortex: the input from low threshold mechanoreceptors and cutaneous receptors primarily reach areas 3b and 1 [222 - 230], whereas muscle vibration produces Ia afferent input that reaches both area 3a [231 - 233] and area 4 of the motor cortex directly [234]; area 2 is reached from either deep or cutaneous afferent inputs [235] (Fig. **29**). Additionally, using electrophysiological mapping methods, a further functional segregation within area 3b of monkeys has been suggested: indeed, consistently with the evidences that different low-threshold mechanoreceptor afferents elicit distinct sensations of pressure (evoked by stimulation below 2 Hz), tapping/flutter (evoked by stimulation between 2-40 Hz) and vibration (evoked by stimulation between 40-200 Hz) [236, 237], numerous psychophysical studies show that independent processing pathways mediate these three different sensations, suggesting that there is some degree of segregation in their central projections to somatosensory cortex [238 - 242].

These experimental findings in turn are consistent with the traditional neurophysiological knowledge on the principal sensory tracts, summarized in Table **4** and, with regard to the posterior (dorsal) columns pathway, in Fig. (**30**).

Thus, *muscle spindle inputs could potentially have a stronger and more selective influence on the motor cortex than those from cutaneous inputs*. From this point of view, the duration of the vibration stimulus (3 up to 5 weeks) seems to be important, as shown in studies by Bosco *et al.* [243, 244]. Whatever the mechanism, it appears that small-amplitude vibration may be a more sensitive test of the input/output relations of the cortex than electrical nerve stimulation [214].

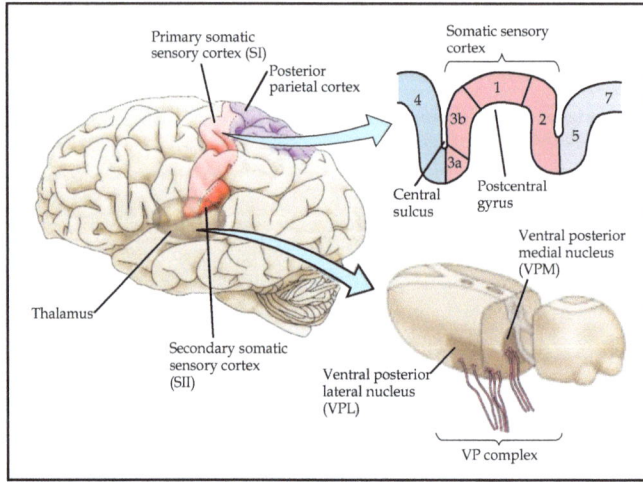

Fig. (29).   Cortical and thalamic projection of proprioceptive system. From: Purves D, Augustine GJ, Fitzpatrick D, Hall WC, LaMantia AS, McNamara JO, Williams SM, Eds. Neuroscience. 3rd ed. Sunderland (MA): Sinauer Associates 2004; 8: p. 204.

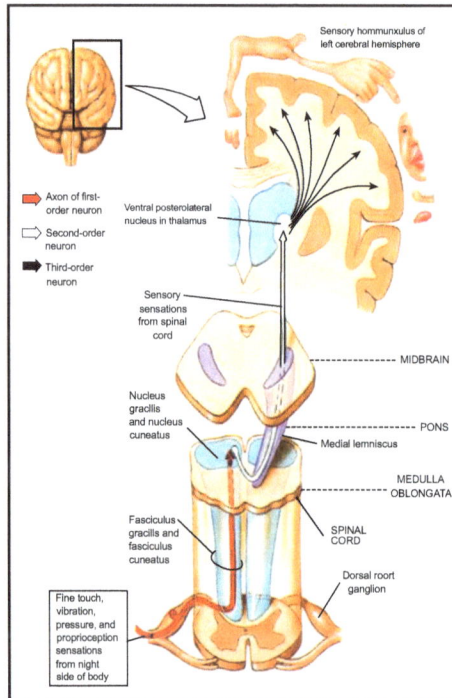

Fig. (30).   Posterior column-medial lemniscus pathway. From: Martini FH, Timmons MJ, Tallitsch RB. Human Anatomy. 7th ed. Pearson Benjamin Cummings 2012.

It has been also demonstrated that *vibrations of certain frequency, magnitude, duration and direction are able to ensure that the mechanoreceptors generate action potentials of the same frequency of the applied stimulation (driving phenomenon)* [245, 246]; a repeated stimulation by means of evoked action potentials of defined frequency is able to selectively recruit precise nerve networks, according to a long-term (months) potentiation phenomenon.

Table 4. Principal ascending (sensory) tracts and the sensory information they provide.

Principal Ascending (Sensory) Tracts and the Sensory Information They Provide						
		Location of Neuron Cell Bodies				
Tract	Sensations	First-Order	Second-Order	Third-Order	Final Destination	Site of Crossover
POSTERIOR COLUMNS						
Fasciculus gracilis	Proprioception, fine touch, pressure, and vibration from levels inferior to T_6	Dorsal root ganglia of lower body; axons enter CNS in dorsal roots and ascend within fasciculus gracilis	Nucleus gracilis of medulla oblongata: axons cross over before entering medial lemniscus	Ventral posterolateral nucleus of thalamus	Primary sensory cortex on side opposite stimulus	Axons of second-order neurons, before joining medial lemniscus
Fasciculus cuneatus	Proprioception, fine touch, pressure, and vibration from levels at or superior to T_6	Dorsal root ganglia of upper body; axons enter CNS in dorsal roots and ascend within fasciculus cuneatus	Nucleus cuneatus of medulla oblongata: axons cross over before entering medial lemniscus	Ventral posterolateral nucleus of thalamus	As above	As above
SPINOTHALAMIC TRACT						
Lateral spinothalamic tracts	Pain and temperature sensations	Dorsal root ganglia; axons enter CNS in dorsal roots and enter posterior gray horn	In posterior gray horn: axons enter lateral spinothalamic tract	Ventral posterolateral nucleus of thalamus	Primary sensory cortex on side opposite stimulus	Axons of second-order neurons, at level of entry
Anterior spinothalamic tracts	Crude touch and pressure sensations	As above	In posterior gray horn: axons enter anterior spinothalamic tract on opposite side	As above	As above	As above
SPINOCEREBELLAR TRACTS						
Posterior spinocerebellar tracts	Proprioception	Dorsal root ganglia; axons enter CNS in dorsal roots	In posterior gray horn: axons enter posterior spinocerebellar tract on same side	Not present	Cerebellar cortex on side of stimulus	None
Anterior spinocerebellar tracts	Proprioception	As above	In same spinal segment: axons enter anterior spinocerebellar tract on same or opposite side	Not present	Cerebellar cortex, primarily on side of stimulus	Axons of most second-order neurons cross before entering tract and then cross again within cerebellum

Modified from: Martini FH, Timmons MJ, Tallitsch RB. Human Anatomy. 7th ed. Pearson Benjamin Cummings 2012.

The long-term potentiation provides the base for the application of vibration in some of the most common neurological diseases associated with motor impairment conditions: cerebral palsy, multiple sclerosis, Parkinson's disease, stroke, spinal cord injury. A systematic review by del Pozo-Cruz *et al.* concluded that there is moderate evidence that one session of WBV has positive effects on strength, whereas there is a weak level of evidence that it could improve proprioception and health-related quality of life measures in neurological patients. With respect to long-term effects, there is minor evidence from the studies with the best methodological quality that WBV improves strength, proprioception, gait, and balance [247]. Ahlborg *et al.* performed the only study which measured the effect of WBV on spasticity in diplegic adults with cerebral palsy using the modified Ashworth's scale; the authors reported a decrement in hypertonia after 8 weeks of WBV compared with resistance training, but this change was significant (p = 0.031) only for knee extensors muscles [248]. The application of vibrations in neurorehabilitation has been greatly promoted by the development of focal vibration systems, as described below.

FROM WHOLE-BODY TO FOCAL VIBRATION

The long-term potentiation also provides the base for the modulation of pain transmission. The analgesic effect of vibration is attributed to influencing the "gate" proposed by Melzack and Wall in their "gate control" theory of pain. According to this theory, the stimulation of the Aβ afferent fibers causes the inhibition of the nociceptive fibers by the activation of the inhibitory interneurons in the lamina II (substantia gelatinosa) of the spinal cord dorsal horn [249]. So, the physiology of pain transmission would have a common anatomical pathway with that of Ia afferent fiber of the muscle spindle, as illustrated in Fig. (**31**).

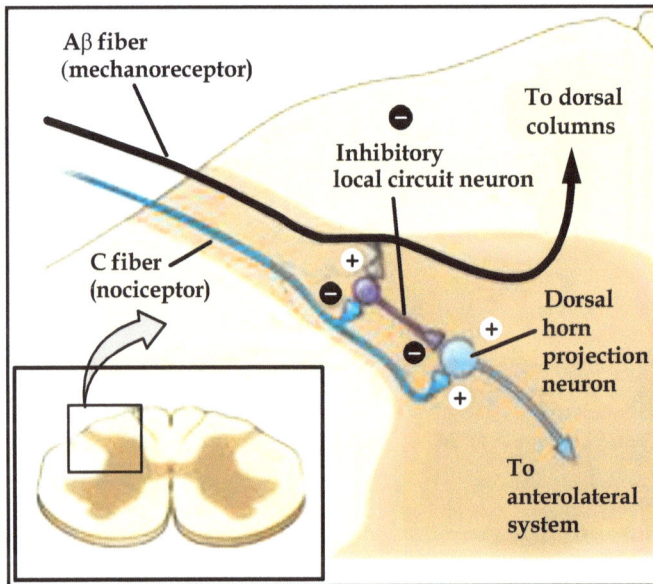

Fig. (31). The anatomo-physiological substrate for the "gate control" theory of pain.

This application has been made possible with the development of systems of focal vibration. Treatment devices for pain have some obvious advantages over pharmaceutical treatments, particularly that nothing has to be ingested and the side effect profile is arguably to be much less; it is also arguably that they are cheaper than pharmaceutical management and can be used in conjunction with those rehabilitation treatments for which there is evidence of efficacy [250]. To relieve pain, since the 1980s vibrations were delivered by electromechanical vibrators driven by a generator the signal of which was amplified by a power amplifier, and were primarily used for musculoskeletal acute and chronic pain and in painful conditions of neurogenic origin [251 - 256]. After attempts to develop systems based on solenoid valves and even on internal combustion engines, in the early 2000s the technologies available to produce focal vibration exploit the principle of the connecting rod, the eccentrics or the electromagnetism. The systems with solenoid valves produce vibrations at high frequency (even over 100 Hz) but at low amplitude; on the contrary, the systems with connecting rod produce vibrations of adequate amplitude but at maximum frequency of 60-70 Hz. The systems based on the eccentrics in direct contact of the treated district dissipate energy in all directions, and for frequencies higher than 70 Hz minimize the amplitude; the electromagnetic systems produce vibrations of adequate intensity at frequencies of 100 Hz, but manifest problems of hysteresis at frequencies exceeding 100 Hz. The modern systems can deliver wave frequencies up to 300 Hz, thus allowing the full stimulation of the Pacinian corpuscles – not obtainable with the frequencies delivered by the whole body vibrating plates – and therefore inducing a long-term potentiation of selected nerve networks.

Among the novel focal vibration devices, *EndoSphères Therapy*® (Fenix s.n.c., Montesilvano, Italy) consists of a cylinder contained in a head of 55 rotating silicone spheres arranged in a honeycomb structure; an electronic system allows to rotate the cylinder with variable speed, generating a wide range of vibratory frequencies (40-254 Hz) transmitted through the rotation of the spheres to the tissue on which it is applied with suitable pressure (Fig. **32**).

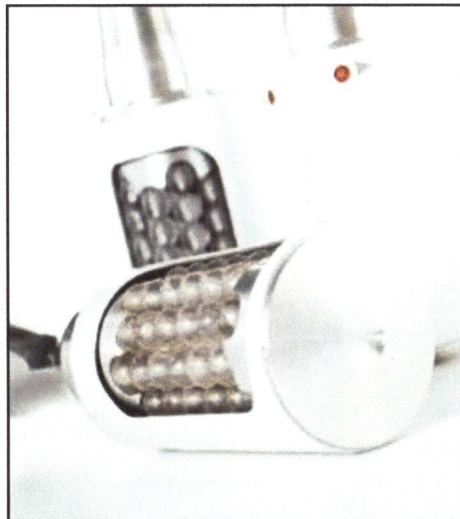

Fig. (32). *EndoSphères Therapy*® (Fenix s.n.c., Montesilvano, Italy). From: www.fenixgroup.it.

The pressure and the particular arrangement of the spheres exert rhythmic compressor and lifting of the superficial tissues, acting as a sort of "vascular gymnastics" on microcirculation of the treated districts, improving perfusion and lymphatic drainage, and following increase in local temperature and oxygenation, reshuffle of interstitial fibrosis, resolution of local lymphatic stasis, lymphedema and painful panniculosis, remodeling of the fat compartment and dermis (Fig. **33**).

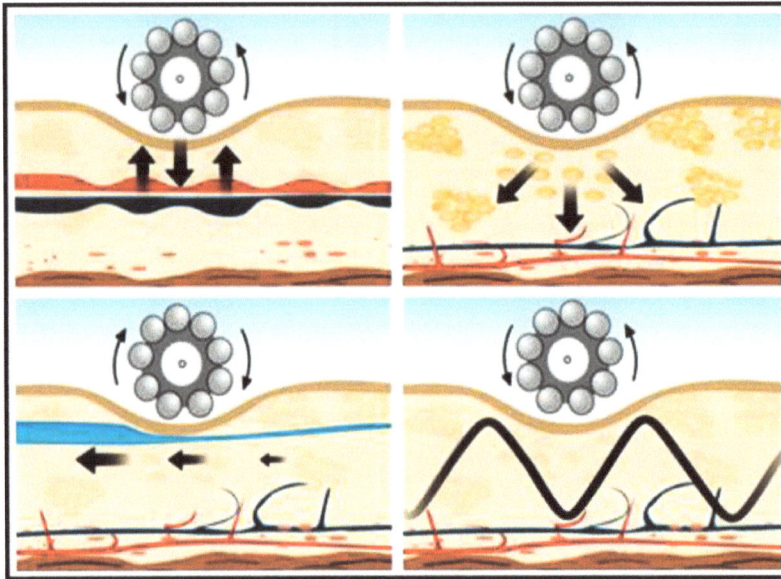

Fig. (33). The four actions of *EndoSphères Therapy*®: from left to right and top to bottom, the "vascular gymnastics", the "tissue re-compactation", the lymphatic drainage, and the analgesic effect. Modified from: www.fenixgroup.it.

Due to the particular shape of the produced wave, the *radial shock wave* can be considered a unique form of vibration too. It is a low-to-medium-energy shock wave (less than 0.1 mJ/mm^2) generated through the acceleration of a projectile pneumatically propelled inside a barrel in the hand piece of the device. Once the projectile impacts the tip of the applicator (that constitutes the focus), the high kinetic energy is transferred directly to the skin, on which the applicator is directly placed, and then transmitted radially (hence the expression "radial waves") to the target zone [257], scattering and damping by the third power of the penetration depth in the tissue while deepening up to 3.5 cm, without focusing the shock wave field in the tissue. Indeed, compared to the conventional focused shock wave – whose focus is centered on the target site instead of on the tip of the applicator (Fig. **34**) and whose wave shows a higher peak and a very short rise in pressure (Fig. **35**) – the propagation of radial shock wave is limited to the most superficial (but larger) areas of the body (see Chapter 4). Therefore, this technique has some limitations for treatment of deep soft tissue or bone injuries, instead providing potential advantages in applications like skin conditions and calcifying tendinopathies [258 - 269], and being used to treat the painful region rather than a painful point, as in plantar fasciitis [270 - 276].

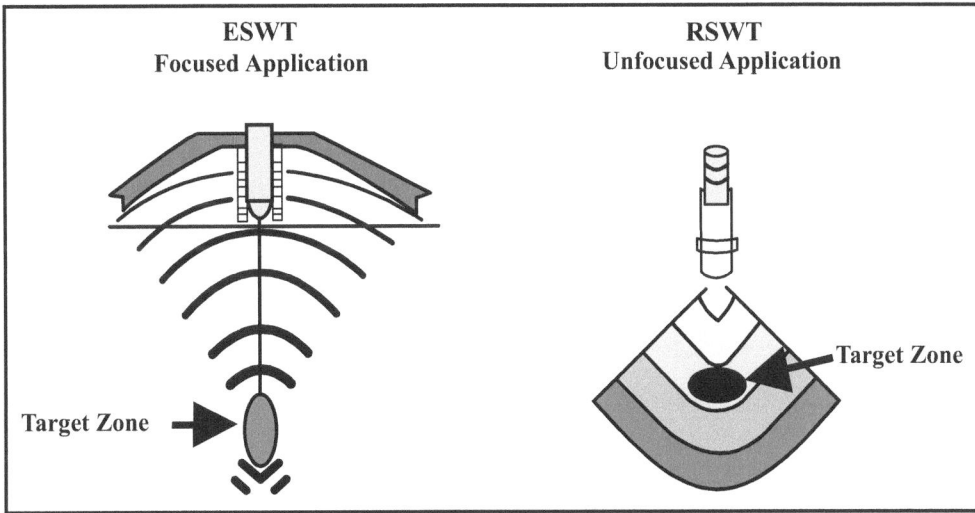

Fig. (34). Wave propagation of extracorporeal shock wave (ESW, left) and radial shock wave (RSW, right). From: Cacchio A, Paoloni M, Barile A, *et al*. Effectiveness of radial shock-wave therapy for calcific tendinitis of the shoulder: single-blind, randomized clinical study. Phys Ther 2006; 86(5): 672-82.

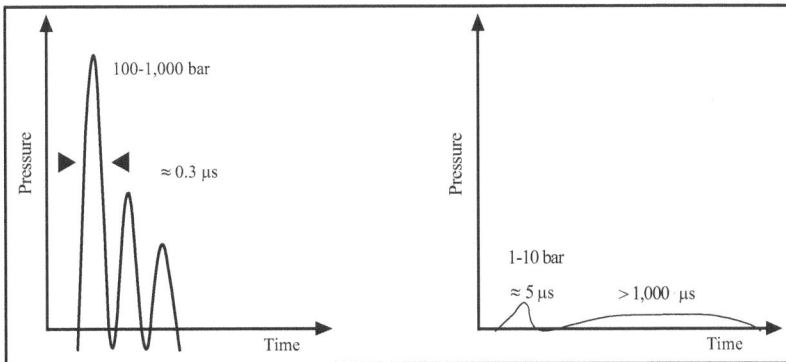

Fig. (35). Physical characteristics of extracorporeal shock wave (left) and radial shock wave (right). From: Cacchio A, Paoloni M, Barile A, *et al*. Effectiveness of radial shock-wave therapy for calcific tendinitis of the shoulder: single-blind, randomized clinical study. Phys Ther 2006; 86(5): 672-82.

Another device developed to produce vibratory waves with particular shape is *Synergy VissThe so-modified acoustic wave assumes acoustic* (Synergy Viss

Human Tecar® Unibell srl, Calco, Italy). It consists of a 32,000-revolution turbine with a flow rate of 35 m³/hour able to generate air waves with a pressure up to 250 mbar, and of a flow modulator which makes air vibrate with a pressure up to 630 mbar and a frequency up to 980 Hz (however, frequency within 300 Hz is recommended) producing mechano-acoustic waves (Fig. **36**).

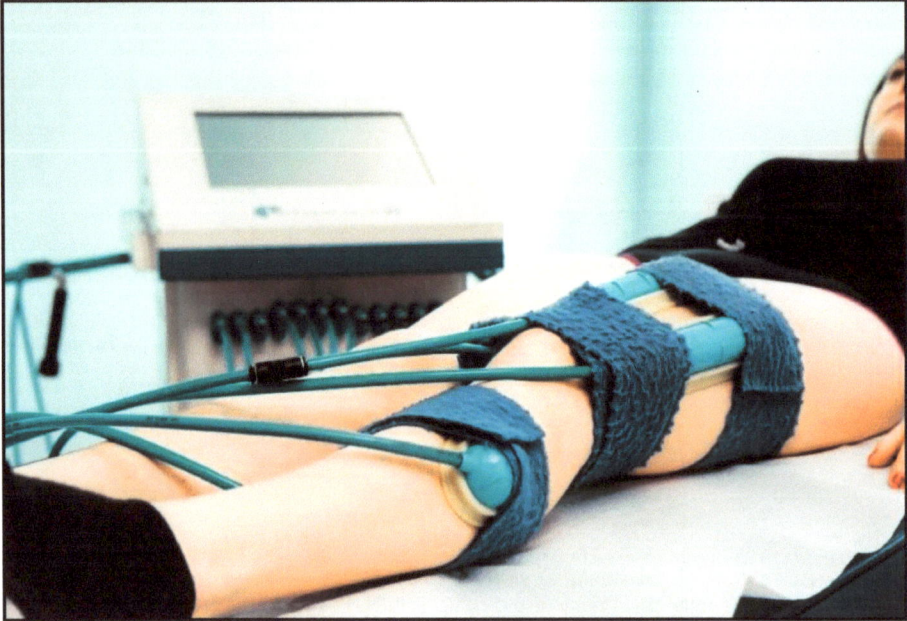

Fig. (36). *Synergy Viss* (Synergy Viss Human Tecar® Unibell srl, Calco, Italy). From: www.riabilitazioneunich.it.

The so-modified acoustic wave assumes acoustic wave assumes a sinusoidal enlarged periodic waveform as a square wave type, in which the amplitude alternates at a steady frequency between fixed minimum and maximum values, with the same duration at minimum and maximum and an ideally instantaneous transition between minimum to maximum (Fig. **37**). This allows to reach the maximum wave amplitude instantly and to maintain it on constant values, as well as to stimulate the mechanoreceptors in a continuous manner throughout the duration of the maximum.

Within the broad range of frequencies available by means of the currently marketed focal vibration devices, several major effects can be distinguished depending on the selected frequency: muscle relaxation around 50 Hz, inhibition of spasticity at 100 Hz, pain relief at 200 Hz, muscle training up to 300 Hz [277].

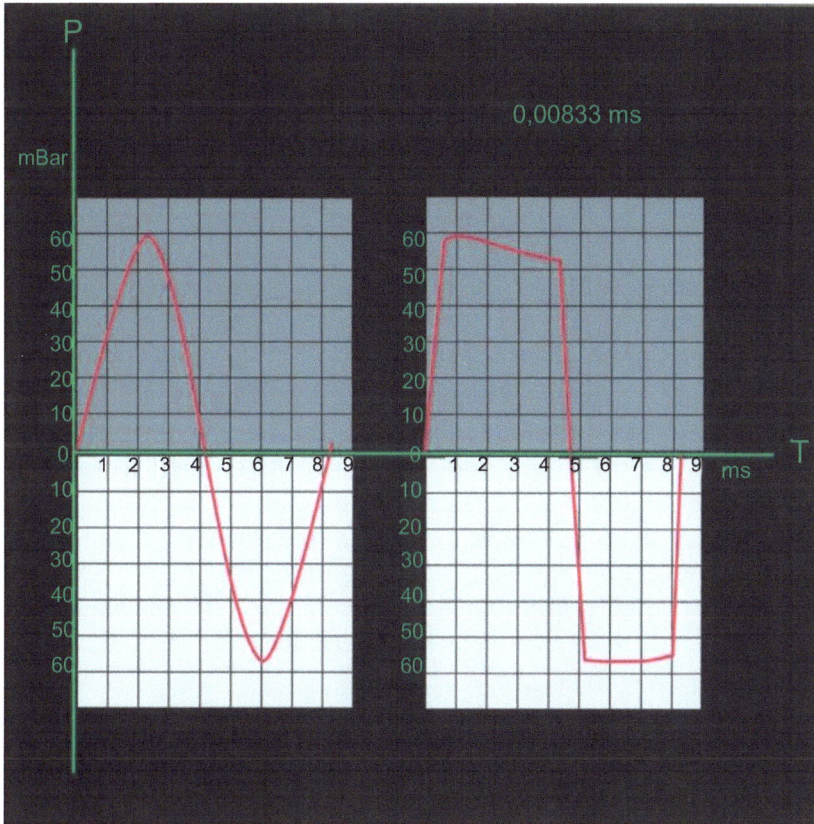

Fig. (37). Sinusoidal and sinusoidal enlarged periodic waveform as a square wave type.

Using low-frequency focal vibration, the muscle relaxation effect is unique in rate and effectiveness of interrupting the "pain-contracture-pain" vicious circle. In an experimental rehabilitation protocol, Saggini *et al.* have identified that a local 90-Hz vibration treatment versus infiltrative therapy with lidocaine is safe and effective in myofascial syndrome of the upper trapezius muscle: in patients receiving vibration therapy there was a significant improvement in pain and muscle elasticity, tone and stiffness, which remained constant at follow-up, whereas patients treated with lidocaine infiltration showed a significant improvement of the stiffness at follow-up, highlighting that vibrations are a valid therapeutic tool for the treatment of musculoskeletal pain and that a protocol of at least 8 weeks lets achieve a therapeutic outcome more efficiently and with a lower onset of pain in patients [278, 279].

Otherwise, using high-frequency focal vibration, the same authors reached the normalization of the basal tone in two heads of the quadriceps femoris muscle (rectus femoris and vastus medialis) in ten sporting subjects [280]. In another study, sarcopenic thigh muscles submitted to local vibrational training at 300 Hz showed no increment in fiber or muscle size but changes in genetic and molecular expression [281], and serum level of growth hormone, creatine phosphokinase (increase) and cortisol (decrease) [282]. These findings are consistent with those of Kvorning *et al.* (acute increase in levels of growth hormone, decrease in levels of cortisol, no effect on levels of testosterone [283]) and of Bosco *et al.* (acute increase in concentration of growth hormone and testosterone, decrease in levels of cortisol [190]) after WBVT. However, with regard to the last study it must be noted that Marco Cardinale stated that «the results of this preliminary study have been used by many companies to advertise WBVT as a way to boost anabolic hormones, reduce stress, and accelerate muscle remodelling. For this reason, it is important to recognize that the study has many limitations, the primary one being the absence of a control condition. Also, not all studies have shown acute increases in strength/power performances and hormone concentrations» [65]. Indeed, the matter is still debated, since in the face of these studies other investigations reported no improvement with similar WBVT protocols (ten 26- or 30-Hz-frequency, 4-mm-amplitude, 17-g-acceleration vibration series of 60-s duration with 60-s rest between each treatment and with 5 or 6 minutes of rest after the first five series) [284, 285].

Using the focused mechano-acoustic vibration at 300 Hz, it has been also shown that a 12-week training is equivalent to a global sensorimotor and a resistance training (60-80% of maximum theoretical force, 10-12 repetitions for 3 sets, 2 sessions per week) in improving balance, with a reduction of sway area and of ellipse surface, and in increasing the length of half-step and reducing the width of the support at the gait analysis, with reduction of the risk of falls in the sarcopenic elderly subjects enrolled in the study [286]. Improvement in static and dynamic baropodometry and stabilometry have been also reported in patients suffering from progressive supranuclear palsy, an atypical parkinsonism clinically characterized by prominent axial extrapyramidal motor symptoms with frequent falls and poor response to L-dopa, in which a valid therapeutic option can be represented by a rehabilitation program combining the use of *Vibration Sound System*® and of a dynamic antigravity postural system (*SPAD*®, a device for body weight relief and postural schema realignment consisting of a machinery designed to reduce, modify, and influence the force of gravity acting on the body during the gait on a treadmill) 3 sessions per week for 2 months [287]. De Nunzio *et al.* reported that in patients with Parkinson's disease vibration increases the stride length, cadence and velocity while walking, especially when applied on erectores spinae muscles, decrease the stance and swing time, increase the width of support base when applied on soleus or tibialis anterior but not on erectores spinae muscles, probably because of vibration of the erectores spinae muscles increments in the antero-posterior or medio-lateral oscillations of the center of mass, while vibration on the tibialis anterior and soleus muscles alternates muscles activation enhancing medio-lateral shift of weight [288].

Therefore, *in the same ways as WBV, nowadays the application field of the focused vibrations has been expanded from musculoskeletal to common neurological disorders, in which is well tolerated, effective and easy to use, without side effects.*

In neurorehabilitation, focal vibration is used as a versatile tool for several purposes:

- *to improve gait*. Focal vibration can be applied over different muscle groups to improve gait and, therefore, it is a useful tool for gait rehabilitation. Particularly:
  - *in Parkinson's disease*, the erectores spinae, lumbar paraspinal and quadriceps muscles vibration during walking can improve stride length and walking velocity [288, 289]; also vibration on the sole can improve gait, decreasing stride variability and increasing in speed [290]. Moreover, within a postural rehabilitation program, vibratory stimulation could constitute a valid tool – as much as visual and auditory cues – to reach a sort of "corticalization" of the gait cycle automatism, hindering its progressive impairment,
  - *in stroke*, tibialis anterior and gluteus medius muscles vibration can increase gait speed [291]; on the other side, vibration on tibialis anterior and peroneus longus improved foot support in the stance phase and increased gait speed in stroke [292],
  - *in spinal cord injury*, rectus femoris muscle vibration can be useful because it increases proximal muscle activity in the stance phase, allowing support of weight during gait training [293]; on the other side, if patients with incomplete SCI are still not able to realize gait training, at lying position to train steplike movement with tensor fascia latae muscle vibration could be a good alternative [294, 295];
- *to reduce spasticity*, a frequent and limiting problem in neurorehabilitation. Spasticity may restrict range of movement, impair dexterity and cause abnormal postures and pain interfering with daily living activities or maintenance of hygiene. To reduce spasticity during daily living activities is of practical utility, since focal vibration reduces spasticity successfully in the applied muscle independent from the underlying neurological disease or disorder. Focal vibration combined with physiotherapy might be useful for functional improvement in stroke patients, such as performing movements with the affected arm or improving stability of the entire hemiparetic arm during goal-directed movements [296 - 303]. Nowadays, there are no studies on functional

improvement of the upper limb with focal vibration in multiple sclerosis nor in spinal cord injury [304];

- *to enhance attention in hemineglect.* Neck muscle vibration is able even to create a kinesthetic illusion that allows an improvement in task performance and spatial postural control, body sensation and orientation in the external environment, as well as in visual exploration trained tasks, such as reading [305 - 308].

CONCLUDING REMARKS

In conclusion, the use of vibration has an important place in the history of rehabilitation with physical means. From Charcot's initial observations, a long way has been gone, and despite the adverse effects observed in subjects improperly exposed to vibratory sources for various reasons, human intelligence has developed various devices able to appropriately modulate the effects of this type of physical energy. Nonetheless, little is known about its exact mechanism(s) of action, and many potential applications need to be explored, taking care to ensure adequate size samples in the studies, accurately select the type of patients to enroll, and ensure the presence of a control group, always respecting the up-to-date protocols, in order to eventually codify the role of vibration therapy in physical and rehabilitation medicine.

CONFLICT OF INTEREST

The author (editor) declares no conflict of interest, financial or otherwise.

ACKNOWLEDGEMENTS

Declared none.

REFERENCES

[1]   Wolff J. Das Gesetz der Transformation der Knochen. Berlin: Hirschwald 1892. [Maquet P, Furlong R (trans). The Law of Bone Remodeling. Berlin: Springer 1986]

[2]   Mountcastle VB, Rose J. Touch and Kinesthesis in Neurophysiology. 1959.

[3]   Mountcastle VB, Talbot WH, Sakata H, Hyvärinen J. Cortical neuronal mechanisms in flutter-vibration studied in unanesthetized monkeys. Neuronal periodicity and frequency discrimination. J Neurophysiol 1969; 32(3): 452-84.
[PMID: 4977839]

[4]   Johansson RS, Vallbo ÅB. Tactile sensory coding in the glabrous skin of the human hand. Trends Neurosci 1983; 6: 27-32.
[http://dx.doi.org/10.1016/0166-2236(83)90011-5]

[5]   Pease DC, Quilliam TA. Electron microscopy of the pacinian corpuscle. J Biophys Biochem Cytol 1957; 3(3): 331-42.
[http://dx.doi.org/10.1083/jcb.3.3.331] [PMID: 13438918]

[6]   Cauna N, Mannan G. The structure of human digital pacinian corpuscles (*corpus cula lamellosa*) and its functional significance. J Anat 1958; 92(1): 1-20.
[PMID: 13513492]

[7]   Shanthaveerappa TR, Bourne GH. New observations on the structure of the Pacinian corpuscle and its relation to the perineural epithelium of peripheral nerves. Am J Anat 1963; 112: 97-109.
[http://dx.doi.org/10.1002/aja.1001120107] [PMID: 13976797]

[8]   LaMotte RH, Mountcastle VB. Capacities of humans and monkeys to discriminate vibratory stimuli of different frequency and amplitude: a correlation between neural events and psychological measurements. J Neurophysiol 1975; 38(3): 539-59.
[PMID: 1127456]

[9]   Loewenstein WR, Skalak R. Mechanical transmission in a Pacinian corpuscle. An analysis and a theory. J Physiol 1966; 182(2): 346-78.
[http://dx.doi.org/10.1113/jphysiol.1966.sp007827] [PMID: 5942033]

[10]   Biswas A, Manivannan M, Srinivasan MA. Multiscale layered biomechanical model of the pacinian corpuscle. IEEE Trans Haptics 2015; 8(1): 31-42.
[http://dx.doi.org/10.1109/TOH.2014.2369416] [PMID: 25398182]

[11]   Biswas A, Manivannan M, Srinivasan MA. Vibrotactile sensitivity threshold: nonlinear stochastic mechanotransduction model of the Pacinian Corpuscle. IEEE Trans Haptics 2015; 8(1): 102-13.
[http://dx.doi.org/10.1109/TOH.2014.2369422] [PMID: 25398183]

[12]   Knibestöl M. Stimulus-response functions of rapidly adapting mechanoreceptors in human glabrous skin area. J Physiol 1973; 232(3): 427-52.
[http://dx.doi.org/10.1113/jphysiol.1973.sp010279] [PMID: 4759677]

[13]   Knibestöl M. Stimulus-response functions of slowly adapting mechanoreceptors in the human glabrous skin area. J Physiol 1975; 245(1): 63-80.
[http://dx.doi.org/10.1113/jphysiol.1975.sp010835] [PMID: 1127614]

[14]   Knibestöl M, Vallbo ÅB. Single unit analysis of mechanoreceptor activity from the human glabrous skin. Acta Physiol Scand 1970; 80(2): 178-95.
[http://dx.doi.org/10.1111/j.1748-1716.1970.tb04783.x] [PMID: 5475340]

[15]   Johansson RS, Vallbo ÅB. Tactile sensibility in the human hand: relative and absolute densities of four types of mechanoreceptive units in glabrous skin. J Physiol 1979; 286: 283-300.
[http://dx.doi.org/10.1113/jphysiol.1979.sp012619] [PMID: 439026]

[16]   Kennedy PM, Inglis JT. Distribution and behaviour of glabrous cutaneous receptors in the human foot sole. J Physiol 2002; 538(Pt 3): 995-1002.
[http://dx.doi.org/10.1113/jphysiol.2001.013087] [PMID: 11826182]

[17]   Magnusson M, Enbom H, Johansson R, Pyykkö I. Significance of pressor input from the human feet in anterior-posterior postural control. The effect of hypothermia on vibration-induced body-sway. Acta Otolaryngol 1990; 110(3-4): 182-8.
[http://dx.doi.org/10.3109/00016489009122535] [PMID: 2239205]

[18]   Kavounoudias A, Roll R, Roll JP. The plantar sole is a dynamometric map for human balance control. Neuroreport 1998; 9(14): 3247-52.
[http://dx.doi.org/10.1097/00001756-199810050-00021] [PMID: 9831459]

[19]   Kavounoudias A, Roll R, Roll JP. Specific whole-body shifts induced by frequency-modulated vibrations of human plantar soles. Neurosci Lett 1999; 266(3): 181-4.
[http://dx.doi.org/10.1016/S0304-3940(99)00302-X] [PMID: 10465703]

[20]   Fitzpatrick R, Rogers DK, McCloskey DI. Stable human standing with lower-limb muscle afferents providing the only sensory input. J Physiol 1994; 480(Pt 2): 395-403.
[http://dx.doi.org/10.1113/jphysiol.1994.sp020369] [PMID: 7869254]

[21] Allum JH, Bloem BR, Carpenter MG, Hulliger M, Hadders-Algra M. Proprioceptive control of posture: a review of new concepts. Gait Posture 1998; 8(3): 214-42.
[http://dx.doi.org/10.1016/S0966-6362(98)00027-7] [PMID: 10200410]

[22] Lestienne F, Soechting J, Berthoz A. Postural readjustments induced by linear motion of visual scenes. Exp Brain Res 1977; 28(3-4): 363-84.
[PMID: 885185]

[23] Bronstein AM, Buckwell D. Automatic control of postural sway by visual motion parallax. Exp Brain Res 1997; 113(2): 243-8.
[http://dx.doi.org/10.1007/BF02450322] [PMID: 9063710]

[24] Lacour M, Borel L. Vestibular control of posture and gait. Arch Ital Biol 1993; 131(2-3): 81-104.
[PMID: 8338392]

[25] Horak FB, Shupert CL, Dietz V, Horstmann G. Vestibular and somatosensory contributions to responses to head and body displacements in stance. Exp Brain Res 1994; 100(1): 93-106.
[http://dx.doi.org/10.1007/BF00227282] [PMID: 7813657]

[26] Hlavačka F, Krizková M, Horak FB. Modification of human postural response to leg muscle vibration by electrical vestibular stimulation. Neurosci Lett 1995; 189(1): 9-12.
[http://dx.doi.org/10.1016/0304-3940(95)11436-Z] [PMID: 7603629]

[27] Hlavačka F, Mergner T, Križková M. Control of the body vertical by vestibular and proprioceptive inputs. Brain Res Bull 1996; 40(5-6): 431-4.
[http://dx.doi.org/10.1016/0361-9230(96)00138-4] [PMID: 8886370]

[28] Roll JP, Roll R. From eye to foot: a proprioceptive chain involved in postural control. In: Amblard B, Berthoz A, Clarac F, Eds. Posture and Gait: Development Adaptation and Modulation. Amsterdam: Elsevier 1988; pp. 155-64.

[29] Gurfinkel VS, Ivanenko YuP , Levik YuS , Babakova IA. Kinesthetic reference for human orthograde posture. Neuroscience 1995; 68(1): 229-43.
[http://dx.doi.org/10.1016/0306-4522(95)00136-7] [PMID: 7477928]

[30] Orma EJ. The effects of cooling the feet and closing the eyes on standing equilibrium, different patterns of standing equilibrium in young adult men and women. Acta Physiol Scand 1957; 38(3-4): 288-97.
[http://dx.doi.org/10.1111/j.1748-1716.1957.tb01392.x] [PMID: 13410627]

[31] Asai H, Fujiwara K, Toyama H, Yamashina T, Tachino K, Nara I. The influence of foot soles cooling on standing postural control analyzed by tracking the center of foot pressure. In: Woollacoot M, Horak F, Eds. Posture and Gait: Control Mechanisms. Eugene, OR: University of Oregon Books 1992; Vol. II: pp. 151-4.

[32] Perry SD, McIlroy WE, Maki BE. The role of plantar cutaneous mechanoreceptors in the control of compensatory stepping reactions evoked by unpredictable, multi-directional perturbation. Brain Res 2000; 877(2): 401-6.
[http://dx.doi.org/10.1016/S0006-8993(00)02712-8] [PMID: 10986360]

[33] Nurse MA, Nigg BM. The effect of changes in foot sensation on plantar pressure and muscle activity. Clin Biomech (Bristol, Avon) 2001; 16(9): 719-27.
[http://dx.doi.org/10.1016/S0268-0033(01)00090-0] [PMID: 11714548]

[34] Eils E, Nolte S, Tewes M, Thorwesten L, Völker K, Rosenbaum D. Modified pressure distribution patterns in walking following reduction of plantar sensation. J Biomech 2002; 35(10): 1307-13.
[http://dx.doi.org/10.1016/S0021-9290(02)00168-9] [PMID: 12231276]

[35] Stål F, Fransson PA, Magnusson M, Karlberg M. Effects of hypothermic anesthesia of the feet on vibration-induced body sway and adaptation. J Vestib Res 2003; 13(1): 39-52.
[PMID: 14646023]

[36]   McKeon PO, Hertel J. Diminished plantar cutaneous sensation and postural control. Percept Mot Skills 2007; 104(1): 56-66.
[http://dx.doi.org/10.2466/pms.104.1.56-66] [PMID: 17450964]

[37]   Hong SL, Manor B, Li L. Stance and sensory feedback influence on postural dynamics. Neurosci Lett 2007; 423(2): 104-8.
[http://dx.doi.org/10.1016/j.neulet.2007.06.043] [PMID: 17673367]

[38]   Patel M, Fransson PA, Johansson R, Magnusson M. Foam posturography: standing on foam is not equivalent to standing with decreased rapidly adapting mechanoreceptive sensation. Exp Brain Res 2011; 208(4): 519-27.
[http://dx.doi.org/10.1007/s00221-010-2498-6] [PMID: 21120458]

[39]   Do MC, Bussel B, Breniere Y. Influence of plantar cutaneous afferents on early compensatory reactions to forward fall. Exp Brain Res 1990; 79(2): 319-24.
[http://dx.doi.org/10.1007/BF00608241] [PMID: 2323379]

[40]   Thoumie P, Do MC. Changes in motor activity and biomechanics during balance recovery following cutaneous and muscular deafferentation. Exp Brain Res 1996; 110(2): 289-97.
[http://dx.doi.org/10.1007/BF00228559] [PMID: 8836692]

[41]   Mauritz KH, Dietz V. Characteristics of postural instability induced by ischemic blocking of leg afferents. Exp Brain Res 1980; 38(1): 117-9.
[http://dx.doi.org/10.1007/BF00237939] [PMID: 6965370]

[42]   Diener HC, Dichgans J, Guschlbauer B, Mau H. The significance of proprioception on postural stabilization as assessed by ischemia. Brain Res 1984; 296(1): 103-9.
[http://dx.doi.org/10.1016/0006-8993(84)90515-8] [PMID: 6713202]

[43]   Horak FB, Nashner LM, Diener HC. Postural strategies associated with somatosensory and vestibular loss. Exp Brain Res 1990; 82(1): 167-77.
[http://dx.doi.org/10.1007/BF00230848] [PMID: 2257901]

[44]   Wu G, Chiang JH. The significance of somatosensory stimulations to the human foot in the control of postural reflexes. Exp Brain Res 1997; 114(1): 163-9.
[http://dx.doi.org/10.1007/PL00005616] [PMID: 9125462]

[45]   Okubo J, Watanabe I, Baron JB. Study on influences of the plantar mechanoreceptor on body sways. Agressologie 1980; 21(D): 61-9.
[PMID: 7294286]

[46]   Hulliger M. The mammalian muscle spindle and its central control. Rev Physiol Biochem Pharmacol 1984; 101: 1-110.
[http://dx.doi.org/10.1007/BFb0027694] [PMID: 6240757]

[47]   Vallbo ÅB, al-Falahe NA. Human muscle spindle response in a motor learning task. J Physiol 1990; 421: 553-68.
[http://dx.doi.org/10.1113/jphysiol.1990.sp017961] [PMID: 2140862]

[48]   Boyd IA. The isolated mammalian muscle spindle. Trends Neurosci 1980; 3(11): 258-65.
[http://dx.doi.org/10.1016/0166-2236(80)90096-X]

[49]   Heckmann CJ, Gorassini MA, Bennett DJ. Persistent inward currents in motoneuron dendrites: implications for motor output. Muscle Nerve 2005; 31(2): 135-56.
[http://dx.doi.org/10.1002/mus.20261] [PMID: 15736297]

[50]   Bianconi R, van der MEULEN J. The response to vibration of the end organs of mammalian muscle spindles. J Neurophysiol 1963; 26: 177-90.
[PMID: 13968075]

[51]   Lance JW. The reflex effects of muscle vibration. Proc Aust Assoc Neurol 1966; 4: 49-56.
[PMID: 5966202]

[52] Hagbarth KE, Eklund G. Tonic vibration reflexes (TVR) in spasticity. Brain Res 1966; 2(2): 201-3.
[http://dx.doi.org/10.1016/0006-8993(66)90029-1] [PMID: 5968925]

[53] Eklund G, Hagbarth KE. Normal variability of tonic vibration reflexes in man. Exp Neurol 1966; 16(1): 80-92.
[http://dx.doi.org/10.1016/0014-4886(66)90088-4] [PMID: 5923486]

[54] Eklund G, Hagbarth KE. Motor effects of vibratory muscle stimuli in man. Electroencephalogr Clin Neurophysiol 1965; 19: 619.

[55] Hagbarth KE, Eklund G. Motor effects of vibratory muscle stimuli in man. In: Granit R, Ed. Proceedings of the First Nobel Symposium. Stockholm: Almqvist and Wiksell 1966; pp. 177-86.

[56] De Gail P, Lance JW, Neilson PD. Differential effects on tonic and phasic reflex mechanisms produced by vibration of muscles in man. J Neurol Neurosurg Psychiatry 1966; 29(1): 1-11.
[http://dx.doi.org/10.1136/jnnp.29.1.1] [PMID: 5910574]

[57] Lance JW, de Gail P, Neilson PD. Tonic and phasic spinal cord mechanisms in man. J Neurol Neurosurg Psychiatry 1966; 29: 535-44.
[http://dx.doi.org/10.1136/jnnp.29.6.535]

[58] Rushworth G, Young RR. The effect of vibration on tonic and phasic reflexes in man. J Physiol 1966; 185: 63P-4P.

[59] Hagbarth KE, Eklund G. The effects of muscle vibration in spasticity, rigidity, and cerebellar disorders. J Neurol Neurosurg Psychiatry 1968; 31(3): 207-13.
[http://dx.doi.org/10.1136/jnnp.31.3.207] [PMID: 5684025]

[60] De Domenico G. Tonic vibratory reflex. What is it? Can we use it? Physiotherapy 1979; 65(2): 44-8.
[PMID: 441188]

[61] Nigg BM, Wakeling JM. Impact forces and muscle tuning: a new paradigm. Exerc Sport Sci Rev 2001; 29(1): 37-41.
[http://dx.doi.org/10.1097/00003677-200101000-00008] [PMID: 11210446]

[62] Wakeling JM, Nigg BM. Modification of soft tissue vibrations in the leg by muscular activity. J Appl Physiol 2001; 90(2): 412-20.
[PMID: 11160036]

[63] Wakeling JM, Von Tscharner V, Nigg BM, Stergiou P. Muscle activity in the leg is tuned in response to ground reaction forces. J Appl Physiol 2001; 91(3): 1307-17.
[PMID: 11509530]

[64] Nigg BM. Impact forces in running. Curr Opin Orthop 1997; 8: 43-7.
[http://dx.doi.org/10.1097/00001433-199712000-00007]

[65] Cardinale M, Wakeling J. Whole body vibration exercise: are vibrations good for you? Br J Sports Med 2005; 39(9): 585-9.
[http://dx.doi.org/10.1136/bjsm.2005.016857] [PMID: 16118292]

[66] Rack PM, Westbury DR. The short range stiffness of active mammalian muscle and its effect on mechanical properties. J Physiol 1974; 240(2): 331-50.
[http://dx.doi.org/10.1113/jphysiol.1974.sp010613] [PMID: 4424163]

[67] Wakeling JM, Nigg BM. Soft-tissue vibrations in the quadriceps measured with skin mounted transducers. J Biomech 2001; 34(4): 539-43.
[http://dx.doi.org/10.1016/S0021-9290(00)00203-7] [PMID: 11266679]

[68] Ettema GJ, Huijing PA. Frequency response to rat gastrocnemius medialis in small amplitude vibrations. J Biomech 1994; 27(8): 1015-22.
[http://dx.doi.org/10.1016/0021-9290(94)90218-6] [PMID: 8089156]

[69]   Kawai M, Brandt PW. Sinusoidal analysis: a high resolution method for correlating biochemical reactions with physiological processes in activated skeletal muscles of rabbit, frog and crayfish. J Muscle Res Cell Motil 1980; 1(3): 279-303.
[http://dx.doi.org/10.1007/BF00711932] [PMID: 6971874]

[70]   Wakeling JM, Nigg BM, Rozitis AI. Muscle activity in the lower extremity damps the soft tissue vibrations which occur in response to pulsed and continuous vibrations. J Appl Physiol 2002; 93(3): 1093-103.
[http://dx.doi.org/10.1152/japplphysiol.00142.2002] [PMID: 12183507]

[71]   Adamo DE, Martin BJ, Johnson PW. Vibration-induced muscle fatigue, a possible contribution to musculoskeletal injury. Eur J Appl Physiol 2002; 88(1-2): 134-40.
[http://dx.doi.org/10.1007/s00421-002-0660-y] [PMID: 12436281]

[72]   Necking LE, Lundborg G, Friden J. Hand muscle weakness in long-term vibration exposure. J Hand Surg [Br] 2002; 27(6): 520-5.
[http://dx.doi.org/10.1054/jhsb.2002.0810] [PMID: 12475507]

[73]   Bongiovanni LG, Hagbarth KE, Stjernberg L. Prolonged muscle vibration reducing motor output in maximal voluntary contractions in man. J Physiol 1990; 423: 15-26.
[http://dx.doi.org/10.1113/jphysiol.1990.sp018008] [PMID: 2388149]

[74]   Dupuis H, Jansen G. Immediate effects of vibration transmitted to the hand. In: Bianchi G, Frolvlov KV, Oledzky A, Eds. Proceedings of the International CISM-IFToMM-WHO Symposium. Amsterdam: Elsevier 1981; pp. 76-86.
[http://dx.doi.org/10.1016/S0166-1116(09)70140-2]

[75]   Gauthier GM, Roll JP, Martin B, Harlay F. Effects of whole-body vibrations on sensory motor system performance in man. Aviat Space Environ Med 1981; 52(8): 473-9.
[PMID: 7259700]

[76]   Wasserman DE, Taylor W. Lessons from hand-arm vibration syndrome research. Am J Ind Med 1991; 19(4): 539-46.
[http://dx.doi.org/10.1002/ajim.4700190411] [PMID: 2035552]

[77]   Craven BC. Effectiveness of Vibration and Standing Versus Standing Alone for the Treatment of Osteoporosis for People With Spinal Cord Injury 2005.

[78]   Armstrong TJ, Fine LJ, Radwin RG, Silverstein BS. Ergonomics and the effects of vibration in hand-intensive work. Scand J Work Environ Health 1987; 13(4): 286-9.
[http://dx.doi.org/10.5271/sjweh.2049] [PMID: 3324309]

[79]   Johanning E, Wilder DG, Landrigan PJ, Pope MH. Whole-body vibration exposure in subway cars and review of adverse health effects. J Occup Med 1991; 33(5): 605-12.
[PMID: 1831231]

[80]   Lings S, Leboeuf-Yde C. Whole-body vibration and low back pain: a systematic, critical review of the epidemiological literature 19921999. Int Arch Occup Environ Health 2000; 73(5): 290-7.
[http://dx.doi.org/10.1007/s004200000118] [PMID: 10963411]

[81]   Griffin MJ. Minimum health and safety requirements for workers exposed to hand-transmitted vibration and whole-body vibration in the European Union; a review. Occup Environ Med 2004; 61(5): 387-97.
[http://dx.doi.org/10.1136/oem.2002.006304] [PMID: 15090658]

[82]   Ribot-Ciscar E, Bergenheim M, Albert F, Roll JP. Proprioceptive population coding of limb position in humans. Exp Brain Res 2003; 149(4): 512-9.
[http://dx.doi.org/10.1007/s00221-003-1384-x] [PMID: 12677332]

[83]   Fontana TL, Richardson CA, Stanton WR. The effect of weight-bearing exercise with low frequency, whole body vibration on lumbosacral proprioception: a pilot study on normal subjects. Aust J

Physiother 2005; 51(4): 259-63.
[http://dx.doi.org/10.1016/S0004-9514(05)70007-6] [PMID: 16321133]

[84]   Buckminster Fuller R. Synergetics: Explorations in the Geometry of Thinking. New York: Macmillian Publishing Co. 1975.

[85]   Chen CS, Ingber DE. Tensegrity and mechanoregulation: from skeleton to cytoskeleton. Osteoarthritis Cartilage 1999; 7(1): 81-94.
[http://dx.doi.org/10.1053/joca.1998.0164] [PMID: 10367017]

[86]   Mow VC, Ratcliffe A, Poole AR. Cartilage and diarthrodial joints as paradigms for hierarchical materials and structures. Biomaterials 1992; 13(2): 67-97.
[http://dx.doi.org/10.1016/0142-9612(92)90001-5] [PMID: 1550898]

[87]   Lakes R. Materials with structural hierarchy. Nature 1993; 361: 511-5.
[http://dx.doi.org/10.1038/361511a0]

[88]   Martin RB, Burr DB. Structure, Function, and Adaptation of Compact Bone. New York: Raven Press 1989.

[89]   Silbert JE. Advances in the biochemistry of proteoglycans. In: Uitto J, Perejda AJ, Eds. Connective Tissue Disease: Molecular Pathology of the Extracellular Matrix. New York: Marcel Dekker 1987; pp. 83-98.

[90]   Bachrach NM, Valhmu WB, Stazzone E, Ratcliffe A, Lai WM, Mow VC. Changes in proteoglycan synthesis of chondrocytes in articular cartilage are associated with the time-dependent changes in their mechanical environment. J Biomech 1995; 28(12): 1561-9.
[http://dx.doi.org/10.1016/0021-9290(95)00103-4] [PMID: 8666595]

[91]   Mow VC, Ratcliffe A. Structure and function of articular cartilage. In: Mow VC, Hayes WC, Eds. Basic Orthopaedic Biomechanics. Philadelphia: Lippincott-Raven 1997; pp. 113-77.

[92]   Guilak F, Sah RL, Setton LA. Physical regulation of cartilage metabolism. In: Mow VC, Hayes WC, Eds. Basic Orthopaedic Biomechanics. Philadelphia: Lippincott-Raven 1997; pp. 179-208.

[93]   Guilak F, Jones WR, Ting-Beall HP, Lee GM. The deformation behavior and mechanical properties of chondrocytes in articular cartilage. Osteoarthritis Cartilage 1999; 7(1): 59-70.
[http://dx.doi.org/10.1053/joca.1998.0162] [PMID: 10367015]

[94]   Wang JH. Mechanobiology of tendon. J Biomech 2006; 39(9): 1563-82.
[http://dx.doi.org/10.1016/j.jbiomech.2005.05.011] [PMID: 16000201]

[95]   Birk DE, Silver FH, Trelstad RL. Matrix assembly. In: Hay ED, Ed. Cell Biology of Extracellular Matrix. 2nd ed. New York: Academic Press 1991; pp. 221-54.
[http://dx.doi.org/10.1007/978-1-4615-3770-0_8]

[96]   Elliott DH. Structure and function of mammalian tendon. Biol Rev Camb Philos Soc 1965; 40: 392-421.
[http://dx.doi.org/10.1111/j.1469-185X.1965.tb00808.x] [PMID: 14340913]

[97]   Silver FH, Kato YP, Ohno M, Wasserman AJ. Analysis of mammalian connective tissue: relationship between hierarchical structures and mechanical properties. J Long Term Eff Med Implants 1992; 2(2-3): 165-98.
[PMID: 10171619]

[98]   Silver FH, Christiansen DL, Snowhill PB, Chen Y. Role of storage on changes in the mechanical properties of tendon and self-assembled collagen fibers. Connect Tissue Res 2000; 41(2): 155-64.
[http://dx.doi.org/10.3109/03008200009067667] [PMID: 10992161]

[99]   Ingber D. Integrins as mechanochemical transducers. Curr Opin Cell Biol 1991; 3(5): 841-8.
[http://dx.doi.org/10.1016/0955-0674(91)90058-7] [PMID: 1931084]

[100]   Ingber D. How cells (might) sense microgravity. FASEB J 1999; 13 (Suppl.): S3-S15.
[PMID: 10352140]

[101] Wang N, Tolić-Nørrelykke IM, Chen J, *et al.* Cell prestress. I. Stiffness and prestress are closely associated in adherent contractile cells. Am J Physiol Cell Physiol 2002; 282(3): C606-16.
[http://dx.doi.org/10.1152/ajpcell.00269.2001] [PMID: 11832346]

[102] Stamenović D, Mijailovich SM, Tolić-Nørrelykke IM, Chen J, Wang N. Cell prestress. II. Contribution of microtubules. Am J Physiol Cell Physiol 2002; 282(3): C617-24.
[http://dx.doi.org/10.1152/ajpcell.00271.2001] [PMID: 11832347]

[103] Ingber DE, Jamieson JD. Cells as tensegrity structures: architectural regulation of histodifferentiation by physical forces transduced over basement membrane. In: Andersson L, Gahmberg C, Ekblom P, Eds. Gene expression during normal and malignant differentiation. San Diego: Academic Press 1985; pp. 13-32.

[104] Danowski BA. Fibroblast contractility and actin organization are stimulated by microtubule inhibitors. J Cell Sci 1989; 93(Pt 2): 255-66.
[PMID: 2482296]

[105] Heidemann SR, Buxbaum RE. Tension as a regulator and integrator of axonal growth. Cell Motil Cytoskeleton 1990; 17(1): 6-10.
[http://dx.doi.org/10.1002/cm.970170103] [PMID: 2225090]

[106] Ingber DE, Dike L, Hansen L, *et al.* Cellular tensegrity: exploring how mechanical changes in the cytoskeleton regulate cell growth, migration, and tissue pattern during morphogenesis. Int Rev Cytol 1994; 150: 173-224.
[http://dx.doi.org/10.1016/S0074-7696(08)61542-9] [PMID: 8169080]

[107] Giancotti FG, Ruoslahti E. Integrin signaling. Science 1999; 285(5430): 1028-32.
[http://dx.doi.org/10.1126/science.285.5430.1028] [PMID: 10446041]

[108] Ingber DE. Tensegrity: the architectural basis of cellular mechanotransduction. Annu Rev Physiol 1997; 59: 575-99.
[http://dx.doi.org/10.1146/annurev.physiol.59.1.575] [PMID: 9074778]

[109] Ingber DE. Integrins, tensegrity, and mechanotransduction. Gravit Space Biol Bull 1997; 10(2): 49-55.
[PMID: 11540119]

[110] Ingber DE. Tensegrity and mechanotransduction. J Bodyw Mov Ther 2008; 12(3): 198-200.
[http://dx.doi.org/10.1016/j.jbmt.2008.04.038] [PMID: 19083675]

[111] Charcot J-M. La médicine vibratoire – Application des vibrations rapides et continues a traitement de quelques maladies du système nerveux. Prog Méd 1892; 16: 149-51. [Charcot J-M. Vibratory therapeutics – The application of rapid and continuous vibrations to the treatment of certain diseases of the nervous system. J Nerv Ment Dis 2011; 199(11): 821-7.]

[112] Anonymous . Vibratory Therapeutics. Sci Am 1892; 67(17): 265.
[http://dx.doi.org/10.1038/scientificamerican10221892-265]

[113] Whedon GD, Deitrick JE, Shorr E. Modification of the effects of immobilization upon metabolic and physiologic functions of normal men by the use of an oscillating bed. Am J Med 1949; 6(6): 684-711.
[http://dx.doi.org/10.1016/0002-9343(49)90306-X] [PMID: 18134065]

[114] Rubin CT, McLeod KJ. Promotion of bony ingrowth by frequency-specific, low-amplitude mechanical strain. Clin Orthop Relat Res 1994; (298): 165-74.
[PMID: 8118971]

[115] Rubin C, Xu G, Judex S. The anabolic activity of bone tissue, suppressed by disuse, is normalized by brief exposure to extremely low-magnitude mechanical stimuli. FASEB J 2001; 15(12): 2225-9.
[http://dx.doi.org/10.1096/fj.01-0166com] [PMID: 11641249]

[116] Rubin C, Turner AS, Bain S, Mallinckrodt C, McLeod K. Anabolism. Low mechanical signals strengthen long bones. Nature 2001; 412(6847): 603-4.
[http://dx.doi.org/10.1038/35088122] [PMID: 11493908]

[117] Rubin C, Turner AS, Müller R, *et al.* Quantity and quality of trabecular bone in the femur are enhanced by a strongly anabolic, noninvasive mechanical intervention. J Bone Miner Res 2002; 17(2): 349-57.
[http://dx.doi.org/10.1359/jbmr.2002.17.2.349] [PMID: 11811566]

[118] Rubin C, Recker R, Cullen D, Ryaby J, McCabe J, McLeod K. Prevention of postmenopausal bone loss by a low-magnitude, high-frequency mechanical stimuli: a clinical trial assessing compliance, efficacy, and safety. J Bone Miner Res 2004; 19(3): 343-51.
[http://dx.doi.org/10.1359/JBMR.0301251] [PMID: 15040821]

[119] Verschueren SM, Roelants M, Delecluse C, Swinnen S, Vanderschueren D, Boonen S. Effect of 6-month whole body vibration training on hip density, muscle strength, and postural control in postmenopausal women: a randomized controlled pilot study. J Bone Miner Res 2004; 19(3): 352-9.
[http://dx.doi.org/10.1359/JBMR.0301245] [PMID: 15040822]

[120] van Nes IJ, Geurts AC, Hendricks HT, Duysens J. Short-term effects of whole-body vibration on postural control in unilateral chronic stroke patients: preliminary evidence. Am J Phys Med Rehabil 2004; 83(11): 867-73.
[http://dx.doi.org/10.1097/01.PHM.0000140801.23135.09] [PMID: 15502741]

[121] Ward K, Alsop C, Caulton J, Rubin C, Adams J, Mughal Z. Low magnitude mechanical loading is osteogenic in children with disabling conditions. J Bone Miner Res 2004; 19(3): 360-9.
[http://dx.doi.org/10.1359/JBMR.040129] [PMID: 15040823]

[122] Gilsanz V, Wren TA, Sanchez M, Dorey F, Judex S, Rubin C. Low-level, high-frequency mechanical signals enhance musculoskeletal development of young women with low BMD. J Bone Miner Res 2006; 21(9): 1464-74.
[http://dx.doi.org/10.1359/jbmr.060612] [PMID: 16939405]

[123] Armbrecht G, Belavý DL, Gast U, *et al.* Resistive vibration exercise attenuates bone and muscle atrophy in 56 days of bed rest: biochemical markers of bone metabolism. Osteoporos Int 2010; 21(4): 597-607.
[http://dx.doi.org/10.1007/s00198-009-0985-z] [PMID: 19536451]

[124] Reyes ML, Hernández M, Holmgren LJ, Sanhueza E, Escobar RG. High-frequency, low-intensity vibrations increase bone mass and muscle strength in upper limbs, improving autonomy in disabled children. J Bone Miner Res 2011; 26(8): 1759-66.
[http://dx.doi.org/10.1002/jbmr.402] [PMID: 21491486]

[125] Turner CH, Forwood MR. What role does the osteocyte network play in bone adaptation? Bone 1995; 16(3): 283-5.
[http://dx.doi.org/10.1016/8756-3282(94)00052-2] [PMID: 7786630]

[126] Hert J, Lisková M, Landa J. Reaction of bone to mechanical stimuli. 1. Continuous and intermittent loading of tibia in rabbit. Folia Morphol (Praha) 1971; 19(3): 290-300.
[PMID: 5142775]

[127] Chamay A, Tschantz P. Mechanical influences in bone remodeling. Experimental research on Wolffs law. J Biomech 1972; 5(2): 173-80.
[http://dx.doi.org/10.1016/0021-9290(72)90053-X] [PMID: 5020948]

[128] Lanyon LE, Baggott DG. Mechanical function as an influence on the structure and form of bone. J Bone Joint Surg Br 1976; 58-B(4): 436-43.
[PMID: 1018029]

[129] Burr DB, Schaffler MB, Yang KH, *et al.* Skeletal change in response to altered strain environments: is woven bone a response to elevated strain? Bone 1989; 10(3): 223-33.
[http://dx.doi.org/10.1016/8756-3282(89)90057-4] [PMID: 2803857]

[130] Burger EH, Veldhuijzen JP. Influence of mechanical factors in bone formation, resorption and growth *in vitro*. In: Hall BK, Ed. Bone-Growth-B.Boca Raton (FL): CRC Press 1993; vol. 7: pp. 37-56.

[131] Huiskes R, Hollister SJ. From structure to process, from organ to cell: recent developments of FE-analysis in orthopaedic biomechanics. J Biomech Eng 1993; 115(4B): 520-7.
[http://dx.doi.org/10.1115/1.2895534] [PMID: 8302035]

[132] Harter LV, Hruska KA, Duncan RL. Human osteoblast-like cells respond to mechanical strain with increased bone matrix protein production independent of hormonal regulation. Endocrinology 1995; 136(2): 528-35.
[http://dx.doi.org/10.1210/endo.136.2.7530647] [PMID: 7530647]

[133] Rubin J, Rubin C, Jacobs CR. Molecular pathways mediating mechanical signaling in bone. Gene 2006; 367: 1-16.
[http://dx.doi.org/10.1016/j.gene.2005.10.028] [PMID: 16361069]

[134] Bacabac RG, Smit TH, Van Loon JJ, Doulabi BZ, Helder M, Klein-Nulend J. Bone cell responses to high-frequency vibration stress: does the nucleus oscillate within the cytoplasm? FASEB J 2006; 20(7): 858-64.
[http://dx.doi.org/10.1096/fj.05-4966.com] [PMID: 16675843]

[135] Engler AJ, Sen S, Sweeney HL, Discher DE. Matrix elasticity directs stem cell lineage specification. Cell 2006; 126(4): 677-89.
[http://dx.doi.org/10.1016/j.cell.2006.06.044] [PMID: 16923388]

[136] Discher DE, Mooney DJ, Zandstra PW. Growth factors, matrices, and forces combine and control stem cells. Science 2009; 324(5935): 1673-7.
[http://dx.doi.org/10.1126/science.1171643] [PMID: 19556500]

[137] Reich KM, Gay CV, Frangos JA. Fluid shear stress as a mediator of osteoblast cyclic adenosine monophosphate production. J Cell Physiol 1990; 143(1): 100-4.
[http://dx.doi.org/10.1002/jcp.1041430113] [PMID: 2156870]

[138] Qin YX, Lin W, Rubin C. The pathway of bone fluid flow as defined by *in vivo* intramedullary pressure and streaming potential measurements. Ann Biomed Eng 2002; 30(5): 693-702.
[http://dx.doi.org/10.1114/1.1483863] [PMID: 12108843]

[139] Qin YX, Kaplan T, Saldanha A, Rubin C. Fluid pressure gradients, arising from oscillations in intramedullary pressure, is correlated with the formation of bone and inhibition of intracortical porosity. J Biomech 2003; 36(10): 1427-37.
[http://dx.doi.org/10.1016/S0021-9290(03)00127-1] [PMID: 14499292]

[140] Qin YX, Lam H. Intramedullary pressure and matrix strain induced by oscillatory skeletal muscle stimulation and its potential in adaptation. J Biomech 2009; 42(2): 140-5.
[http://dx.doi.org/10.1016/j.jbiomech.2008.10.018] [PMID: 19081096]

[141] Pollack SR, Salzstein R, Pienkowski D. Streaming potentials in fluid filled bone. Ferroelectrics 1984; 60: 297-309.
[http://dx.doi.org/10.1080/00150198408017530]

[142] Otter M, Shoenung J, Williams WS. Evidence for different sources of stress-generated potentials in wet and dry bone. J Orthop Res 1985; 3(3): 321-4.
[http://dx.doi.org/10.1002/jor.1100030308] [PMID: 4032103]

[143] Salzstein RA, Pollack SR, Mak AF, Petrov N. Electromechanical potentials in cortical boneI. A continuum approach. J Biomech 1987; 20(3): 261-70.
[http://dx.doi.org/10.1016/0021-9290(87)90293-4] [PMID: 3584151]

[144] Salzstein RA, Pollack SR. Electromechanical potentials in cortical boneII. Experimental analysis. J Biomech 1987; 20(3): 271-80.
[http://dx.doi.org/10.1016/0021-9290(87)90294-6] [PMID: 3584152]

[145] Chakkalakal DA. Mechanoelectric transduction in bone. J Mater Res 1989; 4(4): 1034-46.
[http://dx.doi.org/10.1557/JMR.1989.1034]

[146] Scott GC, Korostoff E. Oscillatory and step response electromechanical phenomena in human and bovine bone. J Biomech 1990; 23(2): 127-43.
[http://dx.doi.org/10.1016/0021-9290(90)90347-6] [PMID: 2179217]

[147] Otter MW, Palmieri VR, Wu DD, Seiz KG, MacGinitie LA, Cochran GV. A comparative analysis of streaming potentials *in vivo* and *in vitro*. J Orthop Res 1992; 10(5): 710-9.
[http://dx.doi.org/10.1002/jor.1100100513] [PMID: 1500983]

[148] Cowin SC, Moss-Salentijn L, Moss ML. Candidates for the mechanosensory system in bone. J Biomech Eng 1991; 113(2): 191-7.
[http://dx.doi.org/10.1115/1.2891234] [PMID: 1875693]

[149] Turner CH, Forwood MR, Otter MW. Mechanotransduction in bone: do bone cells act as sensors of fluid flow? FASEB J 1994; 8(11): 875-8.
[PMID: 8070637]

[150] Klein-Nulend J, van der Plas A, Semeins CM, *et al.* Sensitivity of osteocytes to biomechanical stress *in vitro*. FASEB J 1995; 9(5): 441-5.
[PMID: 7896017]

[151] Duncan RL, Turner CH. Mechanotransduction and the functional response of bone to mechanical strain. Calcif Tissue Int 1995; 57(5): 344-58.
[http://dx.doi.org/10.1007/BF00302070] [PMID: 8564797]

[152] Rubin C, Turner AS, Mallinckrodt C, Jerome C, McLeod K, Bain S. Mechanical strain, induced noninvasively in the high-frequency domain, is anabolic to cancellous bone, but not cortical bone. Bone 2002; 30(3): 445-52.
[http://dx.doi.org/10.1016/S8756-3282(01)00689-5] [PMID: 11882457]

[153] Stevens HY, Meays DR, Frangos JA. Pressure gradients and transport in the murine femur upon hindlimb suspension. Bone 2006; 39(3): 565-72.
[http://dx.doi.org/10.1016/j.bone.2006.03.007] [PMID: 16677866]

[154] Pitukcheewanont P, Safani D, Gilsanz V, Rubin C. Short term low level mechanical stimulation increases cancellous and cortical bone density and muscles of females with osteoporosis: A pilot study. 84th Meeting of the Endocrine Society. 19-22 June 2002; San Francisco (CA). 2003; pp. 2-725.

[155] Garman R, Gaudette G, Donahue LR, Rubin C, Judex S. Low-level accelerations applied in the absence of weight bearing can enhance trabecular bone formation. J Orthop Res 2007; 25(6): 732-40.
[http://dx.doi.org/10.1002/jor.20354] [PMID: 17318899]

[156] Judex S, Lei X, Han D, Rubin C. Low-magnitude mechanical signals that stimulate bone formation in the ovariectomized rat are dependent on the applied frequency but not on the strain magnitude. J Biomech 2007; 40(6): 1333-9.
[http://dx.doi.org/10.1016/j.jbiomech.2006.05.014] [PMID: 16814792]

[157] Sehmisch S, Galal R, Kolios L, *et al.* Effects of low-magnitude, high-frequency mechanical stimulation in the rat osteopenia model. Osteoporos Int 2009; 20(12): 1999-2008.
[http://dx.doi.org/10.1007/s00198-009-0892-3] [PMID: 19283328]

[158] Frost HM. Laws of bone structure. Springfield, IL: Charles C. Thomas 1964.

[159] Frost HM. A determinant of bone architecture. The minimum effective strain. Clin Orthop Relat Res 1983; (175): 286-92.
[PMID: 6839601]

[160] Frost HM. The mechanostat: a proposed pathogenic mechanism of osteoporoses and the bone mass effects of mechanical and nonmechanical agents. Bone Miner 1987; 2(2): 73-85.
[PMID: 3333019]

[161] Frost HM. Bone mass and the mechanostat: a proposal. Anat Rec 1987; 219(1): 1-9.
[http://dx.doi.org/10.1002/ar.1092190104] [PMID: 3688455]

[162] Frost HM. Skeletal structural adaptations to mechanical usage (SATMU): 1. Redefining Wolffs law: the bone modeling problem. Anat Rec 1990; 226(4): 403-13.
       [http://dx.doi.org/10.1002/ar.1092260402] [PMID: 2184695]

[163] Frost HM. Skeletal structural adaptations to mechanical usage (SATMU): 2. Redefining Wolffs law: the remodeling problem. Anat Rec 1990; 226(4): 414-22.
       [http://dx.doi.org/10.1002/ar.1092260403] [PMID: 2184696]

[164] Frost HM. Perspectives: bones mechanical usage windows. Bone Miner 1992; 19(3): 257-71.
       [http://dx.doi.org/10.1016/0169-6009(92)90875-E] [PMID: 1472896]

[165] Frost HM. Perspectives: a proposed general model of the mechanostat (suggestions from a new skeletal-biologic paradigm). Anat Rec 1996; 244(2): 139-47.
       [http://dx.doi.org/10.1002/(SICI)1097-0185(199602)244:2<139::AID-AR1>3.0.CO;2-X]   [PMID: 8808388]

[166] Frost HM. Strain and other mechanical influences on bone strength and maintenance. Curr Opin Orthop 1997; 8: 60-70.
       [http://dx.doi.org/10.1097/00001433-199710000-00010]

[167] Frost HM, Ferretti JL, Jee WS. Perspectives: some roles of mechanical usage, muscle strength, and the mechanostat in skeletal physiology, disease, and research. Calcif Tissue Int 1998; 62(1): 1-7.
       [http://dx.doi.org/10.1007/s002239900384] [PMID: 9405724]

[168] Frost HM. From Wolffs law to the mechanostat: a new face of physiology. J Orthop Sci 1998; 3(5): 282-6.
       [http://dx.doi.org/10.1007/s007760050054] [PMID: 9732563]

[169] Frost HM. From Wolffs law to the Utah paradigm: insights about bone physiology and its clinical applications. Anat Rec 2001; 262(4): 398-419.
       [http://dx.doi.org/10.1002/ar.1049] [PMID: 11275971]

[170] Frost HM. Bones mechanostat: a 2003 update. Anat Rec A Discov Mol Cell Evol Biol 2003; 275(2): 1081-101.
       [http://dx.doi.org/10.1002/ar.a.10119] [PMID: 14613308]

[171] Frost HM. A 2003 update of bone physiology and Wolffs Law for clinicians. Angle Orthod 2004; 74(1): 3-15.
       [PMID: 15038485]

[172] Skerry TM. One mechanostat or many? Modifications of the site-specific response of bone to mechanical loading by nature and nurture. J Musculoskelet Neuronal Interact 2006; 6(2): 122-7.
       [PMID: 16849820]

[173] Hughes JM, Petit MA. Biological underpinnings of Frosts mechanostat thresholds: the important role of osteocytes. J Musculoskelet Neuronal Interact 2010; 10(2): 128-35.
       [PMID: 20516629]

[174] Carter DR. Mechanical loading histories and cortical bone remodeling. Calcif Tissue Int 1984; 36 (Suppl. 1): S19-24.
       [http://dx.doi.org/10.1007/BF02406129] [PMID: 6430518]

[175] Fyhrie DP, Carter DR. A unifying principle relating stress to trabecular bone morphology. J Orthop Res 1986; 4(3): 304-17.
       [http://dx.doi.org/10.1002/jor.1100040307] [PMID: 3734938]

[176] Carter DR, Fyhrie DP, Whalen RT. Trabecular bone density and loading history: regulation of connective tissue biology by mechanical energy. J Biomech 1987; 20(8): 785-94.
       [http://dx.doi.org/10.1016/0021-9290(87)90058-3] [PMID: 3654678]

[177] Carter DR. Mechanical loading history and skeletal biology. J Biomech 1987; 20(11-12): 1095-109.
       [http://dx.doi.org/10.1016/0021-9290(87)90027-3] [PMID: 3323201]

[178] Carter DR, Orr TE, Fyhrie DP. Relationships between loading history and femoral cancellous bone architecture. J Biomech 1989; 22(3): 231-44.
[http://dx.doi.org/10.1016/0021-9290(89)90091-2] [PMID: 2722894]

[179] Beaupré GS, Orr TE, Carter DR. An approach for time-dependent bone modeling and remodelingtheoretical development. J Orthop Res 1990; 8(5): 651-61.
[http://dx.doi.org/10.1002/jor.1100080506] [PMID: 2388105]

[180] Qin YX, Rubin CT, McLeod KJ. Nonlinear dependence of loading intensity and cycle number in the maintenance of bone mass and morphology. J Orthop Res 1998; 16(4): 482-9.
[http://dx.doi.org/10.1002/jor.1100160414] [PMID: 9747791]

[181] Rubin CT, Lanyon LE. Regulation of bone formation by applied dynamic loads. J Bone Joint Surg Am 1984; 66(3): 397-402.
[http://dx.doi.org/10.2106/00004623-198466030-00012] [PMID: 6699056]

[182] Rubin CT, Lanyon LE. Regulation of bone mass by mechanical strain magnitude. Calcif Tissue Int 1985; 37(4): 411-7.
[http://dx.doi.org/10.1007/BF02553711] [PMID: 3930039]

[183] Cardinale M, Bosco C. The use of vibration as an exercise intervention. Exerc Sport Sci Rev 2003; 31(1): 3-7.
[http://dx.doi.org/10.1097/00003677-200301000-00002] [PMID: 12562163]

[184] Totosy de Zepetnek JO, Giangregorio LM, Craven BC. Whole-body vibration as potential intervention for people with low bone mineral density and osteoporosis: a review. J Rehabil Res Dev 2009; 46(4): 529-42.
[http://dx.doi.org/10.1682/JRRD.2008.09.0136] [PMID: 19882487]

[185] Rubin C, Pope M, Fritton JC, Magnusson M, Hansson T, McLeod K. Transmissibility of 15-hertz to 35-hertz vibrations to the human hip and lumbar spine: determining the physiologic feasibility of delivering low-level anabolic mechanical stimuli to skeletal regions at greatest risk of fracture because of osteoporosis. Spine 2003; 28(23): 2621-7.
[http://dx.doi.org/10.1097/01.BRS.0000102682.61791.C9] [PMID: 14652479]

[186] Abercromby AF, Amonette WE, Layne CS, McFarlin BK, Hinman MR, Paloski WH. Variation in neuromuscular responses during acute whole-body vibration exercise. Med Sci Sports Exerc 2007; 39(9): 1642-50.
[http://dx.doi.org/10.1249/mss.0b013e318093f551] [PMID: 17805098]

[187] Abercromby AF, Amonette WE, Layne CS, McFarlin BK, Hinman MR, Paloski WH. Vibration exposure and biodynamic responses during whole-body vibration training. Med Sci Sports Exerc 2007; 39(10): 1794-800.
[http://dx.doi.org/10.1249/mss.0b013e3181238a0f] [PMID: 17909407]

[188] Bosco C, Colli R, Introini E, *et al.* Adaptive responses of human skeletal muscle to vibration exposure. Clin Physiol 1999; 19(2): 183-7.
[http://dx.doi.org/10.1046/j.1365-2281.1999.00155.x] [PMID: 10200901]

[189] Bosco C, Cardinale M, Tsarpela O. Influence of vibration on mechanical power and electromyogram activity in human arm flexor muscles. Eur J Appl Physiol Occup Physiol 1999; 79(4): 306-11.
[http://dx.doi.org/10.1007/s004210050512] [PMID: 10090628]

[190] Bosco C, Iacovelli M, Tsarpela O, *et al.* Hormonal responses to whole-body vibration in men. Eur J Appl Physiol 2000; 81(6): 449-54.
[http://dx.doi.org/10.1007/s004210050067] [PMID: 10774867]

[191] Kerschan-Schindl K, Grampp S, Henk C, *et al.* Whole-body vibration exercise leads to alterations in muscle blood volume. Clin Physiol 2001; 21(3): 377-82.
[http://dx.doi.org/10.1046/j.1365-2281.2001.00335.x] [PMID: 11380538]

[192] Torvinen S, Kannu P, Sievänen H, *et al.* Effect of a vibration exposure on muscular performance and body balance. Randomized cross-over study. Clin Physiol Funct Imaging 2002; 22(2): 145-52.
[http://dx.doi.org/10.1046/j.1365-2281.2002.00410.x] [PMID: 12005157]

[193] Torvinen S, Sievänen H, Järvinen TA, Pasanen M, Kontulainen S, Kannus P. Effect of 4-min vertical whole body vibration on muscle performance and body balance: a randomized cross-over study. Int J Sports Med 2002; 23(5): 374-9.
[http://dx.doi.org/10.1055/s-2002-33148] [PMID: 12165890]

[194] Torvinen S, Kannus P, Sievänen H, *et al.* Effect of four-month vertical whole body vibration on performance and balance. Med Sci Sports Exerc 2002; 34(9): 1523-8.
[http://dx.doi.org/10.1097/00005768-200209000-00020] [PMID: 12218749]

[195] Torvinen S, Kannus P, Sievänen H, *et al.* Effect of 8-month vertical whole body vibration on bone, muscle performance, and body balance: a randomized controlled study. J Bone Miner Res 2003; 18(5): 876-84.
[http://dx.doi.org/10.1359/jbmr.2003.18.5.876] [PMID: 12733727]

[196] Delecluse C, Roelants M, Verschueren S. Strength increase after whole-body vibration compared with resistance training. Med Sci Sports Exerc 2003; 35(6): 1033-41.
[http://dx.doi.org/10.1249/01.MSS.0000069752.96438.B0] [PMID: 12783053]

[197] Roelants M, Delecluse C, Goris M, Verschueren S. Effects of 24 weeks of whole body vibration training on body composition and muscle strength in untrained females. Int J Sports Med 2004; 25(1): 1-5.
[http://dx.doi.org/10.1055/s-2003-45238] [PMID: 14750005]

[198] Bush JA, Blog GL, Kang J, Faigenbaum AD, Ratamess NA. Effects of quadriceps strength after static and dynamic whole-body vibration exercise. J Strength Cond Res 2015; 29(5): 1367-77.
[http://dx.doi.org/10.1519/JSC.0000000000000709] [PMID: 25268289]

[199] Srinivasan S, Weimer DA, Agans SC, Bain SD, Gross TS. Low-magnitude mechanical loading becomes osteogenic when rest is inserted between each load cycle. J Bone Miner Res 2002; 17(9): 1613-20.
[http://dx.doi.org/10.1359/jbmr.2002.17.9.1613] [PMID: 12211431]

[200] Hettinger T. Der einfluss sinusförmiger schwingungen auf die skelettmuskulatur. Int Z Angew Physiol 1956; 16(3): 192-7. [Influence of sinusoidal oscillations on skeletal musculature].
[PMID: 13376175]

[201] Johnston RM, Bishop B, Coffey GH. Mechanical vibration of skeletal muscles. Phys Ther 1970; 50(4): 499-505.
[PMID: 5434954]

[202] Nazarov V, Spivak G. Development of athlete's strength abilities by means of biomechanical stimulation method. Theory Prac Phys Culture 1985; 12: 445-50.

[203] Samuelson B, Jorfeldt L, Ahlborg B. Influence of vibration on endurance of maximal isometric contraction. Clin Physiol 1989; 9(1): 21-5.
[http://dx.doi.org/10.1111/j.1475-097X.1989.tb00952.x] [PMID: 2706913]

[204] Roelants M, Delecluse C, Verschueren SM. Whole-body-vibration training increases knee-extension strength and speed of movement in older women. J Am Geriatr Soc 2004; 52(6): 901-8.
[http://dx.doi.org/10.1111/j.1532-5415.2004.52256.x] [PMID: 15161453]

[205] Bosco C, Colli R, Cardinale M, *et al.* The effect of whole body vibration on mechanical behavior of skeletal muscle and hormonal profile. In: Lyritis GR, Ed. Musculo skeletal interactions: basic and clinical aspects. Athens: Hylonome Editions 1999; 2: pp. 67-76.

[206] de Ruiter CJ, van der Linden RM, van der Zijden MJ, Hollander AP, de Haan A. Short-term effects of whole-body vibration on maximal voluntary isometric knee extensor force and rate of force rise. Eur J

Appl Physiol 2003; 88(4-5): 472-5.
[http://dx.doi.org/10.1007/s00421-002-0723-0] [PMID: 12527980]

[207] Bosco C, Cardinale M, Tsarpela O, *et al.* The influence on whole body vibration on jumping performance. Biol Sport 1998; 15(3): 157-64.

[208] Burke JR, Schutten MC, Koceja DM, Kamen G. Age-dependent effects of muscle vibration and the Jendrassik maneuver on the patellar tendon reflex response. Arch Phys Med Rehabil 1996; 77(6): 600-4.
[http://dx.doi.org/10.1016/S0003-9993(96)90302-0] [PMID: 8831479]

[209] Lebedev MA, Poliakov AV. [Analysis of the interference electromyogram of human soleus muscle after exposure to vibration]. Neirofiziologiia 1991; 23(1): 57-65.
[PMID: 2034299]

[210] Rittweger J, Beller G, Felsenberg D. Acute physiological effects of exhaustive whole-body vibration exercise in man. Clin Physiol 2000; 20(2): 134-42.
[http://dx.doi.org/10.1046/j.1365-2281.2000.00238.x] [PMID: 10735981]

[211] Burke RE, Rymer WZ. Relative strength of synaptic input from short-latency pathways to motor units of defined type in cat medial gastrocnemius. J Neurophysiol 1976; 39(3): 447-58.
[PMID: 181542]

[212] Bongiovanni LG, Hagbarth KE. Tonic vibration reflexes elicited during fatigue from maximal voluntary contractions in man. J Physiol 1990; 423: 1-14.
[http://dx.doi.org/10.1113/jphysiol.1990.sp018007] [PMID: 2388146]

[213] Ribot-Ciscar E, Rossi-Durand C, Roll JP. Muscle spindle activity following muscle tendon vibration in man. Neurosci Lett 1998; 258(3): 147-50.
[http://dx.doi.org/10.1016/S0304-3940(98)00732-0] [PMID: 9885952]

[214] Steyvers M, Levin O, Van Baelen M, Swinnen SP. Corticospinal excitability changes following prolonged muscle tendon vibration. Neuroreport 2003; 14(15): 1901-5.
[http://dx.doi.org/10.1097/00001756-200310270-00004] [PMID: 14561917]

[215] Rosenkranz K, Rothwell JC. Differential effect of muscle vibration on intracortical inhibitory circuits in humans. J Physiol 2003; 551(Pt 2): 649-60.
[http://dx.doi.org/10.1113/jphysiol.2003.043752] [PMID: 12821723]

[216] Rosenkranz K, Rothwell JC. The effect of sensory input and attention on the sensorimotor organization of the hand area of the human motor cortex. J Physiol 2004; 561(Pt 1): 307-20.
[http://dx.doi.org/10.1113/jphysiol.2004.069328] [PMID: 15388776]

[217] Roick H, von Giesen HJ, Benecke R. On the origin of the postexcitatory inhibition seen after transcranial magnetic brain stimulation in awake human subjects. Exp Brain Res 1993; 94(3): 489-98.
[http://dx.doi.org/10.1007/BF00230207] [PMID: 8359263]

[218] Hanajima R, Ugawa Y, Terao Y, *et al.* Paired-pulse magnetic stimulation of the human motor cortex: differences among I waves. J Physiol 1998; 509(Pt 2): 607-18.
[http://dx.doi.org/10.1111/j.1469-7793.1998.607bn.x] [PMID: 9575308]

[219] Werhahn KJ, Kunesch E, Noachtar S, Benecke R, Classen J. Differential effects on motorcortical inhibition induced by blockade of GABA uptake in humans. J Physiol 1999; 517(Pt 2): 591-7.
[http://dx.doi.org/10.1111/j.1469-7793.1999.0591t.x] [PMID: 10332104]

[220] Sanger TD, Garg RR, Chen R. Interactions between two different inhibitory systems in the human motor cortex. J Physiol 2001; 530(Pt 2): 307-17.
[http://dx.doi.org/10.1111/j.1469-7793.2001.0307l.x] [PMID: 11208978]

[221] Ilić TV, Meintzschel F, Cleff U, Ruge D, Kessler KR, Ziemann U. Short-interval paired-pulse inhibition and facilitation of human motor cortex: the dimension of stimulus intensity. J Physiol 2002; 545(Pt 1): 153-67.
[http://dx.doi.org/10.1113/jphysiol.2002.030122] [PMID: 12433957]

[222] Paul RL, Merzenich M, Goodman H. Representation of slowly and rapidly adapting cutaneous mechanoreceptors of the hand in Brodmanns areas 3 and 1 of *Macaca mulatta.* Brain Res 1972; 36(2): 229-49.
[http://dx.doi.org/10.1016/0006-8993(72)90732-9] [PMID: 4621596]

[223] Merzenich MM, Kaas JH, Sur M, Lin CS. Double representation of the body surface within cytoarchitectonic areas 3b and 1 in SI in the owl monkey (*Aotus trivirgatus*). J Comp Neurol 1978; 181(1): 41-73.
[http://dx.doi.org/10.1002/cne.901810104] [PMID: 98537]

[224] Sur M, Wall JT, Kaas JH. Modular segregation of functional cell classes within the postcentral somatosensory cortex of monkeys. Science 1981; 212(4498): 1059-61.
[http://dx.doi.org/10.1126/science.7233199] [PMID: 7233199]

[225] Sur M, Nelson RJ, Kaas JH. Representations of the body surface in cortical areas 3b and 1 of squirrel monkeys: comparisons with other primates. J Comp Neurol 1982; 211(2): 177-92.
[http://dx.doi.org/10.1002/cne.902110207] [PMID: 7174889]

[226] Sretavan D, Dykes RW. The organization of two cutaneous submodalities in the forearm region of area 3b of cat somatosensory cortex. J Comp Neurol 1983; 213(4): 381-98.
[http://dx.doi.org/10.1002/cne.902130403] [PMID: 6300198]

[227] Sur M, Wall JT, Kaas JH. Modular distribution of neurons with slowly adapting and rapidly adapting responses in area 3b of somatosensory cortex in monkeys. J Neurophysiol 1984; 51(4): 724-44.
[PMID: 6716121]

[228] Sur M, Garraghty PE, Bruce CJ. Somatosensory cortex in macaque monkeys: laminar differences in receptive field size in areas 3b and 1. Brain Res 1985; 342(2): 391-5.
[http://dx.doi.org/10.1016/0006-8993(85)91144-8] [PMID: 4041845]

[229] Kaas JH, Pons TP. The somatosensory system of primates. Comp Primate Biol 1988; 4: 421-68.

[230] Chen LM, Friedman RM, Ramsden BM, LaMotte RH, Roe AW. Fine-scale organization of SI (area 3b) in the squirrel monkey revealed with intrinsic optical imaging. J Neurophysiol 2001; 86(6): 3011-29.
[PMID: 11731557]

[231] Phillips CG, Powell TP, Wiesendanger M. Projection from low-threshold muscle afferents of hand and forearm to area 3a of baboons cortex. J Physiol 1971; 217(2): 419-46.
[http://dx.doi.org/10.1113/jphysiol.1971.sp009579] [PMID: 5097607]

[232] Heath CJ, Hore J, Phillips CG. Inputs from low threshold muscle and cutaneous afferents of hand and forearm to areas 3a and 3b of baboons cerebral cortex. J Physiol 1976; 257(1): 199-227.
[http://dx.doi.org/10.1113/jphysiol.1976.sp011364] [PMID: 820853]

[233] Jones eg, Porter R. What is area 3a? Brain Res 1980; 203(1): 1-43.
[http://dx.doi.org/10.1016/0165-0173(80)90002-8] [PMID: 6994855]

[234] Hore J, Preston JB, Cheney PD. Responses of cortical neurons (areas 3a and 4) to ramp stretch of hindlimb muscles in the baboon. J Neurophysiol 1976; 39(3): 484-500.
[PMID: 133213]

[235] Pons TP, Garraghty PE, Cusick CG, Kaas JH. The somatotopic organization of area 2 in macaque monkeys. J Comp Neurol 1985; 241(4): 445-66.
[http://dx.doi.org/10.1002/cne.902410405] [PMID: 4078042]

[236] Torebjörk HE, Ochoa JL. Specific sensations evoked by activity in single identified sensory units in man. Acta Physiol Scand 1980; 110(4): 445-7.
[http://dx.doi.org/10.1111/j.1748-1716.1980.tb06695.x] [PMID: 7234450]

[237] Ochoa J, Torebjörk E. Sensations evoked by intraneural microstimulation of single mechanoreceptor units innervating the human hand. J Physiol 1983; 342: 633-54.
[http://dx.doi.org/10.1113/jphysiol.1983.sp014873] [PMID: 6631752]

[238] Verrillo RT. Temporal summation in vibrotactile sensitivity. J Acoust Soc Am 1965; 37: 843-6.
[http://dx.doi.org/10.1121/1.1909458] [PMID: 14285445]

[239] Talbot WH, Darian-Smith I, Kornhuber HH, Mountcastle VB. The sense of flutter-vibration: comparison of the human capacity with response patterns of mechanoreceptive afferents from the monkey hand. J Neurophysiol 1968; 31(2): 301-34.
[PMID: 4972033]

[240] Labs SM, Gescheider GA, Fay RR, Lyons CH. Psychophysical tuning curves in vibrotaction. Sens Processes 1978; 2(3): 231-47.
[PMID: 749204]

[241] Gescheider GA, Sklar BF, Van Doren CL, Verrillo RT. Vibrotactile forward masking: psychophysical evidence for a triplex theory of cutaneous mechanoreception. J Acoust Soc Am 1985; 78(2): 534-43.
[http://dx.doi.org/10.1121/1.392475] [PMID: 4031252]

[242] Bolanowski SJ Jr, Gescheider GA, Verrillo RT, Checkosky CM. Four channels mediate the mechanical aspects of touch. J Acoust Soc Am 1988; 84(5): 1680-94.
[http://dx.doi.org/10.1121/1.397184] [PMID: 3209773]

[243] Bosco C. Adaptive response of human skeletal muscle to simulated hypergravity condition. Acta Physiol Scand 1985; 124(4): 507-13.
[http://dx.doi.org/10.1111/j.1748-1716.1985.tb00042.x] [PMID: 4050478]

[244] Bosco C. The effects of extra-load permanent wearing on morphological and functional characteristics of leg extensor muscles 1992. Thesis,Universitè Jean-Monnet de Saint Etienne France

[245] Seidel H. Myoelectric reactions to ultra-low frequency and low-frequency whole body vibration. Eur J Appl Physiol Occup Physiol 1988; 57(5): 558-62.
[http://dx.doi.org/10.1007/BF00418462] [PMID: 3396572]

[246] Lebedev MA, Polyakov AV. Analysis of surface EMG of human soleus muscle subjected to vibration. J Electromyogr Kinesiol 1992; 2(1): 26-35.
[http://dx.doi.org/10.1016/1050-6411(92)90005-4] [PMID: 20870524]

[247] del Pozo-Cruz B, Adsuar JC, Parraca JA, del Pozo-Cruz J, Olivares PR, Gusi N. Using whole-body vibration training in patients affected with common neurological diseases: a systematic literature review. J Altern Complement Med 2012; 18(1): 29-41.
[http://dx.doi.org/10.1089/acm.2010.0691] [PMID: 22233167]

[248] Ahlborg L, Andersson C, Julin P. Whole-body vibration training compared with resistance training: effect on spasticity, muscle strength and motor performance in adults with cerebral palsy. J Rehabil Med 2006; 38(5): 302-8.
[http://dx.doi.org/10.1080/16501970600680262] [PMID: 16931460]

[249] Melzack R, Wall PD. Pain mechanisms: a new theory. Science 1965; 150(3699): 971-9.
[http://dx.doi.org/10.1126/science.150.3699.971] [PMID: 5320816]

[250] Barker KL, Elliott CJ, Sackley CM, Fairbank JC. Treatment of chronic back pain by sensory discrimination training. A Phase I RCT of a novel device (FairMed) *vs.* TENS. BMC Musculoskelet Disord 2008; 9: 97.
[http://dx.doi.org/10.1186/1471-2474-9-97] [PMID: 18588702]

[251] Lundeberg T, Ottoson D, Håkansson S, Meyersson BA. Vibratory stimulation for the control of intractable chronic orofacial pain. 1983.

[252] Lundeberg T. The pain suppressive effect of vibratory stimulation and transcutaneous electrical nerve stimulation (TENS) as compared to aspirin. Brain Res 1984; 294(2): 201-9.
[http://dx.doi.org/10.1016/0006-8993(84)91031-X] [PMID: 6608397]

[253] Lundeberg T. Long-term results of vibratory stimulation as a pain relieving measure for chronic pain. Pain 1984; 20(1): 13-23.
[http://dx.doi.org/10.1016/0304-3959(84)90807-8] [PMID: 6436774]

[254] Lundeberg T, Nordemar R, Ottoson D. Pain alleviation by vibratory stimulation. Pain 1984; 20(1): 25-44.
[http://dx.doi.org/10.1016/0304-3959(84)90808-X] [PMID: 6333660]

[255] Lundeberg T, Abrahamsson P, Bondesson L, Haker E. Vibratory stimulation compared to placebo in alleviation of pain. Scand J Rehabil Med 1987; 19(4): 153-8.
[PMID: 3438712]

[256] Guieu R, Tardy-Gervet MF, Roll JP. Analgesic effects of vibration and transcutaneous electrical nerve stimulation applied separately and simultaneously to patients with chronic pain. Can J Neurol Sci 1991; 18(2): 113-9.
[http://dx.doi.org/10.1017/S0317167100031541] [PMID: 1712660]

[257] Gerdesmeyer L, Maier M, Haake M, Schmitz C. Physical-technical principles of extracorporeal shockwave therapy (ESWT). Orthopade 2002; 31(7): 610-7.
[http://dx.doi.org/10.1007/s00132-002-0319-8] [PMID: 12219657]

[258] Rompe JD, Bürger R, Hopf C, Eysel P. Shoulder function after extracorporal shock wave therapy for calcific tendinitis. J Shoulder Elbow Surg 1998; 7(5): 505-9.
[http://dx.doi.org/10.1016/S1058-2746(98)90203-8] [PMID: 9814931]

[259] Scholl J, Lohrer H. Radial shock wave therapy in insertion tendinopathies. Dtsch Z Sportmed 1999; 50(S1): 110-5.

[260] Seil R, Rupp S, Hammer DS, Ensslin S, Gebhardt T, Kohn D. Extracorporeal shockwave therapy in tendinosis calcarea of the rotator cuff: comparison of different treatment protocols. Z Orthop Ihre Grenzgeb 1999; 137(4): 310-5.
[http://dx.doi.org/10.1055/s-2008-1039717] [PMID: 11051015]

[261] Loew M, Daecke W, Kusnierczak D, Rahmanzadeh M, Ewerbeck V. Shock-wave therapy is effective for chronic calcifying tendinitis of the shoulder. J Bone Joint Surg Br 1999; 81(5): 863-7.
[http://dx.doi.org/10.1302/0301-620X.81B5.9374] [PMID: 10530851]

[262] Maier M, Stäbler A, Lienemann A, et al. Shockwave application in calcifying tendinitis of the shoulderprediction of outcome by imaging. Arch Orthop Trauma Surg 2000; 120(9): 493-8.
[http://dx.doi.org/10.1007/s004020000154] [PMID: 11011666]

[263] Rompe JD, Buch M, Gerdesmeyer L, et al. Musculoskeletal shock wave therapy – current database of clinical research. Z Orthop Ihre Grenzgeb 2002; 140(3): 267-74.
[http://dx.doi.org/10.1055/s-2002-32477] [PMID: 12085291]

[264] Maier M, Milz S, Wirtz DC, Rompe JD, Schmitz C. Basic research of applying extracorporeal shockwaves on the musculoskeletal system. An assessment of current status. Orthopade 2002; 31(7): 667-77.
[http://dx.doi.org/10.1007/s00132-002-0328-7] [PMID: 12219666]

[265] Haupt G, Diesch R, Straub T, et al. Radial Shock Wave Therapy in Heel Spurs. Der Niedergelassene Chirurg 2002; 6: 1-6.

[266] Magosch P, Lichtenberg S, Habermeyer P. Radial shock wave therapy in calcifying tendinitis of the rotator cuffa prospective study. Z Orthop Ihre Grenzgeb 2003; 141(6): 629-36.
[PMID: 14679427]

[267] Gerdesmeyer L, Gollwitzer H, Diehl P, Wagner K. Radial extracorporeal shock wave therapy in

orthopaedics. J Miner Stoffwechs 2004; 11: 369.

[268] Spacca G, Necozione S, Cacchio A. Radial shock wave therapy for lateral epicondylitis: a prospective randomised controlled single-blind study. Eura Medicophys 2005; 41(1): 17-25.
[PMID: 16175767]

[269] Cacchio A, Paoloni M, Barile A, *et al.* Effectiveness of radial shock-wave therapy for calcific tendinitis of the shoulder: single-blind, randomized clinical study. Phys Ther 2006; 86(5): 672-82.
[PMID: 16649891]

[270] Straub T, Penninger E, Frölich T, *et al.* Successful therapy of painful fasciitis plantar by radial shock wave: a prospective, multi-centric and placebo-controlled study. Int J Sports Med 1999; 20: 21-3.

[271] Lohrer H, Schöll J, Arentz S, *et al.* Effectiveness of radial shock wave therapy (RSWT) on tennis elbow and plantar fasciitis. Alberta, Canada: Annual Simposium of Canadian Academy of Sport Medicine 2001.

[272] Rompe JD, Schoellner C, Nafe B. Evaluation of low-energy extracorporeal shock-wave application for treatment of chronic plantar fasciitis. J Bone Joint Surg Am 2002; 84-A(3): 335-41.
[http://dx.doi.org/10.2106/00004623-200203000-00001] [PMID: 11886900]

[273] Haupt G, Diesch R, Straub T. Radial shock wave therapy for fasciitis plantaris. Der niedergelassene. Chirurg 2002; 6(4): 36-40.

[274] Gerdesmeyer L, Frey C, Vester J, *et al.* Radial extracorporeal shock wave therapy is safe and effective in the treatment of chronic recalcitrant plantar fasciitis: results of a confirmatory randomized placebo-controlled multicenter study. Am J Sports Med 2008; 36(11): 2100-9.
[http://dx.doi.org/10.1177/0363546508324176] [PMID: 18832341]

[275] Greve JM, Grecco MV, Santos-Silva PR. Comparison of radial shockwaves and conventional physiotherapy for treating plantar fasciitis. Clinics (Sao Paulo) 2009; 64(2): 97-103.
[http://dx.doi.org/10.1590/S1807-59322009000200006] [PMID: 19219314]

[276] Shaheen AM. Comparison of three different treatment protocols of low-energy radial extracorporeal shock wave therapy for management of chronic plantar fasciitis. Indian J Physiother Occup Ther 2010; 4(1): 8-12.

[277] Buselli P, Messina S, Fontanesi M, *et al.* Vibrazioni a onde meccanosonore. Il fisioterapista 2014; 3: 75-81.

[278] Saggini R, Bellomo RG, Cancelli F, Iodice P. Treatment on myofascial pain syndromes: local acoustic vibration vs local lidocaine injection. J Musculoskel Pain. Haworth Medical Press Publ 2007; (Suppl. 13)15.

[279] Saggini R, Iodice P, Galati V, Marri A, Bellomo RG. Treatment on myofascial pain syndromes: local selective acoustic vibration vs lidocaine injection. J Rehabil Med 2008; (Suppl. 47)94.

[280] Saggini R, Di Pancrazio L, Supplizi M, Bellomo RG. The effect of focused high-frequency vibration at 300 Hz on muscle basal tone. Giornale Italiano di Medicina Riabilitativa 2012; 26(2-3): 46.

[281] Pietrangelo T, Mancinelli R, Toniolo L, *et al.* Effects of local vibrations on skeletal muscle trophism in elderly people: mechanical, cellular, and molecular events. Int J Mol Med 2009; 24(4): 503-12.
[http://dx.doi.org/10.3892/ijmm_00000259] [PMID: 19724891]

[282] Iodice P, Bellomo RG, Gialluca G, Fanò G, Saggini R. Acute and cumulative effects of focused high-frequency vibrations on the endocrine system and muscle strength. Eur J Appl Physiol 2011; 111(6): 897-904.
[http://dx.doi.org/10.1007/s00421-010-1677-2] [PMID: 21063726]

[283] Kvorning T, Bagger M, Caserotti P, Madsen K. Effects of vibration and resistance training on neuromuscular and hormonal measures. Eur J Appl Physiol 2006; 96(5): 615-25.
[http://dx.doi.org/10.1007/s00421-006-0139-3] [PMID: 16482475]

[284] Di Loreto C, Ranchelli A, Lucidi P, *et al.* Effects of whole-body vibration exercise on the endocrine

system of healthy men. J Endocrinol Invest 2004; 27(4): 323-7.
[http://dx.doi.org/10.1007/BF03351056] [PMID: 15233550]

[285] Cardinale M, Leiper J, Erskine J, Milroy M, Bell S. The acute effects of different whole body vibration amplitudes on the endocrine system of young healthy men: a preliminary study. Clin Physiol Funct Imaging 2006; 26(6): 380-4.
[http://dx.doi.org/10.1111/j.1475-097X.2006.00706.x] [PMID: 17042906]

[286] Bellomo RG, Iodice P, Maffulli N, Maghradze T, Coco V, Saggini R. Muscle strength and balance training in sarcopenic elderly: a pilot study with randomized controlled trial. Eur J Inflamm 2013; 11(1): 189-97.
[http://dx.doi.org/10.1177/1721727X1301100118]

[287] Di Pancrazio L, Bellomo RG, Franciotti R, *et al.* Combined rehabilitation program for postural instability in progressive supranuclear palsy. NeuroRehabilitation 2013; 32(4): 855-60.
[PMID: 23867411]

[288] De Nunzio AM, Grasso M, Nardone A, Godi M, Schieppati M. Alternate rhythmic vibratory stimulation of trunk muscles affects walking cadence and velocity in Parkinsons disease. Clin Neurophysiol 2010; 121(2): 240-7.
[http://dx.doi.org/10.1016/j.clinph.2009.10.018] [PMID: 19955020]

[289] Camerota F, Celletti C, Suppa A, *et al.* Focal Muscle Vibration Improves Gait in Parkinson's Disease: A Pilot Randomized, Controlled Trial. Movement Disorders Clinical Practice. 2015. 3, 6, p. 559-566 8 p www.interscience.wiley.com
[http://dx.doi.org/10.1002/mdc3.12323]

[290] Novak P, Novak V. Effect of step-synchronized vibration stimulation of soles on gait in Parkinsons disease: a pilot study. J Neuroeng Rehabil 2006; 3: 9.
[http://dx.doi.org/10.1186/1743-0003-3-9] [PMID: 16674823]

[291] Kawahira K, Higashihara K, Matsumoto S, *et al.* New functional vibratory stimulation device for extremities in patients with stroke. Int J Rehabil Res 2004; 27(4): 335-7.
[http://dx.doi.org/10.1097/00004356-200412000-00015] [PMID: 15573001]

[292] Paoloni M, Mangone M, Scettri P, Procaccianti R, Cometa A, Santilli V. Segmental muscle vibration improves walking in chronic stroke patients with foot drop: a randomized controlled trial. Neurorehabil Neural Repair 2010; 24(3): 254-62.
[http://dx.doi.org/10.1177/1545968309349940] [PMID: 19855076]

[293] Cotey D, Hornby TG, Gordon KE, Schmit BD. Increases in muscle activity produced by vibration of the thigh muscles during locomotion in chronic human spinal cord injury. Exp Brain Res 2009; 196(3): 361-74.
[http://dx.doi.org/10.1007/s00221-009-1855-9] [PMID: 19479245]

[294] Murillo N, Kumru H, Vidal-Samso J, *et al.* Decrease of spasticity with muscle vibration in patients with spinal cord injury. Clin Neurophysiol 2011; 122(6): 1183-9.
[http://dx.doi.org/10.1016/j.clinph.2010.11.012] [PMID: 21172739]

[295] Field-Fote E, Ness LL, Ionno M. Vibration elicits involuntary, step-like behavior in individuals with spinal cord injury. Neurorehabil Neural Repair 2012; 26(7): 861-9.
[http://dx.doi.org/10.1177/1545968311433603] [PMID: 22328683]

[296] Noma T, Matsumoto S, Etoh S, Shimodozono M, Kawahira K. Anti-spastic effects of the direct application of vibratory stimuli to the spastic muscles of hemiplegic limbs in post-stroke patients. Brain Inj 2009; 23(7): 623-31.
[http://dx.doi.org/10.1080/02699050902997896] [PMID: 19557565]

[297] Liepert J, Binder C. Vibration-induced effects in stroke patients with spastic hemiparesis a pilot study. Restor Neurol Neurosci 2010; 28(6): 729-35.
[PMID: 21209488]

[298] Conrad MO, Scheidt RA, Schmit BD. Effects of wrist tendon vibration on targeted upper-arm movements in poststroke hemiparesis. Neurorehabil Neural Repair 2011; 25(1): 61-70.
[http://dx.doi.org/10.1177/1545968310378507] [PMID: 20921324]

[299] Marconi B, Filippi GM, Koch G, *et al.* Long-term effects on cortical excitability and motor recovery induced by repeated muscle vibration in chronic stroke patients. Neurorehabil Neural Repair 2011; 25(1): 48-60.
[http://dx.doi.org/10.1177/1545968310376757] [PMID: 20834043]

[300] Noma T, Matsumoto S, Shimodozono M, Etoh S, Kawahira K. Anti-spastic effects of the direct application of vibratory stimuli to the spastic muscles of hemiplegic limbs in post-stroke patients: a proof-of-principle study. J Rehabil Med 2012; 44(4): 325-30.
[http://dx.doi.org/10.2340/16501977-0946] [PMID: 22402727]

[301] Caliandro P, Celletti C, Padua L, *et al.* Focal muscle vibration in the treatment of upper limb spasticity: a pilot randomized controlled trial in patients with chronic stroke. Arch Phys Med Rehabil 2012; 93(9): 1656-61.
[http://dx.doi.org/10.1016/j.apmr.2012.04.002] [PMID: 22507444]

[302] Tavernese E, Paoloni M, Mangone M, *et al.* Segmental muscle vibration improves reaching movement in patients with chronic stroke. A randomized controlled trial. NeuroRehabilitation 2013; 32(3): 591-9.
[PMID: 23648613]

[303] Paoloni M, Tavernese E, Fini M, *et al.* Segmental muscle vibration modifies muscle activation during reaching in chronic stroke: A pilot study. NeuroRehabilitation 2014; 35(3): 405-14.
[PMID: 25227540]

[304] Murillo N, Valls-Sole J, Vidal J, Opisso E, Medina J, Kumru H. Focal vibration in neurorehabilitation. Eur J Phys Rehabil Med 2014; 50(2): 231-42.
[PMID: 24842220]

[305] Karnath HO, Christ K, Hartje W. Decrease of contralateral neglect by neck muscle vibration and spatial orientation of trunk midline. Brain 1993; 116(Pt 2): 383-96.
[http://dx.doi.org/10.1093/brain/116.2.383] [PMID: 8461972]

[306] Schindler I, Kerkhoff G, Karnath HO, Keller I, Goldenberg G. Neck muscle vibration induces lasting recovery in spatial neglect. J Neurol Neurosurg Psychiatry 2002; 73(4): 412-9.
[http://dx.doi.org/10.1136/jnnp.73.4.412] [PMID: 12235310]

[307] Johannsen L, Ackermann H, Karnath HO. Lasting amelioration of spatial neglect by treatment with neck muscle vibration even without concurrent training. J Rehabil Med 2003; 35(6): 249-53.
[http://dx.doi.org/10.1080/16501970310009972] [PMID: 14664313]

[308] Kamada K, Shimodozono M, Hamada H, Kawahira K. Effects of 5 minutes of neck-muscle vibration immediately before occupational therapy on unilateral spatial neglect. Disabil Rehabil 2011; 33(23-24): 2322-8.
[http://dx.doi.org/10.3109/09638288.2011.570411] [PMID: 21486139]

CHAPTER 3

The Applied Mechanical Vibration as Ultrasound Energy

Rosa Grazia Bellomo[1,*], **Simona Maria Carmignano**[2] and **Raoul Saggini**[3]

[1] *Physical and Rehabilitation Medicine, Department of Medical Oral and Biotechnological Sciences, "Gabriele d'Annunzio" University, Chieti-Pescara, Italy*

[2] *School of Specialty in Physical and Rehabilitation Medicine, "Gabriele d'Annunzio" University, Chieti-Pescara, Italy*

[3] *Physical and Rehabilitation Medicine, Department of Medical Oral and Biotechnological Sciences, Director of the School of Specialty in Physical and Rehabilitation Medicine, "Gabriele d'Annunzio" University, Chieti-Pescara, Italy; National Coordinator of Schools of Specialty in Physical and Rehabilitation Medicine*

Abstract: Ultrasound is a form of mechanical energy transmitted through and into biological tissues as an acoustic pressure wave at frequencies higher than that of the upper limit of human hearing, and it is used widely in medicine as a therapeutic, operative, and diagnostic tool.

Therapeutic US has a frequency range of 0.75-3 MHz, with most machines set at a frequency of 1 or 3 MHz.

Ultrasound can produce many effects other than just the potential heating effect, acting as a mechanotransduction, a complex biological process that involves the spatial and temporal orchestration of numerous cell types, hundreds if not thousands of genes, and the intricate organization of the extracellular matrix. The intensity or power density of the ultrasound can be adjusted depending on the desired effect and the target tissue.

Keywords: Aesthetic applications, Cavitation, Dosimetry, Non-thermal effects, Phonophoresis, Reparative and Regenerative medicine, Thermal effects, Ultrasound.

INTRODUCTION

Methods to generate and detect ultrasound (US) first became available in the United States in the 19th century; however, the first large-scale application of US was for navigation of submarines during World War II. In the SONAR, a short

* **Corresponding authors Rosa Grazia Bellomo:** Physical and Rehabilitation Medicine, Department of Medical Oral and Biotechnological Sciences, "Gabriele d'Annunzio" University, Chieti-Pescara, Italy; Tel: 03908713555306; Fax: 03909713553224; E-mail: rosa.bellomo@unich.it

Raoul Saggini (Ed.)
All rights reserved-© 2017 Bentham Science Publishers

pulse of US is sent from a submarine through the water, and a detector picks up the echo of the signal. Sound waves are sent out, they returned to the sender "ping" qualities.

In the 1920s it was also observed that extremely high-pressure waves were damaging to living tissues. As early as the 1930s, low intensities of therapeutic US were used for the first time in physical medicine to treat soft tissue conditions with mild heating. Today therapeutic US is a commonly used modality in therapy clinics, applied for its deep heating ability. However, therapeutic forms of US that are available in the twenty-first century are capable of many more applications than providing just deep heating.

PHYSICAL CHARACTERISTICS OF US

Sound is a vibration that propagates as a mechanical wave from a source to a receiver (for example, the ear), through a medium such as air or water. US consists of a mechanical vibration very similar to sound wave, its frequency is greater than 20 kilohertz (20,000 hertz), which represents the threshold of human hearing [1]. The wave specific feature is that the particles of the medium oscillate around a position of equilibrium, this generates movements of the collision between a particle and the other generating a series of similar reactions. A desk ornament, sometimes called Newton's cradle (Fig. **1**), illustrates some principles of this type of energy transfer. It consists of a frame with five metal balls suspended through wires from a horizontal bar so that they touch each other at rest. If one lifts and releases the first ball, the mobile will set in motion. When the first ball swings back into place it bumps into the next ball, which in turn bumps into the one after it. In this way, the energy is transferred from ball to ball. Because the last ball is unopposed, it swings out into space; however, when it drops back into line, a new cycle is set in motion [2].

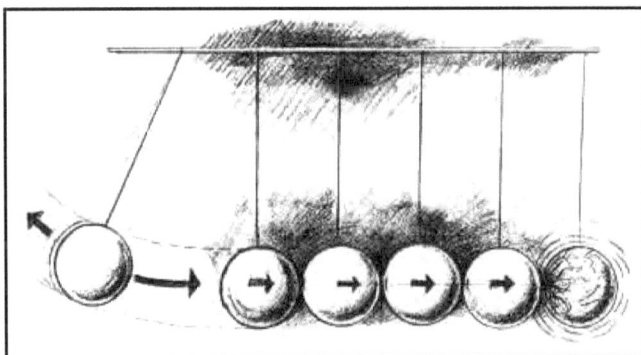

Fig. (1). Newton's cradle. From: http://www.bookvip.net/shock-wave-physics.html.

Waves can travel through media as longitudinal, transverse, and standing waves. When the particles of a medium are compressed and decompressed in the direction that a wave travels, it is termed as longitudinal wave. When particle movement is at right angles to the direction of travel, it is termed as shear or transverse wave (Fig. **2**) [3, 4]. Shear waves propagate or start more readily in solids, and longitudinal waves in liquids and gases.

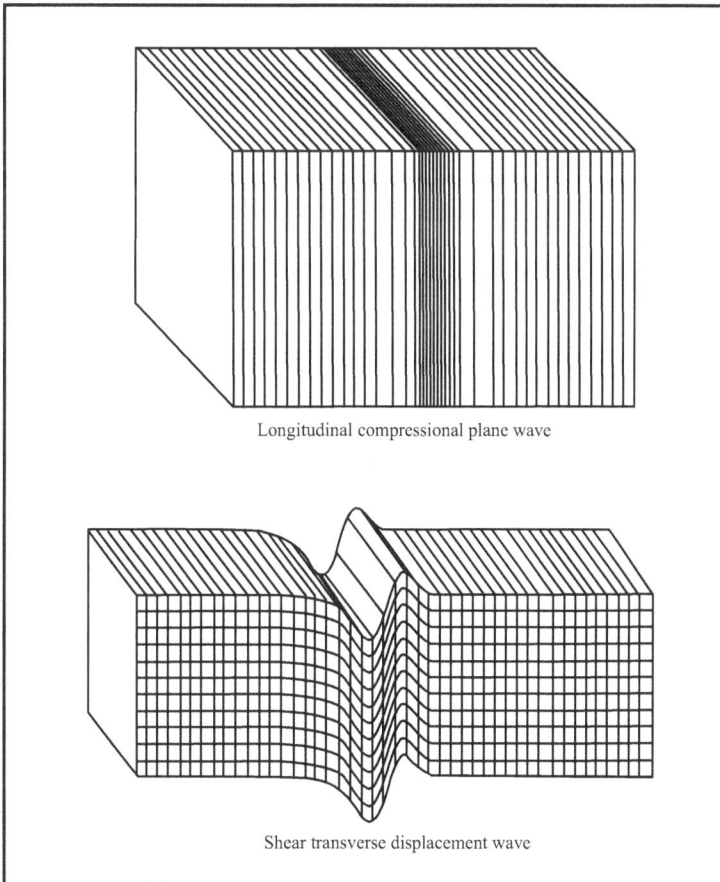

Longitudinal compressional plane wave

Shear transverse displacement wave

Fig. (2). Two examples of acoustic pulses, travelling from left to right. The media on either side of the wave pulse is in the equilibrium position: that the right of the pulse has not yet been disturbed, and that on the left has returned to equilibrium after the oscillations associated with the pulse have damped down. The depicted waves are the longitudinal (compressional) plane wave and the shear (transverse displacement) plane wave. Modified From: Timothy G. Leighton "What is ultrasound?" Progress in Biophysics and Molecular Biology 93 (2007) 3–83.

US can also be defined by the following physical parameters that characterize the wave:

- *Frequency*: It is defined as the number of cycles per second (Hz They are defined ultrasound because the frequency is greater than that perceived by the human ear (15-20,000 Hz). The frequencies used in therapy typically range between 1.0-3.0 MHz [5]. Generally, therapeutic US has a frequency between 0.7-3.3 MHz, to maximize energy absorption at a depth of 2 to 5 cm of soft tissue.
- *Wavelength*: is the distance covered by the wave in an ultrasonic period that is the time (usually measured in seconds) that it takes for one cycle. The period is the reciprocal of frequency:

$$f = 1 / T$$

where f is the frequency, T is the period;

- *Velocity*: it represents the velocity of wave propagation in 'unit of time of the period. It varies depending on the quality of the medium in which they propagate. For example, in a saline solution, the velocity of US is approximately 1500 m/sec compared with approximately 350 m/sec in air (sound waves can travel more rapidly in a more dense medium (from: http://joemanu. free.fr/taratata/) The velocity of US in most tissues is thought to be similar to that in saline. The mathematical representation of the relationship is

$$v = f \cdot \lambda$$

where v is the velocity, f is the frequency and λ is the wavelength;

- *Amplitude*: is the distance to from one peak to other one; it is relative to the amount of energy transported;
- *Intensity*: the intensity registered on a US unit during the delivery of US indicates the intensity delivered during each pulse (W/cm^2), that is the amount of energy flowing in the time unit through a surface of unit area, perpendicular to the direction of wave propagation:

$$I = P / A$$

where P is the ultrasonic power, A is the surface area of transducer. The intensity can range over time if it employs continuous wave or pulsed wave. In particular, the presence of a pulsed field brings a temporal variation, and define a duty cycle, as the ratio between the pulse duration US (in time units) and the length of the period, calculated as a percentage [6, 7] (Fig. **3**).

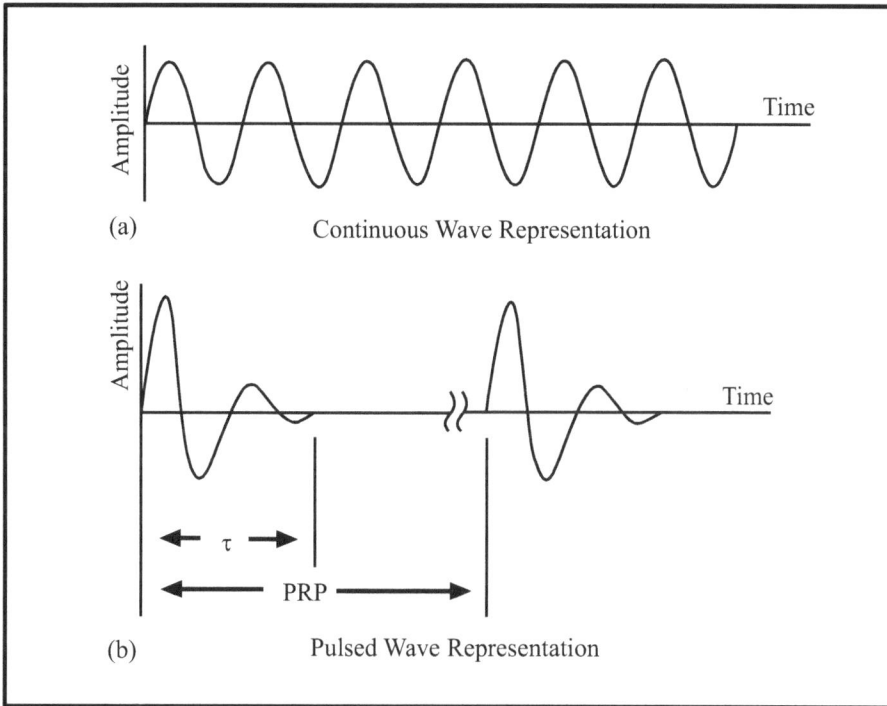

Fig. (3). Schematic representations of continuous wave and pulsed wave US waveforms: (**a**) continuous wave representation and (**b**) pulsed wave representation. From: O'Brien WD Jr. US-biophysics mechanisms. Prog Biophys Mol Biol 2007; 93(1-3): 212-55.

GENERATION OF US

The property to generate electricity in response to a mechanical force or to change shape in response to an electrical current (*piezoelectricity*) was discovered by Paul-Jacques and Pierre Curie in the 1880s [8, 9]. Compressing with a press a quartz crystal, the two scientists observed that the two flattened sides of the crystal had polarized electrically in a manner quite similar to the chemical batteries of the time. The piezoelectric effect consists in the overlapping of two events – one of mechanical nature, the other of electrical origin – and even in the passage from one to another, being a reversible process. Thus, if an electric voltage is applied at the two opposite surfaces of a piezoelectric material block (quartz plates, disks of ceramic material), the material expands or shrinks [10 - 13]. Furthermore, applying an alternating electric field, an alternation of mechanical compressions and expansions is obtained, that is in an acoustic pressure wave [14] (Fig. **4**).

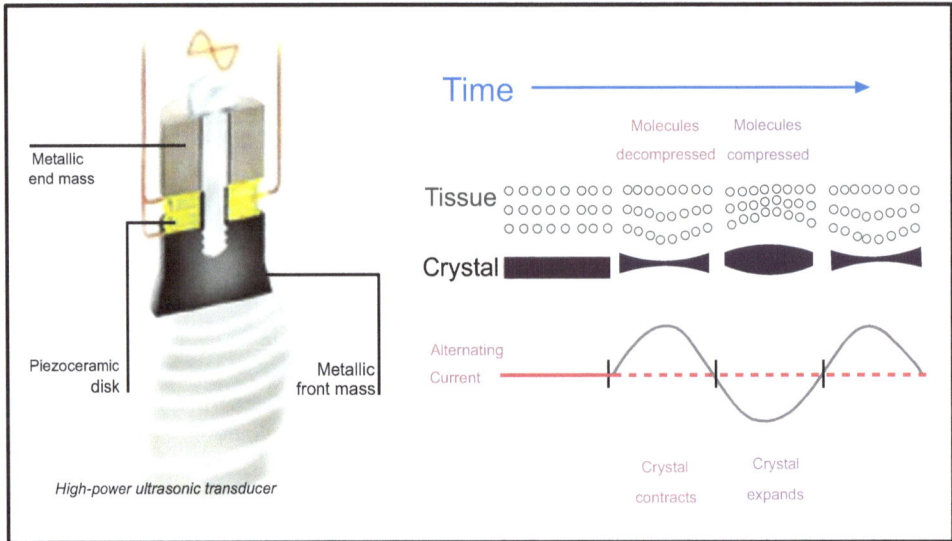

Fig. (4). The phenomenon of piezoelectricity.

The absence of a center of symmetry is a necessary condition to manifest the piezoelectricity, absent in conductive materials and structurally symmetrical. In a crystal, this position occurs when a mechanical action causes appearance of an electric dipole in each molecule, moving the center of the charges positive and negative. The electrostatic balance breaking produces the polarization. The deformed crystal behaves like a condenser to which is applied a difference of potential. If the two faces are connected to an electric circuit is generated and a current. Another necessary condition for the polarization to be successful, is the achievement of Curie temperature during the exposure process to the electric field and the next cooling of the material, always in the presence of the field. By doing so, the domains tend to align in the closest direction to the field, producing a dipole moment.

A common definition of the efficiency of a transducer is the fraction of applied energy that is converted to the desired energy mode.

For a US transducer, this definition of efficiency is described as the *electromechanical coupling coefficient* (Table **1**). If mechanical energy (*i.e.*, pressure) is applied, we obtain

$$k_c^2 = \frac{\text{Mechanical energy converted to electrical energy}}{\text{Applied mechanical energy}}$$

A number of piezoelectric crystals occur in nature (for example, quartz, Rochelle salts, lithium sulphate, tourmaline, and ammonium dihydrogen phosphate); today ceramic materials (such as lead zirconate titanate) and plastic materials (such as polyvinylidene fluoride) have been developed. Nowadays, US transducers are usually made of zirconate titanate because this is the least costly and most efficient piezoelectric material readily available. These materials are most commonly used because the piezoelectric effect is direct, *i.e.* the mechanical input (deformation) produces an electrical output voltage. Polycrystalline materials consisting of a large number of crystal grains are randomly oriented. They exhibit piezoelectric effect only after polarization: application of a high electric field (1-4 kV/mm) that directs the internal electric dipoles in a single direction [15].

Table 1. Properties of selected piezoelectric crystals.

Material	Electromechanical coupling coefficient (K_c)	Curie point (°C)
Quartz	0.11	550
Rochelle salt	0.78	45
Barium titanate	0.30	120
Lead zirconate titanate (PZT-4)	0.70	328
Lead zirconate titanate (PZT-5)	0.70	365

US always need an elastic medium to propagate, whether it be gaseous, liquid or solid against which the US generator is vibrated, producing pressures and dilations that propagate with a speed that is a function of the compression characteristics of matter radiated and which is very different according to the medium (gas, liquid, or solid). When a US wave passes from one medium to another, it is generally assists a phenomena that carried energy by the wave redistribution: a part is reflected and part is transmitted, according to the laws of the classical mechanics.

Each medium crossed is characterized by a complex quantity, the impedance Z, which synthesizes the acoustic characteristics of the medium and quantifies the resistance that the medium itself opposes the passage of sound waves.

The acoustic impedance is defined as the product of the density ρ (kg/m^3) for the propagation velocity c (m/s). So we define:

$$Z = \rho \cdot c$$

The acoustic impedance is the magnitude that describes at a particular frequency how a medium opposes the passage of sound waves [16].

For example, the velocity of sound wave in the air is about 330 meters per second while in liquids is already four or five times higher. Moreover, the density of matter is involved in impedance variation: the impedance increases with the increase of the same density.

Table **2** shows the impedance values for some biological media; in general, the highest values are found in solid matter.

Table 2. The acoustic impedance in various biological media.

Material	Acoustic impedance (rayl)
Muscle	1.70
Fat	1.38
Brain	1.58
Kidney	1.62
Liver	1.65
Blood	1.61
Soft tissue (average)	1.63
Water	1.48
Bone	7.80
Air (NTP)	0.0004

NTP, normal temperature and pressure: 20°C, 1 atm.

The acoustic impedance constitutes an important parameter for various biomedical applications, which gives rise to the practical interest to know its value in different biological media. While for some the values are known with reasonable reliability as the blood, the fat tissues or blood vessels, in others they are subject to considerable variability, consequent indeterminacy of the velocity propagation of the waves: examples are the bones and skin. When a US beam meets the acoustic interface of two media with different acoustic impedances, a part of its energy is reflected and the remaining part continues its path in the middle as a transmitted beam [17]. The maximum transmission of a US wave from one medium to another occurs when the acoustic impedances of the two media are equal.

Much importance are the conditions encountered when a US wave passes in its direction of propagation from one medium to another with different acoustic characteristics. When an ultrasound beam passes through a medium, the energy is undergone to three phenomena: absorption, reflection and diffusion. The attenuation determines energy reduction of the US beam. US is absorbed by the medium if part of the beam energy is converted into heat, this determines an increase in molecular kinetic energy. When the ultrasound beam meets the separation area between two media with different acoustic impedance Z, only part of the beam is transferred from the first to the second medium, while the remaining part is reflected. The diffusion phenomenon, also called "scattering", is related to the size of the defects of media and to the beam speed US, which in turn depends on the frequency of the same. The diffusion occurs for the difference in acoustic impedance between the two media, near the interface between defect and material. The portion of the wave transmitted across the boundary is reduced in power as a result of reflection. Within biological tissues, such boundaries may be formed by any two heterogeneous tissue surfaces such as bone and nerve, muscle and adipose tissue, and many other examples [18] (Fig. **5**).

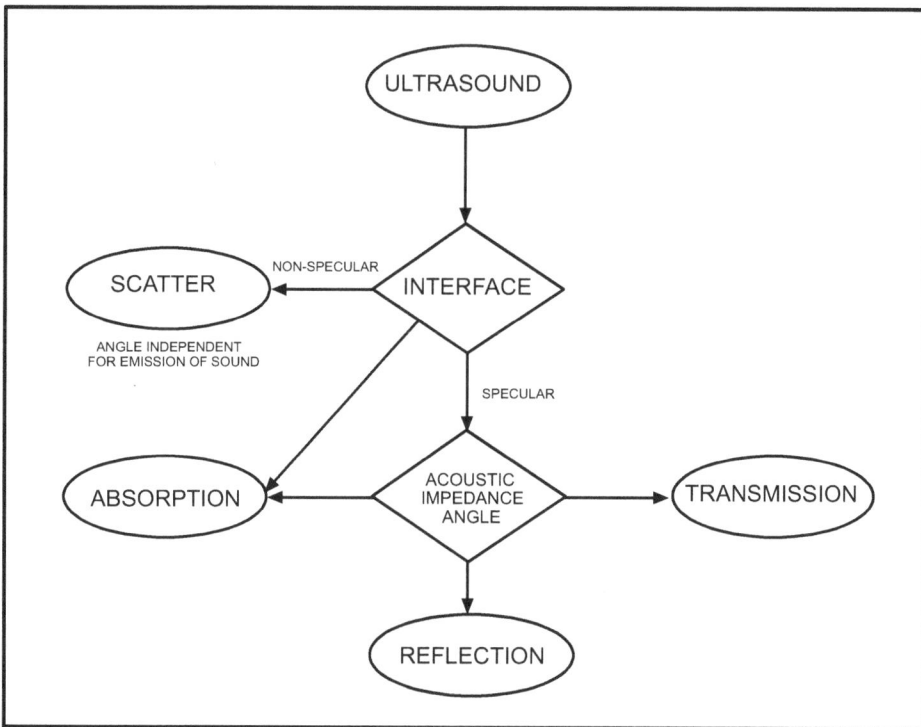

Fig. (5). Summary of interactions of US at boundaries of materials. From: Hendee WR, Ritenour ER. Medical Imaging Physics. 4th ed. Wiley-Liss 2002.

In human tissues US repeatedly encounters boundaries. The acoustic properties of skin, fat, blood vessels, and muscle are similar. When US encounters boundaries between acoustically similar tissues, such as adipose and muscle, the amount of reflection is insignificant to treatment outcome.

The absorption is mainly related to thermo-elastic characteristics and hysteresis of medium in which the propagation takes place. The viscosity and heat conduction can have negative effects on energy transmission, as related movement of the particles in the material. When a wave propagates in a medium, the particles tend to flow relatively to each other to allow the passage of the wave, but the movement is hindered by the viscosity, which leads to the transformation of energy associated part the particles into heat. The models to calculate absorption for homogeneous and isotropic materials are differ from the model for the non-homogeneous materials and anisotropic. The first category belongs to metals, homogeneous materials, such as plastics and coupling fluids. A second category belong the composite materials. Even if, for particular frequencies of the beam (2 to 10 MHz), such materials may appear homogeneous, but they still retain a different absorption model.

The absorption is always associated to dissipation. Therefore, the energy of the US beam is reduced gradually as it passes through the medium. This reduction is called *relaxation energy loss*. During the propagation in a medium, the acoustic wave is subjected to a progressive loss of energy, more properly, it causes a decrease in the intensity in function of the distance from the source.

The attenuation coefficient α describes the attenuation phenomena and it is expressed in units of decibels per centimetre. Many of the values are known only approximately and vary significantly with both the origin and condition of the biologic samples.

The α coefficient therefore, consists of two parts:

$$\alpha = \alpha S + \alpha a$$

where αS is the coefficient relating to the dissemination and αa is that relative absorption.

In soft tissue, the absorption coefficient accounts for 60 to 90% of the attenuation, and scatter accounts for the remainder. The causes are essentially two: the absorption due to on the damping of molecular movement, and the subsequent processing of the same in heat. To absorb is "to take something in", penetrate means "to enter into". "Penetration in US" is the term used to describe the distance from the sound source at which 50% of the original energy remains. As tissues absorb energy from a sound wave, a reduced amount of energy remains to be carried forward by the wave, which lessens its penetration; hence, there is an inverse relationship between absorption and penetration. If energy penetrates deeply into the tissues, then it means it was not absorbed. If energy does not penetrate deeply, then the tissues have absorbed it. The rate at which the beam energy decreases is also a reflection of the attenuation properties of the medium.

However, reflection increase in proportion to the difference in acoustic impedance of the two boundary materials. This means that when US encounters the boundaries in between bone and muscle, some of the acoustical energy is bounced back or reflected into the muscle and surrounding soft tissue and some is transmitted into the bone. The discussion of US reflection above assumes that the US beam strikes the reflecting interface at a right angle. In the body, US impinges upon interfaces at all angles. For any angle of incidence, the angle at which the reflected ultrasonic energy leaves the interface equals the angle of incidence of the US beam; that is:

angle of incidence = angle of reflection

The wave portion that is transmitted across a boundary is also subject to "bending" if the wave meets the boundary at an angle. This is known as refraction.

The greater the difference in impedance at a boundary, the greater the reflection that will occur, and therefore, the smaller the amount of energy that will be transferred [7] (Fig. **6**).

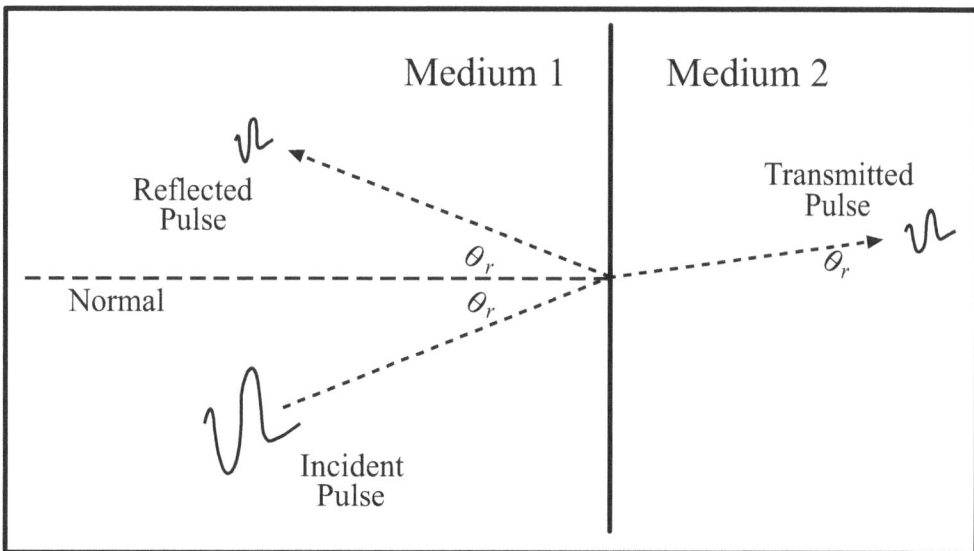

Fig. (6). Reflection and refraction of US at a medium interface.

The dissemination is related to the physical characteristics of the material, in particular to the more or less marked heterogeneity, and acts scattering the beam in multiple directions. Scattering (diffuse reflection) occurs when the incident wave encounters an interface that is not perfectly smooth (for example, surface of visceral organs). The scattered waves result in many different directions [19 - 21] (Fig. **7**).

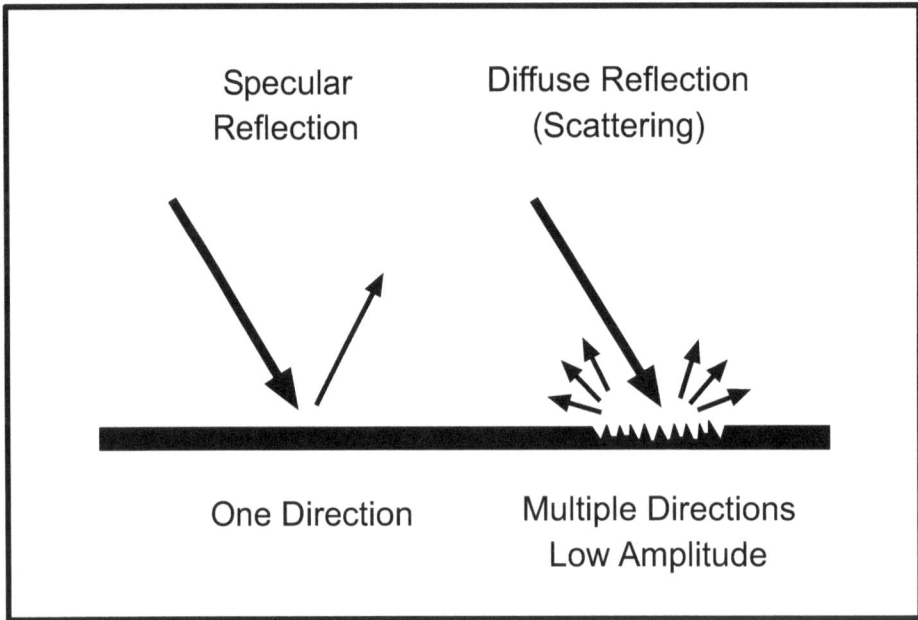

Fig. (7). Reflection and scattering of US at a medium interface.

CHARACTERISTICS OF THERAPEUTIC US

The interaction of US with biological tissue produces energy absorption of that depends on the type of tissue and by the frequency of the waves.

Most medical US equipment operates in the ultrasonic frequency range between 1-15 MHz. Therapeutic US has a frequency range of 0.75-3 MHz, with most machines set at a frequency of 1 or 3 MHz. For most diagnostic applications in abdominal, obstetrical and gynaecological US, and in echocardiography, the frequency range is generally between 2.5-7.5 MHz. For superficial body parts, such as the thyroid and the eye, and peripheral vascular applications where US does not have to penetrate very deeply into the body, higher ultrasonic frequencies in the range of 7.5-15 MHz can be used because ultrasonic attenuation increases with increasing frequency.

In Table **3** are reported some absorption coefficients for tissues crossed by US at frequencies of 1 and 3 MHz.

Table 3. Absorption coefficients of biological tissues.

Tissue	Frequency of 1 MHz	Frequency of 3 MHz
Blood	0.02	0.084
Blood vessels	0.40	1.2
Bone	3.22	-
Skin	0.62	1.86
Cartilage	1.16	3.48
Tendon	1.12	3.36
Muscle	0.76	2.28
Fat	0.14	0.42
Nervous tissue	0.20	0.60
Air (20°C)	2.76	8.28
Water	0.0006	0.0018

Low absorption and high US wave penetration is observed in water and in fat tissue as rich in water (α = 0.14 and 0.42 at 1 and 3 MHz, respectively); therefore it is not produced significant heating when the US wave passes through them. On the contrary, the absorption is higher in the bone tissue and tendons, which are less water-rich. In general, the soft tissues absorb about 10-20% of the power per centimeter, while the adult bone completely absorbs the US beam in a short distance [22]. Thus, US (US) with greater frequency (3 MHz) are absorbed more superficially than those with a lower frequency (1 MHz), which reach greater depths depending on the type of crossed tissue. US at frequency of 1 MHz, absorbed mainly by the tissues to a depth of 3-5 cm [20] and, precisely for this property, as regards for example their physiotherapeutic applications, are recommended for deeper lesions and in patients with more subcutaneous fat. On the contrary, US at frequency of 3 MHz are recommended to more superficial lesions, the depth of 1-2 cm; for this reason, in addition to being used in physiotherapy, they are also used in the aesthetics (medical and non-medical) [23, 24] (Fig. **8**).

The study of biological interaction mechanism between the US and the tissue arises from the spread of ultrasound in diagnosis [25].

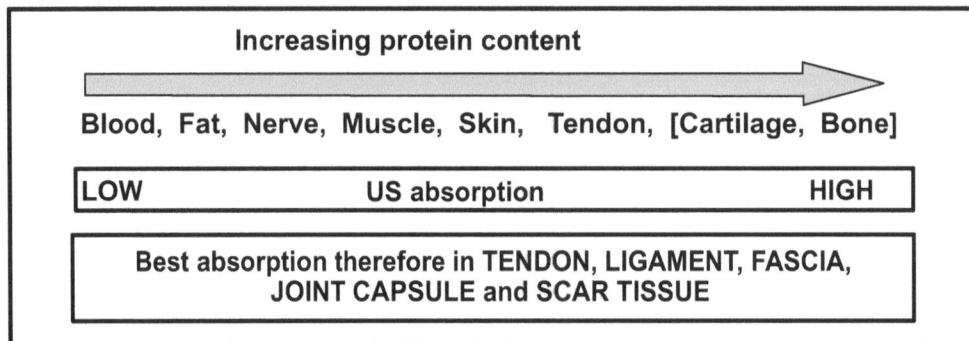

Fig. (8). US at different frequencies and absorption of various tissues. From: Watson T. US in contemporary physiotherapy practice. Ultrasonics 2008; 48(4): 321-9.

More than three decades after the 1880s discovery of the piezoelectric effect by the Curie brothers, the French physicist Paul Langevin developed one of the first uses of US for underwater echo ranging of submerged objects with a quartz crystal at an approximate frequency of 150 kHz [26]. He was, perhaps, the first to observe that ultrasonic energy could have a detrimental effect upon biological material, reporting that *"fish placed in the beam in the neighbourhood of the source operation in a small tank were killed immediately, and certain observers experienced a painful sensation on plunging the hand in this region"* [27], (Langevin, 1920) and also observing the incipient cavitation in water when the source was active.

Another decade passed before a more detailed, experimental study was conducted to investigate Langevin's observations. Although the ultrasonic levels were not specified, Wood and Loomis showed that ultrasonic energy had a range of effects from rupture of *Spirogyra* and *Paramecium* to death of small fishes and frogs by a 1-2-min exposure, the latter also observed by Langevin with a Poulsen arc converter [28].

Many other studies followed on this topic and many authors wrote describing the physical and chemical and biological characteristics of the US; others described their interactions with macromolecules, microorganisms, cells, isolated cells, bacteria, tissues and organs [29].

The ultrasonic exposure conditions of these early works were neither well characterized nor reported, but the exposure levels were undoubtedly high. During the 1930s and 1940s the US are widely applied as its therapeutic modality for the heat generated by the application. However, while it was clear that US could effectively heat tissue, and excess enthusiasm resulted in numerous clinical applications being proposed and tried, the inferior clinical experience caused this modality to fall into disfavor [30]. Later, when it was understood that the heat generated by the US could have a destructive effect on the tissues it is proposed the use of US in surgery. In fact, the possibility of penetrating the surface layers (skin and subcutaneous tissue) and obtain an effect in the deeper layers was exploited for the first time in 1942 [31, 32] in neurosurgery. The surgical application of ultrasound, applying the thermal effect developed in the late 1940s and early 1950s [33]. Since 1952 the US used for the otolaryngologist surgery, to destroy vestibular function to treat the symptoms of Meniere's disease [34, 35].

The greatest expansion in the use of the US took place between the early 1970s and mid-1980s in the diagnostic field, starting with bi-stable, static and ending with grayscale, real-time capabilities. The ability to quantify ultrasonic fields improved considerably. Collaborations between University Started to study the mode of application, the parameters and the effects of the US [36]. In these early years of research, it was thought that the effect to be exploited in therapy was mainly the thermal effect. In 1960, although pulsed US was available, the wave continues in rehabilitation was still using continuous wave output in the range from 0.5 to 1.5 W/cm^2. Then the development of focused US for medical diagnostics and continuing interest in US hyperthermia for treatment of cancer promoted intensive investigation into US effects.

In the 1980s, the pioneering observations by Apfel [37 - 43], Flynn and Church [44, 45] from their mathematical models to describe the dynamic behavior of small bubbles (or micro bubbles) in liquids suggested the strong possibility for transient cavitation (now termed inertial cavitation) to occur from microsecond pulses of US.

One finding of the early research was that US affected tissue growth using very low intensities. This knowledge, generated largely by medical biophysicists, filtered through to physical therapy literature in the early 1980s, leading to a gradual change in practice, in particular, a lowering of treatment dosage. The medical research also gave impetus to research activities led by physical therapists directed specifically toward therapeutic effects of US [46]. It is over years since the interactions between ultra-high frequency sound waves and living tissue were initially studied, and the use of such energy as a form of therapy was first suggested. US has been used to treat a very broad variety of disorders [47 - 56].

Treatment Parameters

Frequency: The number of compression-rarefaction cycles per unit of time, expressed in cycles per second, or Hertz (Hz).

Therapeutic US is usually in the frequency range of 1 to 3 million cycles per second (*i.e.*, 1 to 3 MHz). Increasing the frequency of US causes a decrease in its depth of penetration and concentration of ultrasonic energy in the superficial tissues (Fig. **9**). There is an inverse relationship between penetration and absorption:

$$\uparrow \text{penetration (5 cm)} = \downarrow \text{absorption} = \text{frequency (1 MHz)}$$
$$\downarrow \text{penetration (2.5 cm)} = \uparrow \text{absorption} = \text{frequency (3 MHz)}$$

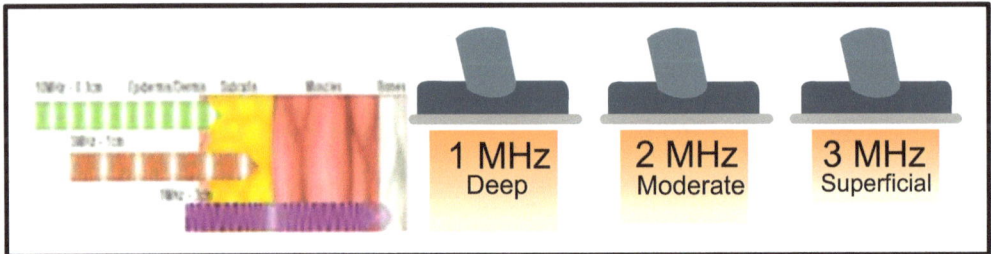

Fig. (9). Frequency of US and depth of penetration.

Intensity: The power per unit area of the sound head, expressed in watts per square centimetre (W/cm^2). The World Health Organization limits the average intensity output by therapeutic US units to 3 W/cm^2.

Power: The amount of acoustic energy, expressed in watts (W), per unit time. In order to characterize exposure, the total power should be specified as well as the following intensities: spatial average temporal average (SATA) intensity; spatial peak temporal peak (SPTP) intensity; spatial peak temporal average (SPTA) intensity; and, if applicable, spatial peak pulse average (SPPA) intensity and spatial average pulse average (SAPA) intensity.

- *Spatial Average, Temporal Average (SATA)*: the average power output of the device over the pulse repetition period divided by a reference, usually that of the transducer face. This measurement of intensity is the most quickly determined.
- *Spatial Peak, Temporal Peak (SPTP)*: the peak intensity at the point in space where the intensity is highest and that occurs when the transducer is emitting. It is highest of the measured intensities.
- *Spatial Peak, Temporal Average (SPTA)*: the peak intensity divided by the transducer surface area, that occurs when the transducer is emitting. This is a measure of the amount of energy delivered to the tissue. The maximal spatial intensity when the sound beam is "on", averaged over the over the period of exposure. It is a measure of the power of the transducer over the pulse repetition period divided by the surface area of the transducer. The SP intensity is usually

two to three times greater than the SA intensity. It is measured in mW/cm².

- *Spatial Peak, Pulse Average (SPPA)*: the average pulse intensity measured at the spatial location where the pulse intensity is maximum.
- *Spatial Average, Pulse Average (SAPA)*: the pulse average intensity averaged over the beam cross sectional area (Figs. **10, 11**).

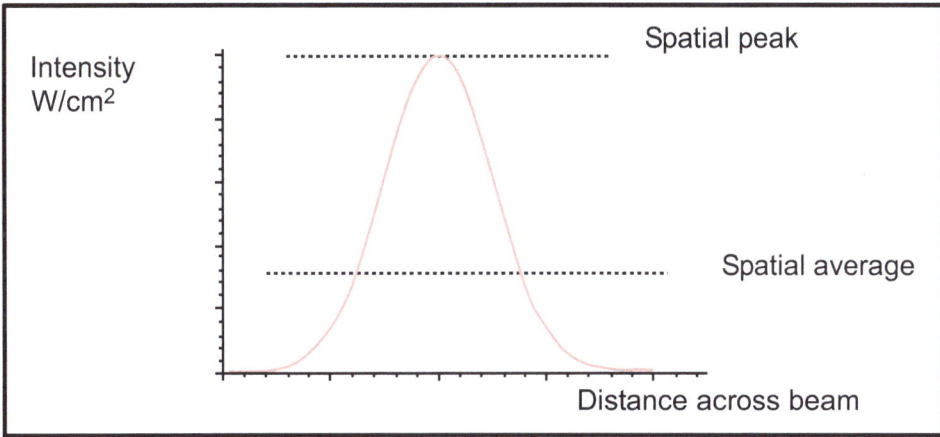

Fig. (10). Intensity and spatial measurements.

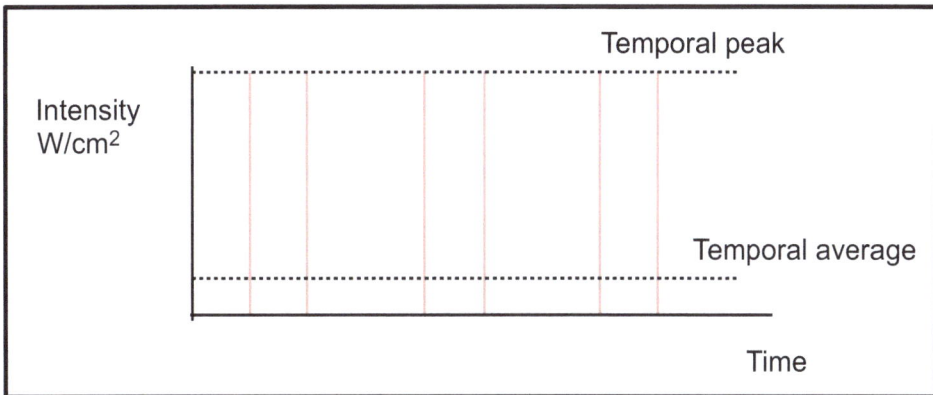

Fig. (11). Intensity and temporal measurements.

Pulse: US can be delivered as continuous or pulsed wave. The continuous mode consists in the continuous delivery of US at a single frequency throughout the treatment period; the pulsed mode consists in the intermittent delivery of US during the treatment period, with a non-constant pressure amplitude (equaling zero for part of the time) (Fig. **12**).

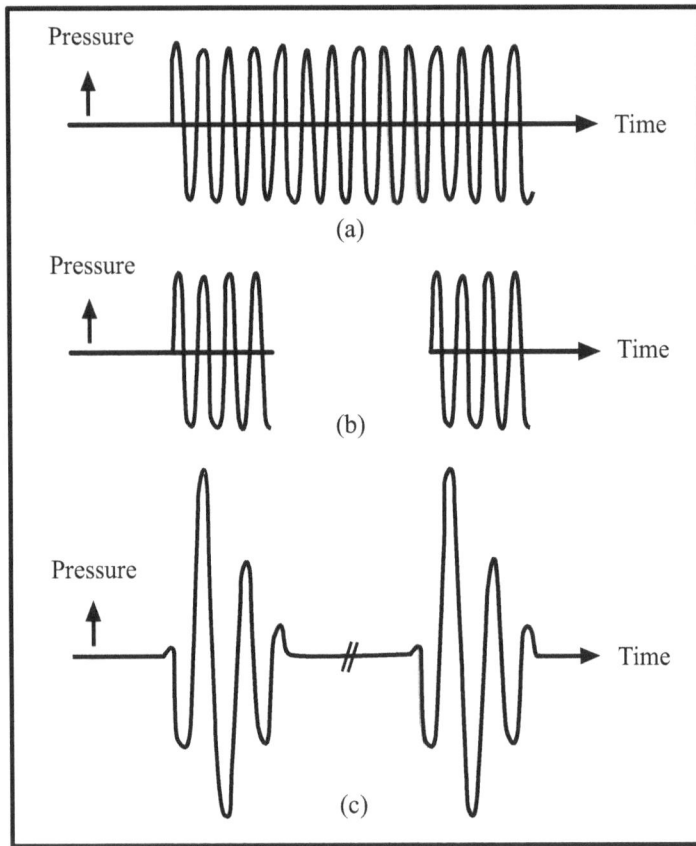

Fig. (12). Low-power US: continuous (**a**), gated continuous (**b**), and pulsed (**c**) wave.

Devices that deliver *continuous US* allow to increase the temperature of the target tissue by 3-8°C within the end of a treatment session (Fig. **13**). The thermal effect generated by continuous US triggers biological changes to occur in the target tissues resulting in the relief of sub-chronic and chronic pain, muscle spasms, and joint contractures.

On the other hand, during the delivery of *pulsed US* no acoustic energy is being emitted between pulses and the US propagates through the medium as small packages of acoustic energy. Pulsed waves can assume any combination of "on"/"off" times. Thus, it is important to specify exactly the time regimen of the pulsed beam. The percentage of "on" time of US output is known as the "duty cycle" (or "duty factor"), which can be expressed as a percentage or as a ratio. Clearly, when output is continuous, the duty cycle is 100%; the output must have an "off" time in this case waves are considered pulsed. For example, if a US unit was programmed to have equaled "on" and "off" periods, this would mean that there would be output for half the time. Typical pulse ratios are 1:1 and 1:4, though others are available; in 1:1 mode the machine offers an output for 2 ms followed by 2-ms rest; in 1:4 mode the 2-ms output is followed by an 8-ms rest period. Fig. (**14**) schematizes the effect of varying the pulse ratio.

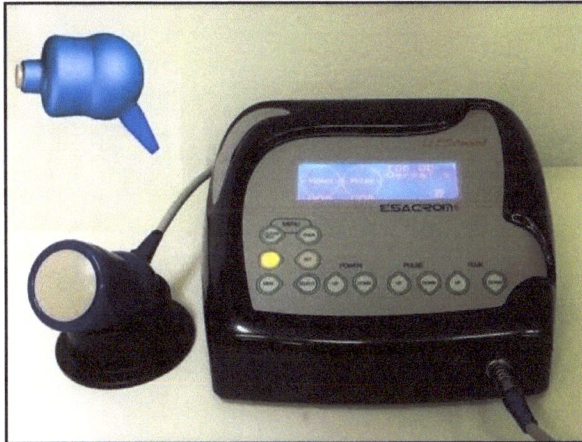

Fig. (13). Low-frequency US shock thermic device – LF Esasound (Esacrom Italy).

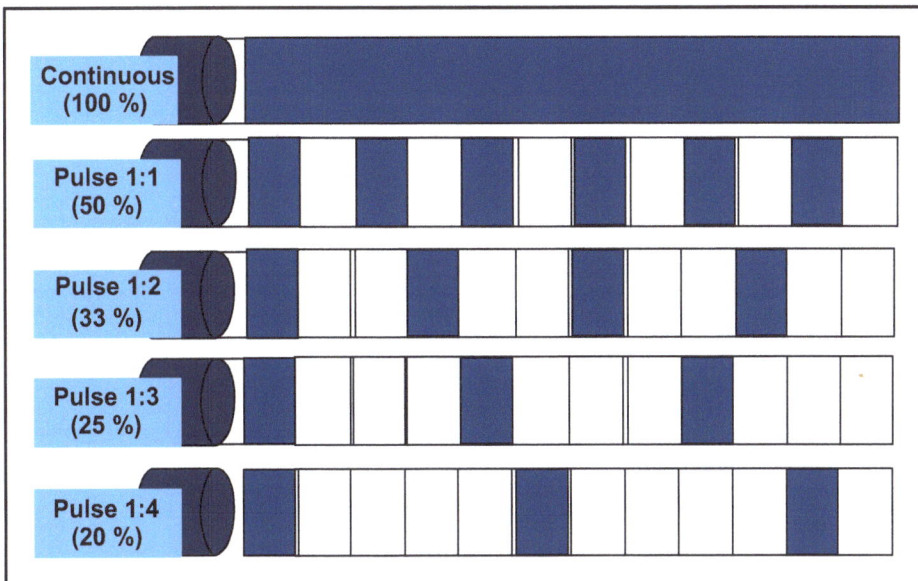

Fig. (14). The diagram illustrates the effect of varying the pulse ratio. Some systems describe their pulsing in terms of a percentage rather than a ratio (1:1 = 50%, 1:4 = 20%, and so on). From: http://www.electrotherapy.org/modality/US-therapy.

Since the sound wave is interrupted, pulsed US produces lesser heating than continuous US at a given intensity, thus minimizing minimizes the thermal effects and having mainly mechanical effects (cavitation, acoustic streaming, micro streaming, increased skin pore size, and increased pore numbers and intercellular space). The newest generation devices work in continuous feedback, always guaranteeing the maximum efficiency of the signal for each treated tissue (Figs. **13**, **15**, **16**).

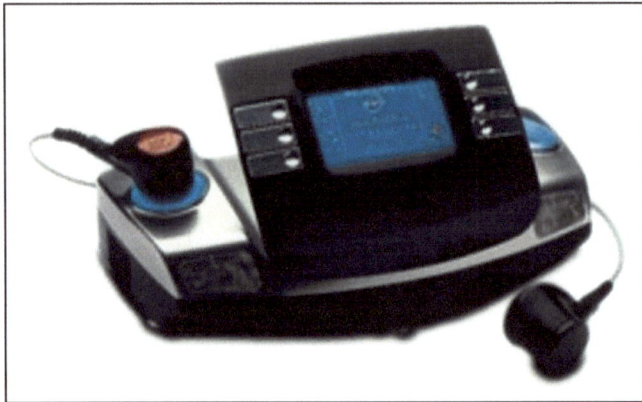

Fig. (15).   Low-frequency pulsed US device *Multicell*® (Medistar s.r.l., Turin, Italy). From: http://www.medistar.it/multicell.html.

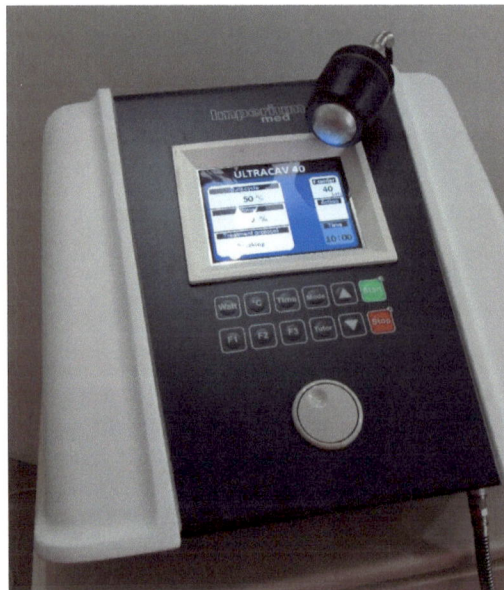

Fig. (16). Low-frequency pulsed US device *Imperium med*®, Brera medical technologies© s.r.l., Ogliastro Cilento, Italy).

Beam Qualities

The importance of being aware of the characteristics of the beam of one's US device is often not fully appreciated [57 - 61].

Some characteristics are of particular importance: the effective radiating area (ERA), Near Field, Far Field, and beam nonuniformity ratio (BNR).

- *Effective Radiating Area (ERA)*: describes the radiating area of the US applicator. This area is usually determined at a distance of 0.5 cm from the transducer face using the same underwater hydrophone mentioned previously. As a rule, the ERA signifies the area of the beam that transmit clinically effective radiation power (5% or more of the maximum intensity in that plane). By this rule, the very low-pressure area around the perimeter of the US beam is not considered to be part of the ERA. The ERA is less than the geometric area of the crystal that emits US. This is due because the crystal is housed inside of the head, making it impossible for the entire head to be part of the ERA. Accurate measurement of the transducer ERA is important because this value is incorporated into the intensity value registered on the device during US treatment (W/cm^2) (Fig. **17**).
- *Near Field* and *Far Field*: the US beam is not uniform and changes in its nature with distance from the transducer. The US beam nearest the treatment head is called the near field (also called the Fresnel region). The behavior of the US in this field is far from regular, with areas of significant interference. The ultrasonic energy in parts of this field can be many times greater than the output set on the machine (possibly as much as 12 to 15 times greater). The size (length) of the near field can be calculated using:

$$r^2 / l$$

r is the radius of the transducer crystal, l is the US wavelength according to the frequency being used (0.5 mm for 3MHz and 1.5 mm for 1.0 MHz). As an example, a crystal with a diameter of 25 mm operating at 1 MHz will have a near field/far field boundary at: boundary = 12.5 mm^2 / 1.5 mm = 10 cm, thus the near field (with greatest interference) extends for approximately 10 cm from the treatment head when using a large treatment head and 1 MHz US. When using higher frequency US, the boundary distance is even greater. Beyond this boundary, lies the Far Field (also called the Fraunhofer region). The US beam in this field is uniform and gently divergent. The hot spots noted in the near field are not significant. For the purposes of therapeutic applications, the far field is effectively out of reach [61].

- *Beam Non-Uniformity Ratio (BNR)*: It describes numerically the ratio of the intensity peaks to the mean intensity in any cross sectional plane. BNR is measured using an underwater microphone known as an acoustical hydrophone. The US applicator is assembled in a tank of degassed water, and the hydrophone moves over the surface of the applicator measuring the output intensity of the US head. A plot of the energy values is produced. BNR varies with distance from the transducer face. The BNR is measured at a fixed point at a distance of 0.5 cm from the transducer surface and it can be an indicator of the quality of the manufacturing process of the head. The result of the measurement is expressed in a ratio compared to 1 (Fig. **18**).

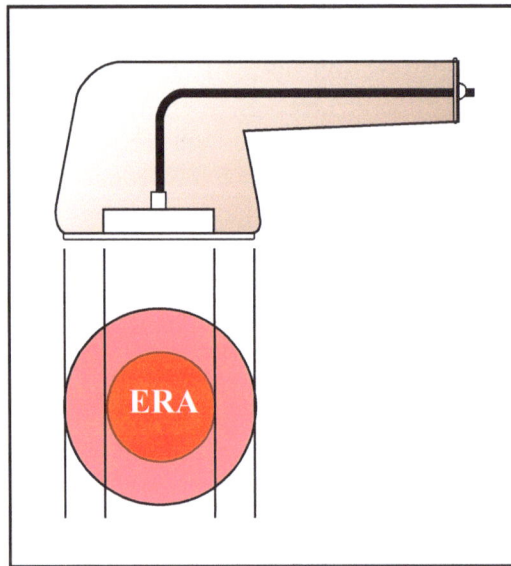

Fig. (17). Effective radiating area (ERA).

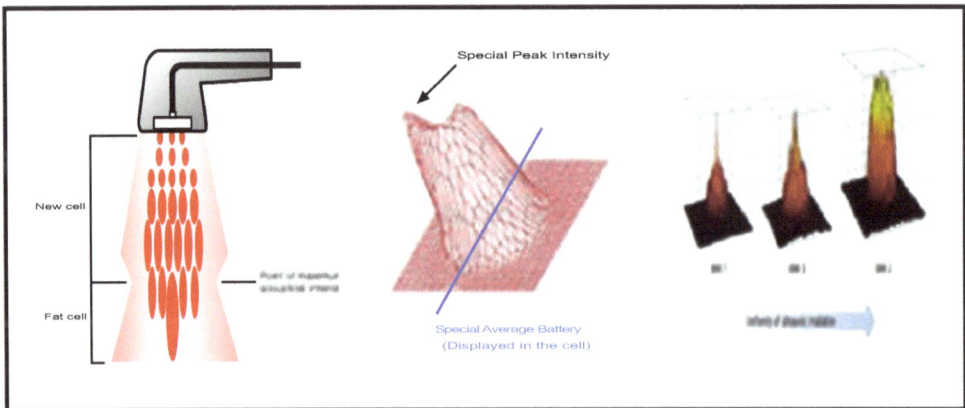

Fig. (18). Description of the amount of variation in the beam. Perfect beam would have a BNR of 1:1. As the smaller the BNR is, the more uniform the US being radiated are, we can see that this is an excellent probe. Generally, minimally acceptable BNR is 8:1 and if it is a BNR ≤ 5 it is considered to be good.

BIOLOGICAL EFFECTS OF US

The basis for this rationale lies in a understanding of the mechanisms by which it is known that US can affect living systems. Such knowledge comes from fundamental laboratory studies [62 - 67].

Biological effects of US are classified as thermal and non-thermal effects [68]. In our opinion, it is incorrect to assume that only one effect is present at any time and that physical therapy treatment may be classified as either thermal (that is, continuous wave exposure) or non-thermal (that is, pulsed exposure). The reality is that the two effects are not separable, and, indeed, it is rarely true that one class of effects may be ignored completely. A notable exception is extra-corporeal lithotripsy, which causes exclusively mechanical bio effects [69].

For all other situations, it is best to assume that non-thermal effects will always be associated by some heating because the interaction between US and tissue is simultaneously thermal and mechanical and there is insufficient evidence as to whether there is a true threshold for bio effects resulting from either mechanism. Conversely, acoustic fields that give rise to heating are always accompanied by non-thermal effects. Pulsing the US beam reduces the temperature rise proportionately to the pulsing ratio; it does not eliminate heating. Nevertheless, it is convenient to classify the effects of insonation as either thermal or non-thermal. Non-thermal effects are those usually associated with cavitation and its associated effects [70 - 72].

Thermal Effects

US is able to produce thermal therapeutic effects.

When the US is propagated in a medium, the acoustic wave amplitude decreases gradually, that is, the US lose their energy and the beam is attenuated due to the absorption and dissipation of the ultrasonic energy. The US produces heat through vibration, shock and friction with the cellular and intercellular structures that make up the tissues traversed. The temperature rise of the medium can cause any chemical or structural changes of biopolymers. This phenomenon is affected by both the characteristics of the US beam that is intensity and frequency, the duration of exposure and the characteristics of the crossed tissues; in particular, the US may be more or less attenuated in function of the difference between the acoustic impedances of the tissues crossed by the sound waves. Heating sets in quickly, but it early settled on a thermal balance due to the faster heat dissipation due to blood flow.

The thermal effect is most evident at the interface level of the tissues and in particular at the level of the periosteum and of the zone of passage between fat and muscle; the periosteum, for its anatomical structure and for the continuity with the bone, absorbs a large amount of energy and is, therefore, seat high heating. The thermal elevation generates, as secondary effects, increase in cellular metabolism and vasodilation; in particular, this latter property is important in the use of therapeutic US in therapy.

In 1987, Dyson suggested that the tissue must reach a temperature of 40°C to 45°C for at least 5 minutes to be therapeutic in nature [22]. Experiments performed with non-perfused tissue demonstrated that US could increase the tissue temperature at a rate of 0.86°C/min (1 W/cm^2, 1 MHz) [6]. Direct *in vivo* measurement of tissue temperature during US treatment has resolved the question of tissue heating. Draper *et al.*, Ashton *et al.*, and Chan *et al.* inserted thermistors to various depths (5 cm or less) and measured the increase in muscle temperature during a 10-minute treatment with either 1-MHz or 3-MHz US [73 - 77].

The use of continuous US (1 MHz, 2.5 W/cm^2) has been tested *in vivo* [78, 79] on laboratory pigs treated on hip demonstrating that the front portion of the articular capsule was increasing the temperature between the first and the second minute of treatment (41°C after 1 minute and 43-44°C after 2 minutes) [79], an intensity of 3.0 W/cm^2 was necessary to determine a temperature increase of between 41-44°C [80]. Literature also reports [79] that it is necessary to increase the intensity of the US from 1.5 W/cm^2 to 3.0 W/cm^2 (0.75 MHz frequency) to obtain the heating of the skin and deep tissue. The authors reported that it is required an intensity of 3.0 W/cm^2 to reach a temperature of 35°C in laboratory pigs, since the interface between muscle and adipose tissue is more extensive.

The ability to homeostasis of organisms to reach an equilibrium condition by counteracting the increase in temperature upon exposure of the US. This mechanism depends on the balance between the loss and heat gain as each temperature rise is contrasted by cooling mechanisms [73 - 75] This mechanism, as shown by Draper *et al.* [73 - 75], acts only partially, because the local and systemic control mechanisms are able to convert the temperature increase in the short time [81] and the key parameter from whom it depends is related to conduction processes in the tissues and dissipation of blood perfusion surrounding; these parameters are difficult to calculate but it is known to be poor in fatty tissue and tendon.

It has been demonstrated, with the use duplex US scans, that if in a saphenous vein is carried out an increase of temperature by a thermal suit (perfused with water at 49 °C) it is determined an increase in the volume and blood flow with a rapid rotation of the warm-blooded, which assisted cooling [82]. *in vivo*, it has been shown, in muscle tissue through the use of radioactive tracers, that warming, including the one led by the US, causes an increase in blood flow that is comparable to that caused by even moderate exercise [83]. Even studies confirm this statement using laser Doppler flowmeter and plethysmography, before and after administration of continuous ultrasound (1.5 W/cm^2 for 5 minutes). The fact that in the literature there are no unique data is linked to the diversity of measurement techniques, probably plethysmography does not measure the tissue-specific changes in blood flow in the tissues such as muscle. Robinson and Buono [84] showed that an intensity of 1.5 W/cm^2 administered for 5 minutes on the forearm does not increase blood flow. " There is still a possibility, however, that US at higher intensities may increase muscle blood flow; in fact, although no increase in muscle blood flow was found at tolerable US intensities, increased muscle blood flow did occur at intolerable US intensities (high-intensity continuous US is intolerable due to pain caused by excessive heating)" [85, 86].

A study carried out using microwave heating to achieve temperatures in excess of 44.5 °C, in muscle tissue, shows that [87]: muscle blood flow increased from a pre-treatment value of 10 ml/min/100 g to 44 ml/min/100 g; however, this increase was far less than the increase from 2 to 4 mL/min/100 g at rest to 80 mL/min/100 g of muscle achieved with extreme exercise. Substantially, often, due to the high intensity of the US required to reach high temperatures, this increase, clinically, never can be reached [88]. The problem is warming due to increased cellular activity. In literature, the increased cell activity and change of enzymatic function is related, erroneously, to the equation of van't Hoff. The issue most discussed it is if the increase in cellular and enzymatic metabolic activities actually translate into an acceleration of the healing process [89 - 95]. It is also generally agreed that the exposure to the US increases the elasticity of the collagen, but, until 1997 only a reported these data. The study was performed *in vivo*, by exposing the knee to US (1.5 W/cm^2 at 1 MHz for 8 minutes) demonstrating an increase,(not statistically significant) of elasticity of the medial and lateral collateral ligaments. Even today, there is a paucity of *in vivo* studies, in contrast with a series of *in vitro* studies of the effect on the extensibility of insonation collagen tissue, usually of rat tail tendons [96, 97]. *In vitro* studies have shown an increase of extensibility after exposure to the US, these data are poorly correlated to human tissues. Reed and Ashikaga [98, 99] suggested that the discrepancy between the results of *in vitro* experiments and their *in vivo* study might have been due to the effect of blood flow on heat dissipation.

Non-thermal Effects

Among the non-thermal effects of US are distinguished mechanical (cavitation and other mechanical effects) and chemical effects.

When it comes to non-thermal effects it is need to talk about the dynamic forces at different frequencies (quasi-stationary defined frequencies up to the acoustic excitation frequency) [100]. A bulk US wave can be defined as a mechanical oscillation of the medium. A frequency of 1 MHz the corresponding wavelength is about 1.5 mm in soft tissues or in culture medium. This wave can activate mechano-transduction inducing oscillatory strains at very high frequency (typically thousands to a few million oscillations per second) compared to physiological strains. The strain amplitudes are a function of the applied intensity, and are typically of the order of for low-intensity US. Secondary, mechanisms at lower frequencies can be triggered, also, by the acoustic radiation force – an oscillatory strain acting at the frequency corresponding to the pulse repetition frequency for pulsed US, resulting in a low frequency cyclic mechanical stimulus.

Among non-thermal effects, the *cavitation effect* is the most widely known. It consists in the formation, growth and implosion of gas bubbles within the fluid subjected to an ultrasonic field. The gas bubbles can be generated and expanding and contracting in tissue when ultrasonic pressure goes to positive peak and negative peak [101, 102] (Fig. **19**).

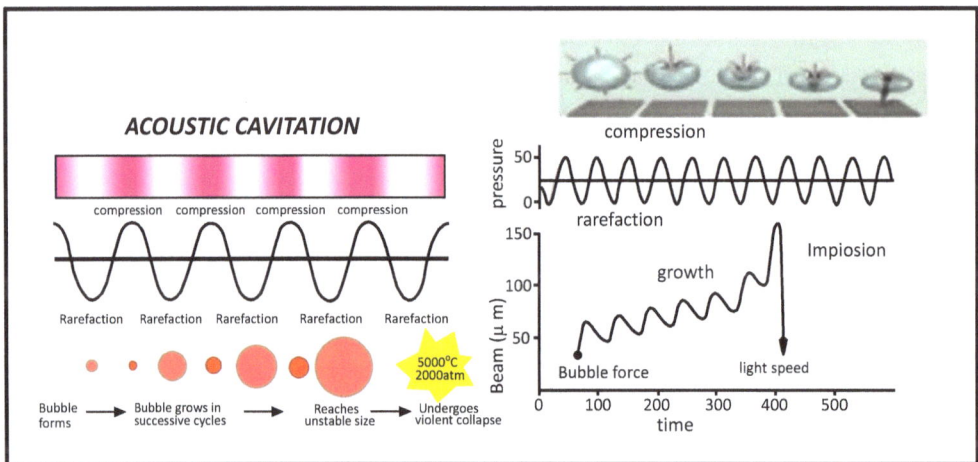

Fig. (19). Cavitation and changes in micro bubbles.

In the fluid components, in the absence of pre-existing bubbles, the process consists of two aspects defined nucleation and successively by driven cavitation activity. The mechanisms for nucleation are quite diverse, ranging from heterogeneous nucleation on imperfectly wetted solid surfaces to transient cavity formation from the absorption of nuclear particles. Despite the cavitation nuclei are not present in human tissues and blood, we assume a priori that nuclei exist and focus instead on the dynamics of an acoustically small (radius) gas bubble in a Newtonian fluid undergoing radial oscillations - all key approximations intended to simplify the model while retaining most of the essential underlying physics [103 - 105]. In particular, within a liquid subjected to the action of a particularly intense ultrasonic field is called "acoustic cavitation, which is generally divided into two categories: inertial (or transient) and non-inertial (or stable) one" [106]. The phenomenon of the "acoustic cavitation" consists of at least three distinct and successive stages: nucleation, bubble growth (expansion), and under proper conditions implosive collapse [107]. The conditions that are established depend on the frequency and amplitude of the applied acoustic pressure, the radius of the bubbles and the properties of the liquid in which they are trapped. This phenomenon occurs in liquids containing air or gas, a fact that obviously facilitates cavitation, but the phenomenon can also occur in a liquid-free gas, if the applied acoustic pressure is larger than the hydrostatic pressure in the liquid [108]. The first phase is characterised by a process identified by the formation of cavitation nuclei generated by micro bubbles; the second phase instead is characterized by the growth of bubbles that expand in relation to the applied wave intensity. Applying high-intensity waves the bubble grows quickly (inertial effect) while if applied to low-intensity growth occurs through "rectified diffusion" "waves (see Fig. **20**), proceeding in a much slower rate and acoustic lasting many more cycles before expansion". When the wave intensity exceeds that of "acoustic cavitation "(typically, a few W/cm^2 for normal exposed to 20 kHz), it appears the third phase of the process, in which bubbles expand up to the maximum energy, and then they implode violently in a so-called "catastrophic collapse". When a bubble is exposed to US, the acoustic pressure acts as an external force, that makes vary the beam, increasing its size. The bubble acts like an oscillating system, with an elasticity which is given by the gas contained within it, and an inertia, which is that of the liquid surrounding the bubble, and that oscillates with the bubble wall itself. The result is, that it has its own frequency, the value of which is inversely proportional to its beam, in equilibrium conditions, when the frequency of the acoustic field, applied approaches the natural frequency of the bubble, this tends to have a resonant behavior and the amplitude of its oscillations depends on how close two frequency values and the value of the applied pressure. In proximity of the resonance, the oscillations take on a characteristic of non-linearity, with generation of higher order harmonics, and with effects that are expressed both in the acoustic field, both in the same medium, sometimes producing chemical and physical modifications. The bubbles into oscillation under the action of the acoustic field may be different; a possibility is the so-called "rectified diffusion", in consequence of which the equilibrium beam of bubble tends to grow with time. This effect occurs at lower acoustic intensity, with development of the cavity in a slow process. The reason is, that during the compression and expansion stages, the gas can diffuse through the surface of the bubble: respectively, towards the outside or towards the inside liquid of the bubble itself, and since the surface area, is larger than that during the expansion respect in the course of the compression, the result is that enters more gas than what comes out. This process corresponds to the *non-inertial (or stable) cavitation*. The micro streaming phenomenon occurs during the stable cavitation. The physical model explains how micro streaming through shear forces may act on the surrounding tissues and in particular on cell membranes by determining their rupture when the intensity is high. A similar effect on cell membranes can also be a result of strenuous exercise. Nevertheless, rupture, even if unimportant from a biologic point of view, occurs because of the body response to an external agent, and therefore it should not be totally dismissed. This phenomenon occurs only with continuous US and for example takes about 1000 cycles so that a bubble arrivals in resonance conditions of 1 MHz [109].

On the contrary, the *inertial (or transient) cavitation* is characterized by a phase of relatively slow expansion of the bubble within the ultrasonic field; the latter is characterized by compression and depression waves. During the phase of negative pressure (depression), one has the enlargement of the bubble and up to a much larger volume than that in equilibrium conditions. During the phase of positive pressure (compression), the enormous pressure exerted on the bubble, the compresses so rapid and violent, until it collapses on itself with consequent implosion and release of energy (Fig. **20**).

With the implosion of gas bubbles, it occurs an emission of large amounts of localized energy, with the achievement of high pressures and temperatures, up to the formation of the so-called "hot spot" (the potential energy given the bubble as it expands to maximum size is concentrated into a heated gas core as the bubble implodes). The instantaneous variations of density, pressure, temperature within the fluid in which propagates the US wave can also produce shock waves (see Chapter 4), explaining the luminescence of a single bubble [110 - 113]. The emission of light from a single bubble, during collapse, has been demonstrated by Lepoint [114], and Hickling [115], who compared the phenomenon with "water freezing" and "micro-plasma formation", from tiny electrified jets projected inside the cavity, respectively. In the "new electrical model" Margulis compared the distortion and splitting of a cavity into small entities to the negative picture of the liquid jet distortion in aerosol sprays [116].

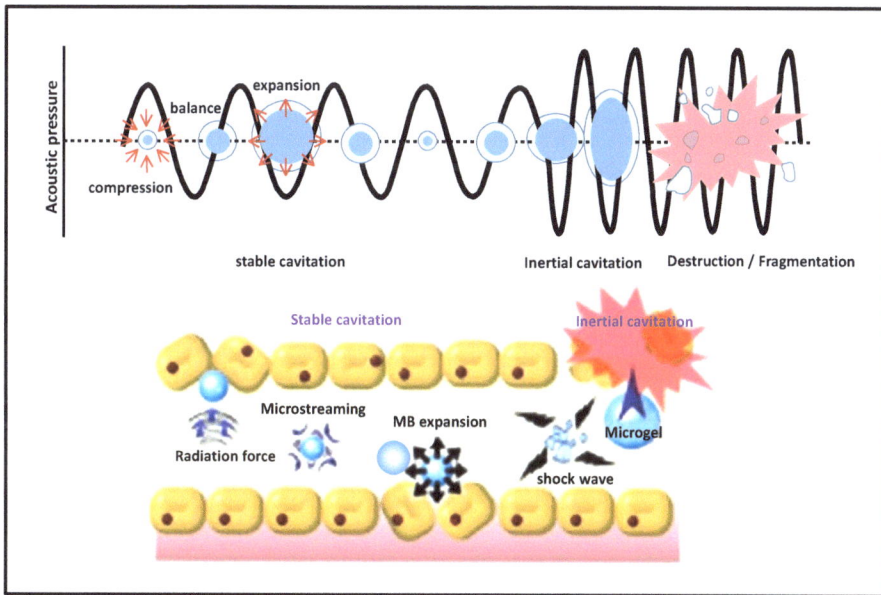

Fig. (20). Stable and inertial cavitation induced by US wave. Adapted from: Liu HL, Fan CH, Ting CY, Yeh CK. Combining micro bubbles and ultrasound for drug delivery to brain tumors: current progress and overview. Theranostics 2014; 4(4): 432-44.

Other Mechanical Effects

The cell membrane is able to absorb mechanical energy from the ultrasonic field, transforming the acoustic energy into mechanical stress by performing a mechanotransduction mechanism, through expansions and contractions of the intermembrane space. The mechanical changes induced are the acoustic streaming and the micro-massage [117].

Acoustic streaming can be defined as a small scale eddying of fluids near a vibrating structure such as cell membranes and the surface of stable cavitation gas bubble [118, 119]. This phenomenon determines the variation of membrane permeability, *i.e.* the variation of membrane permeability to sodium ion causes a change in the membrane potential. Even the transport of calcium ions is changed, the effect of this variation is expressed through a different activation of enzymes related to the metabolic processes of protein synthesis and cell secretion. As a synergistic effect of the final stable cavitation and micro streaming the cell membrane is excited resulting in an increase of the cellular processes. Ultrasound is a trigger process, the real benefits and therapeutic effects are determined by the increase in cellular metabolic activity [72, 120].

Another effect, perhaps overlooked, is the micro-massage, which is a certain effect on the mechanical characteristics of the wave. The mechanical effect of wave, that traveling through tissues, determines the vibration of molecules improving the displacement of the interstitial fluid and therefore the lymphatic drainage. Strong evidences demonstrate this phenomenon. Some experimental studies and theoretical models have highlighted how the effects of the US on biopolymers especially concern the degradation of complex biological structures [121]. Some types of chemical bonds in macromolecules are broken by the impact forces and shear that are generated due to the pressure changes, or following the cavitation phenomena which lead to the formation of radicals. This mechanical action of the US occurs when cells and micro bubbles interact directly. The shear forces, due to the presence of the acoustic wave, can lead to the formation of breaks in the DNA chain. The links that are broken down are typically bonds C–C, C–H and C–O in the structure of the biopolymer. Oxidative stress derived from the production of free radicals can in some cases lead to the modification of nitrogenous bases [122 - 124]. The US action on lipid structures can also occur by means of by mechanical breakage of the membrane areas of micro flow or cavitating micro bubbles that are located near the surface. In particular, it has been investigated the correlation between possible damage to the cell membrane and production of free radicals, induced by therapeutic US of 1 MHz in a population of murine fibroblasts, using the electron parametric resonance (EPR) measurements and the Fourier transform infrared spectroscopy (FTIR). The results demonstrate that exposure of cellular components to the US (such as the phospholipid component of the plasma membrane), modifying the permeability of the membrane itself, without inducing cell death [125]. Some studies of proteins in solution have shown that the actions of the US may lead to the formation of amyloid structures and aggregates [126, 127]. The acoustic field can induce site exposure of the active proteins through a unfolding process or lead to functional changes due to the detachment of a molecular complex. In particular, changes in the secondary structure of membrane proteins may also cause changes in membrane micro viscosity, connected to the sonoporation phenomenon [128]. It is possible to explain both the biological effects induced by cavitation that those induced under non-cavitation, using a model that refers to a direct interaction between the oscillating acoustic pressure and the double layer of the cell membrane. In fact, the literature suggests that the cell membrane is able to absorb mechanical energy from the ultrasonic field, transforming the acoustic energy into mechanical stress, through expansions and contractions of the intermembrane space. In particular, it is conceivable that the space between the two hydrophobic lipid monolayers to inflate and deflate with a certain periodicity when it is exposed to the US [129, 130]. The response of the epithelium depends on the formation of cavitation bubbles as a result of exposure to US: - shape round, elliptical, or parallel ondulate - and dimensions slots (from narrow cavities < 50 nm wide between two neighboring desmosomes to a few μm in width). The cavitation bubbles are observed more frequently around the membranes and between the cells, less frequently is the observation of bubbles around the nucleus, where it can be seen the formation of two laminar fissures that give rise to two membranes that enclose it. Many studies show that following exposure of the US changes the arrangement of the structural membranes of cellular organelles such as mitochondria and endoplasmic reticulum; often the membranes appear interrupted. Further *in vitro* studies performed with layers of skin, which in the last part of exposure were fixed have confirmed these data. These effects were not observed in the untreated controls, excluding the possibility that the observed effects were due to artefacts created by the sampling and fixing process of the treated tissue (for example, dehydration or physical manipulation). The effects vary depending on frequency of application: the cavities are observed in the outer layer and between the most superficial cell layers to 3 MHz, the deeper layers are involved to 1 MHz [131] (Fig. **21**).

The acoustic pressure, which is the mechanical force, oscillates among negative (rarefaction) – in which the two layers of the cell double layer move away from each other, overcoming the forces of molecular attraction, inertial forces of the surrounding water and viscous forces – and the positive (compression) phase, in which the opposite happens during. These expansions and contractions could stimulate the stretch and release cycles in the cell membrane and cytoskeleton, which could activate mechanosensitive proteins, increasing the cell permeability [132]. Based on experimental and theoretical studies the modest acoustic pressures lower than 0.1 MPa can already overcome the forces of attraction between the two lipid layers; in particular, the maximum deformation is proportional to the amplitude of the acoustic pressure and inversely proportional to the square root of the frequency. Results of simulations show that the membrane subjected to US to 1 MHz becomes a mechanical oscillator itself and a source of intracellular cavitation, in a way very similar to a gas bubble in an acoustic field.

Different stages in the interaction between the cell membrane and the ultrasonic field can induce different bio effects on the cell membrane and the cytoskeleton. Mechanical stress through mechanosensitive membrane proteins; produces reversible effects on the cell membrane making pores with an increase of cellular permeability, up to damage of membrane proteins and/or the cytoskeleton. Integrin are critical in mediating the transduction of mechanical forces in most cells studied. The integrins and cadherins (Cell adhesion molecules -CAM) allow cell adhesion fulfilling three main functions: they constitute a physical anchoring system which provides mechanical stability to the tissues; allow the recognition

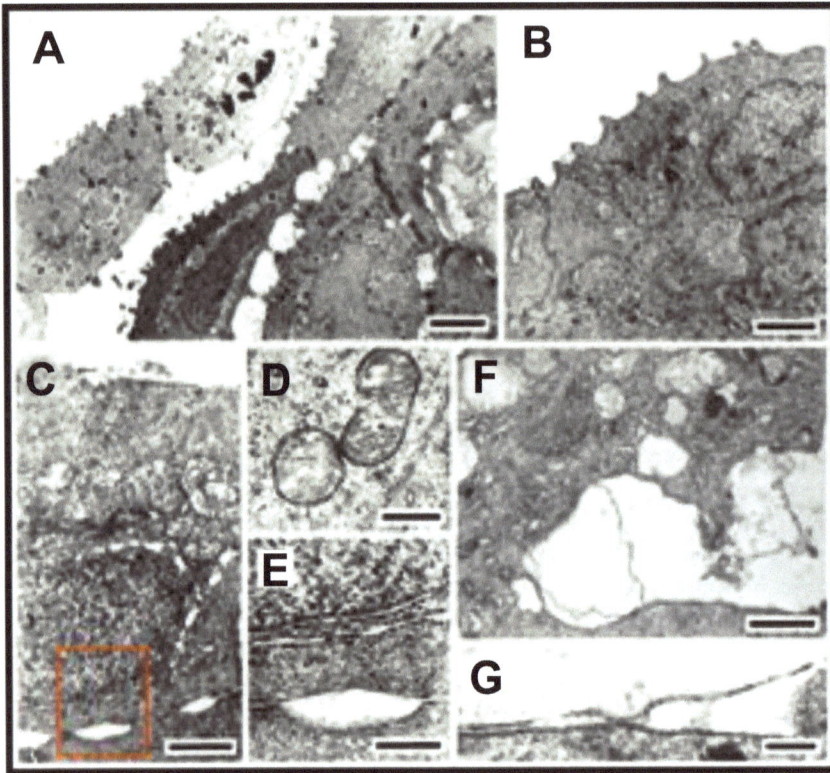

Fig. (21). From: Krasovitski B, Frenkel V, Iger Y. US-induced intercellular space widening in fish epidermis. US Med Biol 2000 Mar;26(3):473-80: "Membrane-localized cavitation following *in vivo* US exposure. The images show transmission electron micrographs of US-exposed fish skin. (A) Outer three layers of skin 2 h after receiving a 1-MHz (1 W·cm^{-2}, 30 s) and then 3-MHz (2.2 W·cm^{-2}, 360 s) exposure. Pocket-shaped gaps are observed between the second and the third layer of cells and to a lesser extent between the third and fourth layers, all of which are still viable (the outer layers are necrosed, evident by compromised apical membrane and reduced electron density). In the cell on the left in the second layer, intracellular gaps are also observed in the endoplasmic reticulum. Larger gaps are also observed where desmosomes are absent (scale bar equals 4 μm). (B) Outer layers of control skin. Outer cells possess micro ridges on their apical surfaces (scale bar equals 2 μm). (C) Outer cell immediately after receiving a 3-MHz (1.7 W·cm^{-2}, 90 s) exposure. Gaps are observed within the intercellular space between the surface cell and the cell immediately beneath it. Gaps are also visible at the nuclear membrane, being larger closer to the apical (upper) side of the cell (scale bar equals 1 μm). (D) Enlargement of box in C. Widening of the two nuclear membranes is shown at the upper part above the pocket-like gap between cells (scale bar equals 0.5 μm). (E) Mitochondria in a second-layer cell immediately after receiving a 3-MHz (2.2 W·cm^{-2}, 90 s) exposure. Disruption of the outer membrane is observed in the mitochondrion on the right, as well as some disruption of the cristae. The cristae in the mitochondrion on the left appear to be completely disrupted (scale bar equals 0.5 μm). (F) Gap between first- and second-layer cells immediately after receiving a 3-MHz (2.2 W·cm^{-2}, 90 s) exposure, where membrane sheets, some intact and some not, bridge between the two cells. Some mitochondria in the outer cell appear to be completely disrupted (scale bar equals 1 μm). (G) Widening of the apical membrane, with some ruptures, of a second-layer cell immediately after receiving a 1-MHz (1.0 W·cm^{-2}, 60 s) exposure. The outer-layer cell has already sloughed off during the exposure (scale bar equals 0.2 μm)."

between cells for formation of tissues; control the differentiation and cell proliferation, enhancing correct growth of tissues both during embryonic development and during the repair processes [133]. The portion of integrins facing the cytoplasmic side of the cell membrane binds actin cytoskeletal contractile molecules. In cells cultured, integrins are concentrated in specific sites of the ventral membrane known as "focal contacts". In these areas converge the ends of terminals actomyosin filaments that are anchored to integrins via a series of cytoskeletal proteins such as talin, the vinculin, paxillin, tensin and the α-actinin. The paxillin and talin interacting directly with the cytoplasmic region of the subunits α and β integrin and, in turn, bind the vinculin and, therefore, the F-actin. As for the cadherins, integrins also exists for a specific molecular form that mediates binding to the membrane of cytokeratin filaments, instead of actin. The integrin involved in this process is the β4 subunit which is localized in the hemidesmosomes, specific adhesion structures of epidermal cells to the basal lamina [134]. The role of integrins in the mechanisms of mechano-transduction is linked to the connections with the extracellular cellular matrix, it seems that the response to mechanical stresses is matrix dependent. Furthermore, under pathological conditions, while certain inflammatory cytokines inhibit the pro-mitogenic effects of mechanical stimulation, other cytokines produced through mechanical stimulation, serve as paracrine transducers of pro-mitogenic stimuli [135 - 137]. For example, the cytokine interleukin-6 (IL-6) is produced in response to mechanical strain in intestinal epithelial cells. Through its gp130 receptor causing ERK1/2 phosphorylation, IL-6 accentuates the mitogenic response triggered by mechanical stimulation [138] (Fig. **22**).

Chemical Effects

The chemical effects caused by the US can be of various types. It is possible locate in the reaction of three distinct parts: the inner area to the bubble of cavitation (gaseous environment), the liquid-bubble interface and the liquid itself. The industry uses many sono-chemical systems with various applications taking advantage of the physical effects of the US as heat, surface activation, and the phase mixing.

The sono-chemical reactions are based on the concept of the acoustic flow mixing that determines the emulsion of liquids that usually are not miscible doing so would it makes the chemical reaction possible. When the system is made of a solid-liquid biphasic medium, catalysis is a consequence of the disruption of the solid by the jetting phenomenon associated with the collapse of cavitation bubbles [139 - 144]. These effects start in the cavities, which are made of micro bubbles filled with vapour of the liquid medium and/or dissolved volatile solutes and gases diffused into them. During the collapse of these cavities, in pure aqueous systems, gaseous water molecules entrapped in expanded micro bubbles, generate reactive oxygen species. Reactive oxygen species may either react in the gas phase or recombine at the cooler gas-liquid interface and/or in the solution bulk, producing in turn other reactive radical species, as hydroxyl radical ($\cdot$OH), hydrogen radical (H$\cdot$), singlet oxygen (O), dioxygen (O$_2$), hydrogen peroxide (H$_2$O$_2$), dihydrogen (H$_2$), hydroperoxyl radical (HO$_2$$\cdot$), and superoxide anion (O$_2^-$) [122 - 124] (Fig. **23**).

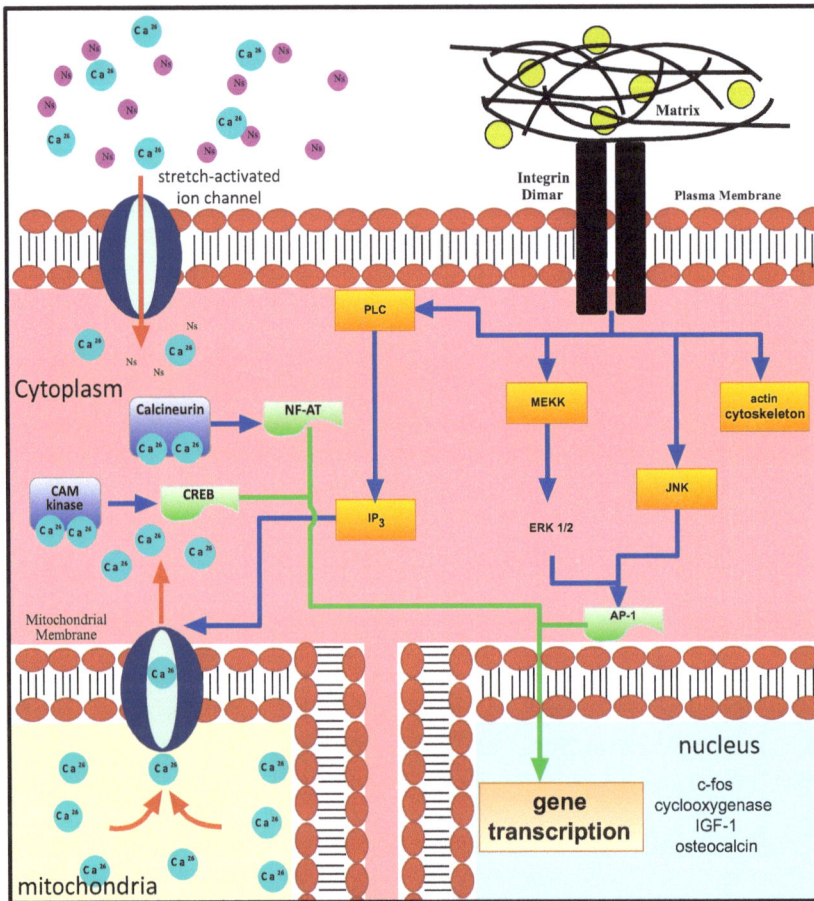

Fig. (22). Mechanisms of mechanotransduction. The forces acting on the surface of molecules activate ion channels, integrins and cadherin initiating mechanosensitivity processes. This induces an intracellular signaling cascade, which includes events such as alterations of the conformation of the proteins (in particular of α-catenin) and recruitment of proteins such as vinculin. The subsequent mechanical response involves the actomyosin cytoskeleton, which can alter cellular contractility. The final result is a potential biological cellular response that will also involve the nuclear transcription and mitochondrial metabolic processes, this response will be felt as a neighbouring cell by the tensile force which will start its cascade molecular process. From: Iqbal J, Zaidi M. Molecular regulation of mechanotransduction. Biochem Biophys Res Commun 2005;328(3):751-5.

Cavitation bubble

H_2O

•H

•OH

Bubble phase

Interfacial layer

H_2O_2 + Substrates

Products

Homolytic cleavage of water (bubble phase)

H_2O → $H\bullet + \bullet OH$

Recombination reactions (interfacial layer)

$2\bullet OH$ → $O + H_2O$

$2\bullet OH$ → H_2O_2

$H_2O + O$ → H_2O_2

Termination reactions (interfacial layer)

$2\bullet H$ → H_2

$2O$ → O_2

$H\bullet + \bullet OH$ → H_2O

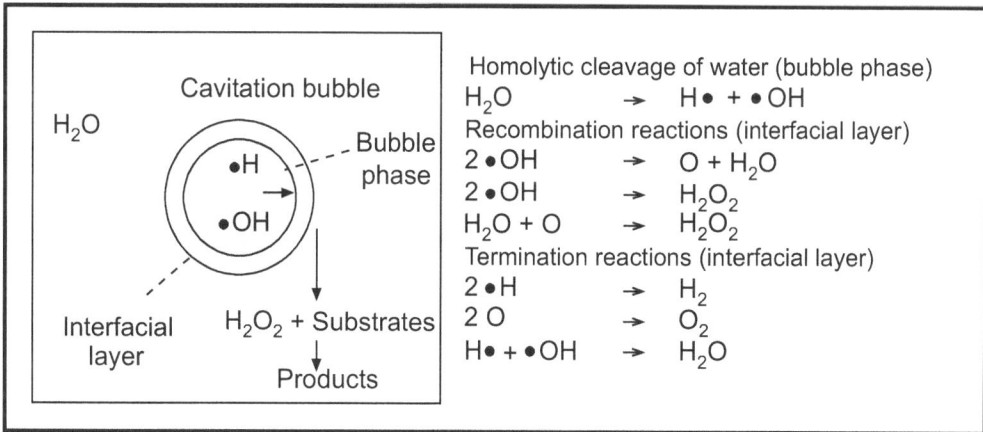

Fig. (23). Simplified reaction scheme illustrating the chemical processes that can occur inside the cavitation bubbles (bubble phase) and at the interfacial layer.

The exposure of cells to intensity of about 0.04 W/cm^2, below the cavitation threshold of, fixed in the literature in 100 mW/cm^2 for 30 minutes to a standard distance- 3 cm transducer, leads to a statistically significant increase of free radicals, which can alter the balance of cell. So it induces peroxidative stress on cell components (such as the phospholipid component of the plasma membrane), by changing the permeability of the same membrane, without inducing cell death [145, 146]. Substantial acceleration forces that cross the tissue after US wave passage determines a chemical action, with the local pH change, and the permeability of cell membranes and molecular changes

DEVICES AND TECHNIQUES OF APPLICATION

US therapy may be administered with several different modes: immersion in direct contact, with fixed or movable the hand piece.

Immersion Treatment

This application mode is useful when the areas to be treated are too small or irregular or when the area is so painful as to prevent direct contact. The part to be treated is immersed in a trough containing water together with the head, placed at a maximum distance of 2-3 cm from the body surface, to avoid an excessive dispersion of the US beam with decrease in therapeutic effectiveness. The treatment heads can normally be immersed fully in the water because it hermetically sealed. For painful areas to direct contact with the head or the parts with bony prominences such as the hands and feet, can be used a underwater treatment. The body part to be treated is immersed in the water and to the massage head is kept in 1-2 cm from the surface of the skin. The head can be used in a fixed position or can be moved in concentric circles holding the surface of the head parallel to the skin surface to minimize the refraction phenomenon. The US wave penetration in tissues varies depending on its frequency of emission, normally comprised between 1-3 MHz. In the first case are, in principle, the treated tissues up to 4-5 cm depth, in the second case up to 1.5 cm. The average intensity of the US for immersion modalities use is 2-3 W/cm^2 for the application to the movable head and is of 0.5-1 W/cm^2 for the fixed head.

The US wave penetration into the tissues varies depending on the application time varies among 5 and 10 minutes in the art fixed head, among 10 and 15 minutes in the immersion and massage mode (Fig. **24**).

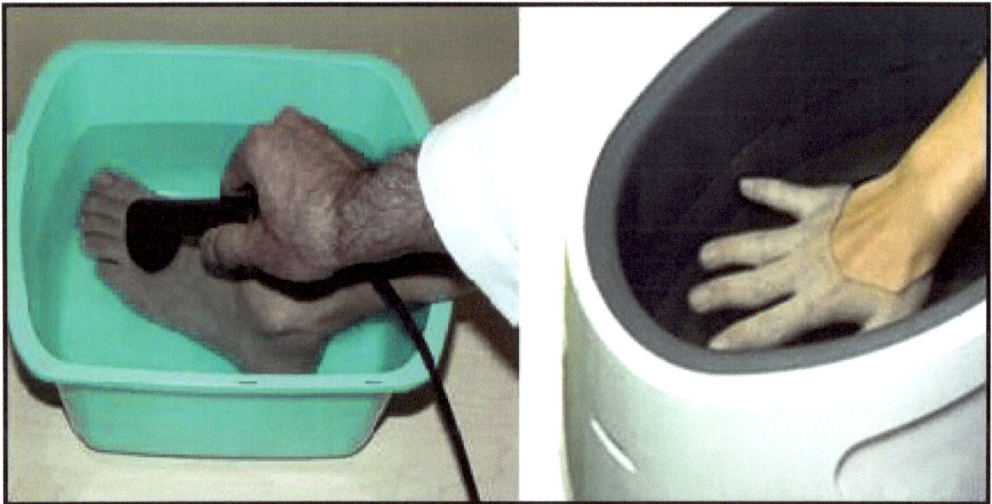

Fig. (24). Devices and techniques of immersion application.

The frequency of the treatment is generally daily, for almost 10 sessions. The use of common water determines dissociation of gas bubbles that accumulate on the patient skin and/or head so the waves are reflected. If it is not possible to avoid the use of common water, it is necessary to frequently remove the gas bubbles from the surface and clean the dispensing area of the head at the end of treatment. For treating in water not without gas, the attenuation of the ultrasonic power is higher than the direct contact for which higher doses are necessary. However, when using gas-free water, the dosage should be the same as that used in direct contact. The water temperature should be around 37°C since the temperature of the body surface is changed is that of the means of coupling both from that of the issuer head. The lower is the water temperature the greater is the heat loss at the cutaneous level and lower the therapeutic effect [148].

Direct Contact Treatment

Most frequently ultrasound application is the direct contact mode that consists in a direct application on skin with hand piece through the interposition of a substance (usually a special conductive gel). The aim is to promote on the one hand the transmission between the head and the skin and on the other hand the adherence, the sliding and the elimination of possible air interposed between the skin and the transducer that could hinder, for its reflective ability, the US wave transmission.

The mode of application in direct contact can be applied to movable or fixed head.

In the *mobile head technique*, the transducer, applied with slight pressure, is made to slide with short movements of 3-4 cm, perpendicular to each other, or with circular movements, having fields of action of 30-50 cm^2 at maximum. In the particularly voluminous joints such as the hip and shoulder of the treatment should be the front, side and rear field side.

In the *fixed head technique*, the transducer is placed on the area to be treated with a stand which supports it and holds it in contact with the skin for the duration of the treatment. With this technique rapid increases in temperature in a very limited area are obtained, while the remaining field is not heated; it is required therefore less power delivery or a pulsed emission. Recently, innovative heads have been introduced the market equipped with thermal sensors, allow to reduce the excessive temperature rise thus providing smooth power delivery of the power on the treated region.

The *mixed-contact mode* with the plastic balloon full of water and gel on the two interfaces has been used for the treatment of ulcers.

Moreover, the application of US can be carried out with a *focused hand piece* that works at a percentage of intensity of 40-60%, for analgesic and muscle relaxant effect, lymphatic drainage and activation of capillary, or a *unfocused hand piece* that works with a high percentage intensity (70-90%), with cavitation and lipolysis effect, and aesthetic and functional improvement (Fig. **25**).

In the first case, since the ultrasonic energy decreases with the distance, due to attenuation, the skin is exposed to a higher intensity than the subcutaneous fat. In case of focused US the ultrasonic the energy is concentrated in a precise subcutaneous area, where produces the lysis of fat cells, instead limiting the damage to the nerves, connective tissue, muscles, blood vessels [149].

THERAPEUTIC APPLICATIONS OF US

In medicine, US can be employed in diagnostics and therapeutics.

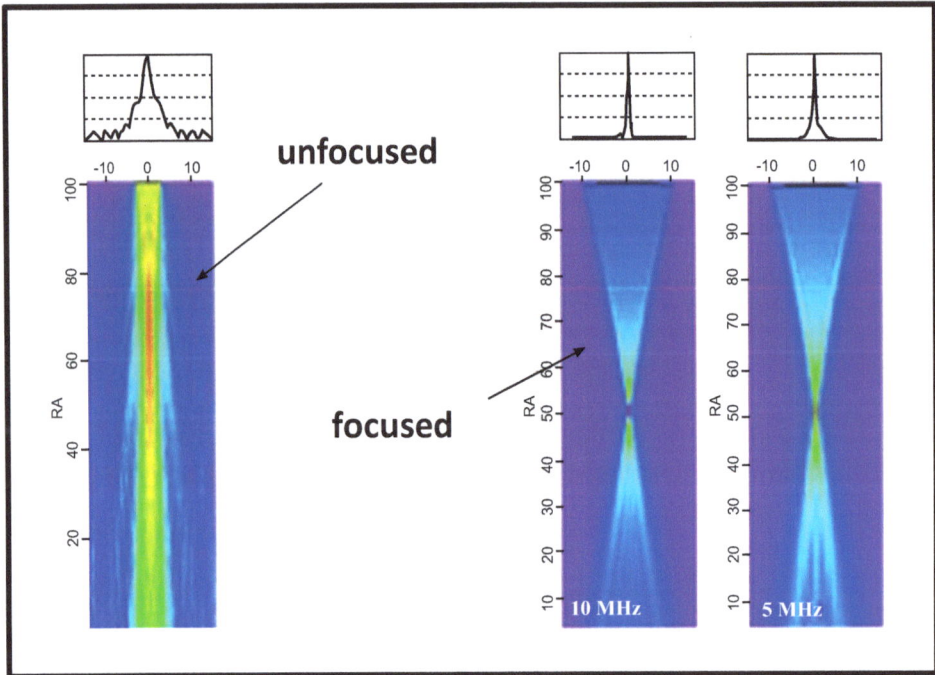

Fig. (25). Low-frequency US: unfocused and focused hand piece.

With regard to diagnostics, the US are typically used in the formation of images for US (abdominal, gynaecological, *etc.*), using the reflections by the US beam in crossing biological tissues.

The US therapy can be conveyed with high-power and low-power US [150, 151]. The first include high-intensity focused US (HIFU) and lithotripsy; the second include physical therapy, pharmaphoresis, sonotransfection, gene therapy. Among low-power US there are those of psychiatric interest; in this case, the US are used in continuous and pulsed regime, with frequencies from 500 kHz to 5 MHz, and intensity of between 0.5 W/cm^2 and 3.0 W/cm^2 (Fig. **26**).

Treatment Protocols For Different Tissues

The choice of parameters to be used play an important role importance in the application because the variation of these parameters influence the absorption and hence the depth of emission with regard to the involvement/achievement of the tissue.

Schematically (Fig. **27**), it can be distinguished:

- a surface layer (skin and adipose tissue);
- an intermediate layer (muscles and tendons);
- a deep layer (bone).

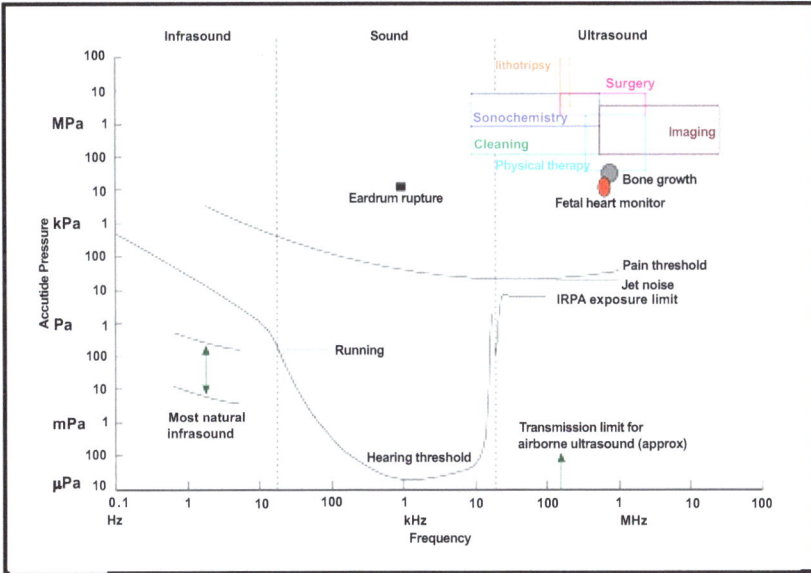

Fig. (26). Sound, infrasound and US application at different frequencies.

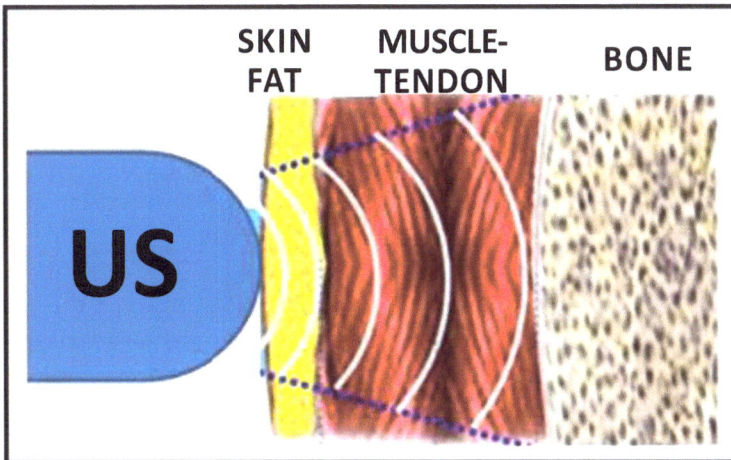

Fig. (27). Different tissues and US therapy.

Before each treatment, it must be considered the anatomical characteristics, the target tissue and the depth related to the anthropometric characteristics, as well as age and sex of the patient. In fact, the distribution of the components (muscle, connective tissue and fat) changes in relation to the physiological senescence, the typical hormonal variations of the different phases of life, and the biological diversity between genders.

Three factors influence the absorption and therefore the depth of emission and the involvement of one or more of the three layers above mentioned:

- the *intensity of the wave*. The energy absorbed by each of the three cell layers is directly proportional to the intensity of the wave: the higher the intensity the higher is the energy that each of the three layers can absorb;
- the *density of the tissue*. In this case it is more dense the tissue and the lower the absorption capacity and therefore penetration;
- the *frequency of the wave*. Because the inverse relationship between penetration and absorption, while the US emitted at frequency of 1 MHz, waves are able to reach the deep (bone) layer, where they reach action depth of about 7 mm. When frequency is 3 MHz waves energy affecting therapeutically effective only, exclusively the surface layers, and the subcutaneous layer, immediately formed by the fat that can be represented with different thickness, depending on the anatomical part and each patient. This layer covers the intermediate cell layer which is constituted by the muscular tissue and tendon tissue from which, in once, it joins the muscles to the skeletal system (deep tissue). Thus, in this intermediate cell layer, where many of the diseases (inflammatory and non) are localized, whether hand by a frequency of 1 MHz is too deep and the other side of the frequency 3 MHz is not able to release enough energy to be therapeutically effective, the optimum frequency for physical reasons is the intermediate one of 2 MHz. Therefore, muscle tissue and the myo-tendinous junction should be treated with an intensity therapeutically appropriate, only through to the frequencies of 2 MHz and 1 MHz. The deep tissue, mainly the bone, which by its nature is able to reflect about two-thirds of the ultrasonic energy and absorbs the remainder. For this reason, the only therapeutically useful frequency is 1 MHz, except in those cases in which for anatomical and morphological reasons the bone tissue is located in the vicinity of the surface tissue (for example, phalanges, epicondyle [152, 153]), for which it is possible to also use the 2 MHz frequency.

Bone

The stimulation of bone growth by physical means has been investigated for many years. Despite at the beginning of the 18th century it was observed that small direct currents acting in the periosteum could induce bone formation, the phenomenon was little or not used until recent times [154].

In 1983, Duarte proposed that US as a safe, non-invasive, and effective method to stimulate bone growth [155]. He applied very low-intensity US, delivered pulsed with a 0.5% duty cycle at approximately 10 W/cm^2 spatial average temporal peak (SATP) intensity, at 4.93 or 1.65 MHz frequency, to 23 rabbit fibulas that were osteotomized and 22 femurs with drilled holes. Treatment was applied for 15 minutes per day, starting 1 day postoperatively, for 4 to 18 days. All animals received bilateral osteotomies and were treated with US unilaterally, so that the contralateral extremity could serve as a control. Treated bones were found to develop callus and trabeculae more rapidly than untreated bones (Fig. **28**).

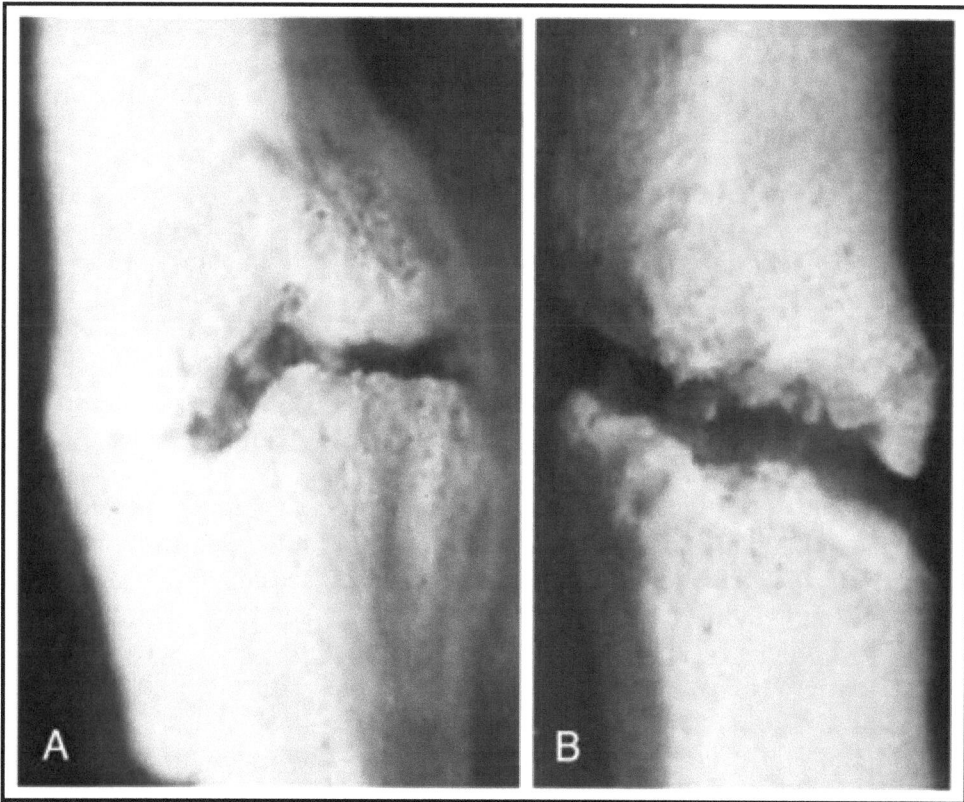

Fig. (28). Fracture healing 13 days after rabbit fibula osteotomy, with (A) and without (B) US application. From: Duarte LR. The stimulation of bone growth by ultrasound. Arch Orthop Trauma Surg 1983; 101: 153-9.

In 1990, Pilla *et al.* evaluated the the effect of US on the rate of fibula osteotomy healing in 139 mature New Zealand white rabbits [156]. Bilateral midshaft fibular osteotomies were made using a 1-mm Gigli saw that US was non-invasively applied to one limb for 20 minutes daily, while the contralateral limb served as a control. US was delivered pulsed with a 20% duty cycle, 0.15 W/cm^2 SATP intensity, 1.5 MHz frequency. Treatment was applied for 20 minutes daily, starting 1 day postoperatively, for 14 to 28 days. Biomechanical healing was accelerated by a factor of 1.7, with treated fractures being as strong as intact bone in 17 days compared with 28 days for control fractures. Maximum strength increases (significant to p ≤ 0.01) ranged from 40 to 85% from postoperative day 14 to 23. These results indicate that biomechanical healing is accelerated by a factor of nearly 1.7.

In 2006, Warden *et al.* treated rats with bilateral femur fractures with active US (1-MHz frequency, 0.5-W/cm^2 intensity, and 20% duty cycle) on one leg and inactive US on the other leg, starting 1 day after fracture, for 5 days a week, 20 minutes a day. At 40 days, the fractures treated with US had increased bone mineral content at the fracture site, a resulting increase in bone size, and 81% greater mechanical strength than placebo-treated fractures [157].

Besides these and other key animal studies, since nowadays the amount of research on US and bone healing has greatly increased, this discussion focuses primarily on randomized placebo-controlled trials in humans. Busse *et al.* conducted a systematic review and meta-analysis to determine effect of US low-intensity on pulsed mode on fracture healing time [158]. The studies included in this systematic review were characterized by the following inclusion criteria: patients of both sexes with one or more fractures, double-blind studies, use of US low-intensity on pulsed mode for at least one of the treatment groups, and the evaluation of fracture healing, determined radiographically. Six human trials that met the inclusion criteria and that examined the effect of US therapy on fracture healing have been identified [159 - 164]. This finding is of considerable importance in that treatment with a low-intensity pulsed US signal may reduce healing time and could yield substantial cost savings and decreases in disability associated with delayed union and non-union of fractures. In all selected studies, the treatment groups received daily 20-min sessions with a US composed of a burst width of 200 μs (± 10%) containing 1.5 MHz (± 5%) sine waves, with a repetition rate of 1 kHz (± 10%) and a spatial average temporal intensity of 30 mW/cm^2 (± 30%). To ensure a standardized signal, each group used the Sonic Accelerated Fracture Healing System (SAFHS 2A) (Exogen, Piscataway, NJ) [165]. Four of the six studies reported positive results [159 - 162]. Three studies were excluded, as one was a repeat analysis of previously presented data [162], and two were performed on patients treated with an intramedullary nail prior to use of US [163, 164]. Three studies [159 - 161], which represents 158 fractures, demonstrated that the time to fracture healing was significantly shorter in the groups treated with low-intensity therapy than in the control groups. The average weighted effect size is 6.41, which translates into an average of 64 days difference in time between the treatment groups and healing control, thus demonstrating the US ability to provide a significant clinical benefit.

Because the complexity of the process of fracture healing and the complexity of the interaction of US with living tissue, there are several ways by which US can influence bone regeneration [166, 167]. Many effects of US on living cells and tissues are known, and provide insights on the biological effects of US on bone. It seems that the biological effect of US on bone is the result of a combination of physical and piezoelectric effects leading to cellular responses where the cell membrane plays an important role (Fig. 29).

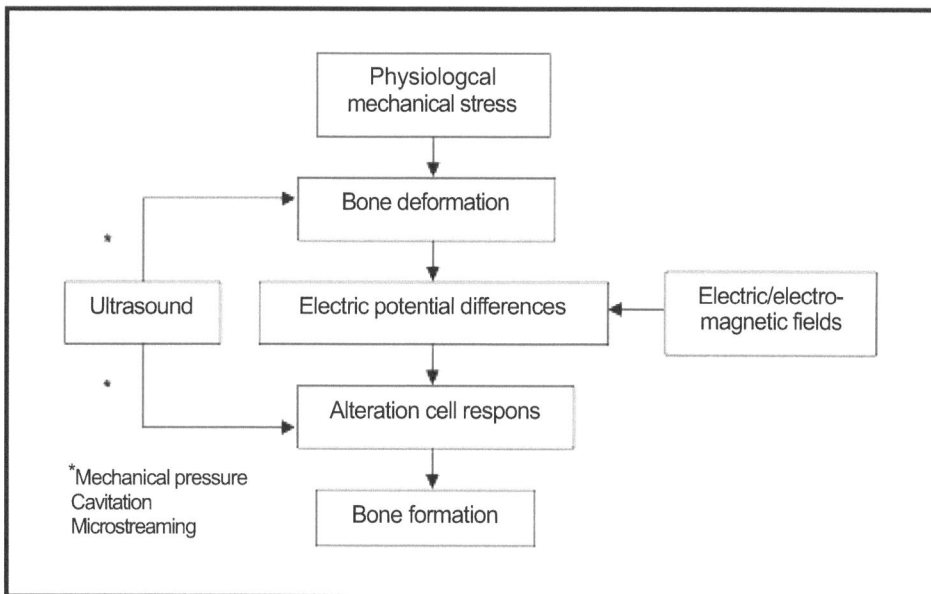

Fig. (29). The basis of biophysical stimulation of bone healing according to Wolff's law in a simplified scheme is depicted. In the case of injury, bone stimulating signals through physiological loading are absent.

Furthermore, US can act on the regeneration process via promotion of cell proliferation, cell pre-conditioning to orient their differentiation during culture [168] or cell transfection [169]. US can modulate the microenvironment by triggering delivery of growth factors or gene expression in engineered cells [170] or by modulating the physical environment by heat deposition or mechanical stimulation [171].

Many *in vitro* studies on cells, involved in inflammation process, have shown that US have an effect in inflammatory, reparative and remodelling phases during the fracture healing process [172, 173]. The typical action of the US in promoting healing is expressed with increase leucocyte adhesion [174] and mast cell degranulation [175], and to stimulate the release of the macrophage-derived fibroblast growth factor [176 - 178]. The scientific evidence shows that the use of the US for the treatment of an acute fracture determines an early reduction of inflammatory phase, favouring the formation of callus. Other studies in animals have shown time reduction of healing and recovery the strength of bone after fractures treated with US. It also may explain why the period of "aggrecan gene expression" seems to occur earlier in the fracture healing process following US treatment. Wu demonstrated in rats applying US therapy (.5 MHz, 50 mW/cm^2, pulsed 1: 4, and a repetition rate 1 kHz for 15 min daily) on bilateral femur fractures that "aggrecan gene expression" was significantly increased only in treated side [179 - 181].

Besides the inflammatory phase, US seems to influence the reparative phase as well. The callus formation, which acts as a repair tissue, is a typical condition that manifests as a result of a trauma or fracture. After approximately 4 weeks of the traumatic event, occurring the first signals, namely the new tissue that has formed, goes to solder the fractured bone fragments, and then change over time in response to the mechanical forces that act on it, becoming stronger and gradually more resistant. There is evidence that US directly stimulates both processes. In chondrocytes, US seems able to increase the intracellular concentration of the second messenger calcium [182] – as well as in fibroblasts [183] – and to stimulate gene expression [184]. Following union, the secondary or definite callus is formed by replacing the newly-developed cartilage by bone through the process of endochondral ossification [185, 186]. US can stimulate osteogenesis as it is demonstrated from animal studies. Numerous studies have shown that the application of the US on the epiphysis of new-born mice and embryonic metatarsal bone *in vitro* can promote the osteogenic process. In particular, it has been shown that by applying US to 30 mW/cm^2 in neonatal mice facilitates the endochondral process [184]. The increase in length of the calcified diaphysis during 7 days of culture In fact, in seven days of culture the diaphysis treated with US stretched out significantly more of the controls. Moreover, even the DNA synthesis is increased after exposure to the US to 1.8 W/cm^2, the histological examination revealed a considerable length greater than the proliferative zone, while the length of the hypertrophic cartilage area was unaffected [185, 186]. Other evidence point to the stimulation of the intramembranous ossification in studies that have shown the healing of fractures after US. Literature reports also controversial data: in fact it is suggested a potential role but the positive effect depends on the medical history, previous treatments, site and type of fracture or bone loss (like bone lengthening), pathology (fresh fracture *vs* delayed unions) and treatment modality (daily treatment duration, intensity, frequency). Therefore, more studies indicate the need of standardization about treatment dose and for further randomized controlled trials [187 - 190]. Current research supports the use of very low-dose US for facilitation of fracture healing. The parameters found to be effective are 1.5 MHz frequency, 0.15 W/cm^2 intensity, 20% duty cycle, for 15 to 20 minutes daily.

Soft Tissues

In soft tissues, earlier resolution of inflammation, accelerated fibrinolysis [191, 192] and angiogenesis have been demonstrated [193, 194] and form the basis for the use of US to promote and accelerate soft tissue healing and decrease oedema and pain [195, 196], particularly in musculoskeletal injuries with a high percentage of collagen fibres.

In fact, US has been reported to be useful in the healing of tendons and ligaments after surgical incision and repair and to be of benefit in tendon injuries. The response of the collagen to the US depends on its piezoelectric characteristics, for which elastic vibrations can induce negative polarization in the area under pressure and positive polarization in the area under tensile strains. This mechanism allows the fibres to orient and align. The flexibility and strength of the tendon, which depend on the biomechanical characteristics, depend on the alignment of the collagen fibers what happens when there is a physiological structural organization of cells between the collagen fibers and the extracellular matrix. The variations in elasticity and strength depend on the time of exposure to the US: Following three minutes of exposure is obtained by the realignment of collagen fibers [197, 198].

Furthermore, the US mechanical strength could serve as extracellular information that is transmitted to the cells, through the rearrangement of cytoskeletal scaffold geometry [199] and stretching of the cationic type receptor channels [200], changes the intracellular signals for the expression of genes that regulate the production of collagen and other extracellular matrix proteins produced by fibroblasts [201 - 204]. For example, in a number of cell types, including mesangial cells [205, 206], smooth muscle cells [207] and cardiac fibroblasts [208, 209] the activation of transforming growth factor beta (TGF-β) by mechanical forces has been demonstrated. It has been shown that mechanical stress induces the expression of TGF-β, which is the most potent activator of collagen production [210]; this biological process is mediated by an autocrine stimulation. Studies on the effect of US on tendon healing, after surgical incision and repair, have yielded more consistently positive results, than those on tendinitis

[211 - 216], with almost all studies showing improved tendon healing after surgical incision despite the use of a wide range of US parameters, including different intensities (0.5 to 2.5 W/cm^2), modes (pulsed or continuous), and treatment durations (3 to 10 minutes). US at 0.5 or 1.0 W/cm^2, continuous, 1 MHz applied daily for the first 9 postoperative days was found to enhance the breaking strength of cut and sutured Achilles tendons in rabbits [217]. The strength of US-treated tendons was greater than that of sham-treated controls, and the strength of those treated with 0.5 W/cm^2 intensity US was greater than that of those treated at 1.0 W/cm^2. Similar benefits were reported from the application of 1.5 W/cm^2, continuous, 1 MHz US for 3 to 4 minutes starting 1 day postoperatively (daily for the first 8 days and every other day thereafter for up to 3 weeks) to repaired Achilles tendons in rats [218]. A more recent study found that both 1 and 2 W/cm^2 applications of continuous 1 MHz US applied for 4 minutes daily resulted in improvements in transected rat Achilles tendon tensile strength after 30 days when compared with controls, and that the higher intensity of 2 W/cm^2 produced better results than an intensity of 1 W/cm^2 [219]. In addition, high-dose pulsed US (2.5 W/cm^2) and 20% duty cycle for 5 minutes 3 times per week was found to improve tensile strength and stiffness in rats with Achilles tendon hemi-tenotomies without surgical repair [220]. One study comparing 1 MHz pulsed and continuous US of 0.5 W/cm^2 applied for 5 minutes, over a period of consecutive days, to transected rat Achilles tendons found that pulsed US resulted in a faster rate of healing than was seen with continuous US [221]. Another study comparing the effects of low-intensity pulsed US and low level laser therapy in the healing of traumatized rat tendons found that both interventions were associated with increased tendon breaking strength compared with controls at 21 days, and that the two together provided no additional benefit. US was applied continuously at an intensity of 0.5 W/cm^2 and a frequency of 1 MHz for 5 minutes daily. Overall, research supports the early use of US for facilitation of tendon healing after rupture with surgical repair. US doses found to be effective for this application are 0.5 to 2.5 W/cm^2 intensity, pulsed or continuous, 1 or 3 MHz frequency for 3 to 5 minutes. Some animal studies show that ruptured ligaments may also benefit from low-intensity US while healing. Sparrow *et al.* found that US applied to transected medial collateral ligaments of rabbits every other day for 6 weeks resulted in an increased proportion of type I collagen and improved biomechanics (ability to resist greater loads and absorb more energy) when compared with ligaments treated with sham US. In this study, continuous US were used with an intensity of 0.3 W/cm^2 at a frequency of 1 MHz for 10 minutes [222]. Warden *et al.* examined the effects of US (1 MHz frequency, 0.5 W/cm^2 intensity, pulsed at 20% duty cycle, for 20 minutes 5 days a week) and a non-steroidal anti-inflammatory drug (NSAID) on ligament healing at 2,4, and 12 weeks, and found that low-intensity pulsed US alone accelerated ligament healing, whereas a NSAID alone delayed ligament healing [223]. A study by Jeremias Júnior *et al.* in rats has shown that, applying ultrasound at low intensity in pulsed mode on tendon lesions surgically induced, it is achieved a significant improvement of the load and tensile strength and a reduction in the lesion area. Low-intensity US parameters and dosage applied: for 5 minutes at 2-W intensity, pulsed a16-Hz frequency, 20% duty cycle, with subaquatic modality [224]. Low-intensity US has been shown to have good results on tensile strength and energy absorption, while unusually high doses promote cell lysis, unstable cavitation, and free radical formation [225, 226].

Because US can penetrate to the depth of most tendons, ligaments, and joint capsules, and because these tissues have high US absorption coefficients, US can be an effective physical agent for heating these tissues before stretching. The deep heating produced by 1 MHz continuous US at 1.0 to 2.5 W/cm^2 has been shown to be more effective in increasing range of motion (ROM) of hip joint in human patients than the superficial heating produced by infrared radiation when applied in conjunction with exercise. In contrast, a study using rats found that both US and infrared radiation when combined with stretching increased ROM to a greater degree than stretching alone after the development of a joint contracture. The similarity in the effectiveness of US and infrared radiation in rats is likely because these animals are so small that, in contrast to the human hip, the low depth of penetration of infrared radiation was sufficient to affect joint mobility. 1-MHz continuous US at 1.5 W/cm applied to the triceps surae muscle combined with static dorsiflexion stretching has been shown to be more effective than static stretching alone at increasing dorsiflexion ROM [227]. However, 1.25 W/cm^2 intensity 3 MHz frequency continuous US applied to normally functioning medial collateral ligaments during a static stretch produced no greater increase in valgus displacement than was produced by stretching alone. This may be because a normally functioning medial collateral ligament can stretch very little without tearing [228]. The increased ROM, observed in some studies in humans, is attributed to increased extensibility of deep and superficial soft tissues resulting from heating by US. The studies described indicate that continuous US of sufficient intensity and duration to increase tissue temperature can increase soft tissue extensibility, thereby reducing soft tissue shortening and increasing articular ROM when applied in conjunction with stretching. The treatment parameters most likely to be effective for this application are 1 or 3 MHz frequency, depending on the tissue depth, at 0.5 to 1.0 W/cm^2 intensity when 3 MHz frequency is used, and at 1.5 to 2.5 W/cm^2 intensity when 1 MHz frequency is used, applied for 5 to 10 minutes. For optimal effect, it is recommended that stretching be applied during heating by US and be maintained for 5 to 10 minutes after US application while the tissue is cooling. Differences in outcomes between the above studies may be due to the use of different treatment parameters and the application of US at different stages of healing. Because applying US with parameters that would increase tissue temperature may aggravate acute inflammation, and because, conversely, pulsed US may be ineffective in the chronic, late stage of recovery if the tissue requires heating to promote more effective stretching or increased circulation, applying US with the same parameters to all patients may obscure any treatment effect. It is recommended that: US should be applied in a pulsed mode at low intensity (0.5 to 1.0 W/cm^2) during the acute phase of tendon inflammation, to minimize the risk of aggravating the condition and to accelerate recovery, and that continuous US at high enough intensity to increase tissue temperature be applied in combination with stretching to assist in the resolution of chronic tendinitis, only if the problem is accompanied by soft tissue shortening due to scarring [229].

Muscle Injuries

Direct traumas or intrinsic factors such as genetic defects or neurological dysfunction can cause injury of the skeletal muscle [230]. There is a slow turnover of muscle fibers as a response to the damages that occur daily during the physiological contractile activity as a result of usury phenomena and mechanical microtear, this was shown in animal studies: 1-2% of myonuclei are replaced every week [231]. In mammals, however, in response to a lesional also severe damage, the muscle responds with a high reparative capacity. Under normal conditions, the regenerated muscle is morphologically and functionally indistinguishable from undamaged muscle. The healing process of muscle tissue is very slow and often depending on the muscle injury does not result in a complete recovery. Because muscle repair is a very slow process and often ineffective in traumatology and sports medicine as well as in rehabilitation one seeks most suitable and clinically appropriate therapy to accelerate and make efficient reparative phase preventing fibrosis [232, 233].

Muscle injuries are a commonly observed conditions, in both sports and non-sports field, despite not require hospitalization, they represent a functional limitation condition especially in athletes resulting in loss of hours of training and high costs for sports societies [234]. The rehabilitation program focuses thus, increasing the normal repair and regenerative processes not only in elite athletes but also in the elderly, in order to achieve a functional improvement and the return to life activities as prior to injury. Therapeutic US is one of the most frequently used treatment modalities for a variety of skeletal muscle injuries.

In spite of over 60 years of a wide range of clinical use, authors affirmed that it is difficult to provide sufficient evidence to establish the clinical efficacy of US therapy, that is for ethical problems related to difficulties in conducting serial muscle biopsies. Although the main aim of the US is to generate an increase of collagen elasticity to reduce the risk of fibrosis and improve ROM, many clinical experiences in the use is related to the reduction of pain associated with the lesion in an attempt to accelerate repair. A systematic review of the literature has shown that the effects of the US are related rather to the non-thermal stimulus, which can produce beneficial effects on the skeletal muscle healing in specific type of musculoskeletal injurie [235 - 237].

It is assumed that repair mechanisms, although are not yet known, as evidenced by recent research, they are determined by changes of permeability of cell membranes induced by US. So, it is theorized that US may influence muscular cellular repair because: (1) it may cause resonance of the cells that may open protein channels, this phenomenon promotes the movement of healing substances; or (2) the mechanical stimulus provided by waves can cause displacement of an inhibitor of a multi-molecular complex, making functional the complex. This leads to the activation of signal transduction pathways involved in healing. The hypothesis of the resonance frequency is based on the knowledge that the mechanical energy of the US is absorbed by proteins, what determines a structural modification for both the single protein that in multimolecular complexes. Moreover, the US wave may induce resonant activity in the protein, modulating the molecule or multi-molecular complex effector function. One can view an enzymatic protein as a physical machine performing a physical function within a cell. Enzymes are commonly found in one of two three-dimensional shapes: an active or inactive conformation; movement between the two conformations requires a change in the state of energy, which is normally accomplished by the addition or removal of a phosphate molecule. Once activated the enzyme is determined by a cascade of events that amplify the signal by determining an effect on cellular metabolism. The ultrasonic wave energy causes variations in the enzyme structural configuration (*i.e*, kinase or phosphatase) and therefore of the entire cell functionality. Another explanation refers instead dissociative effect on multi-molecular complex or to the release of molecules that are physiologically adherent to receptors, which therefore may be triggered (Fig. **30**). Hypothetically, frequency resonance may imply that each different frequency (1 MHz, 3 MHz, 45 kHz, and others) establish a unique resonant or shearing force (or both) [238, 239].

Collectively, studies support the frequency resonance hypothesis "US may modulate signal transduction pathways and gene products associated with the inflammatory response and cells directly involved in the healing response. So, therapeutic US (1 MHz, 3 MHz, and 45 kHz) stimulate cellular and molecular events that are centrally involved in the inflammatory and healing processes" [240 - 243].

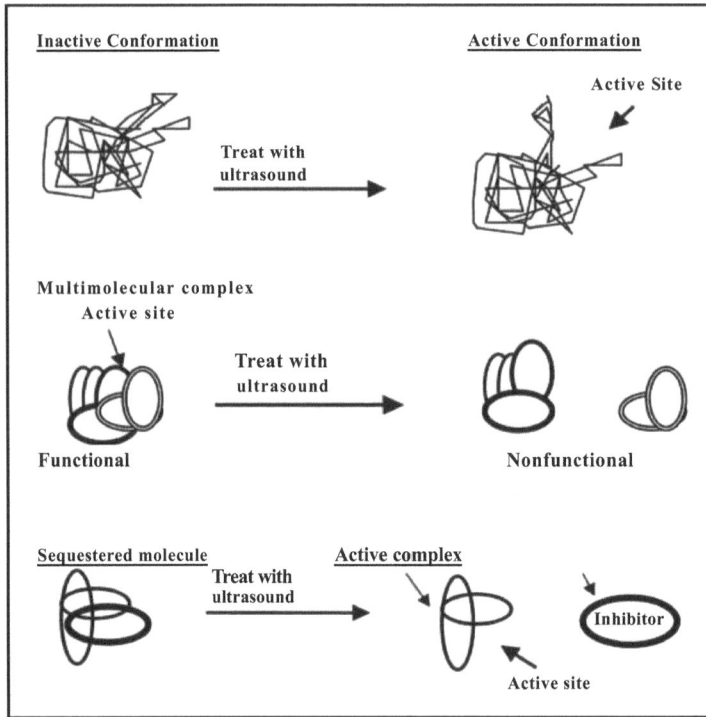

Fig. (30). From: Johns LD. Nonthermal effects of therapeutic ultrasound: the frequency resonance hypothesis. J Athl Train 2002; 37(3): 293-9. The action of the mechanical force, produced by the US, determines a change molecular conformation (active or inactive). This change occurs through the disjunction of complex consisting of multiple molecules or detachment of inhibitory molecules which leads to the activation of cellular transduction signal pathways.

Applying to the muscle cells *in vitro* tensile forces that simulate those *in vivo*, it is possible to observe an increase in the outflow of PGE2 and PGF2α prostaglandins which determines metabolic adaptations, and the growth of muscle cells. Prostaglandins are key messengers in regulating the turnover of muscle protein, also intervening in the secondary bone growth regulating the application of external mechanical forces [244 - 246]. Satellite cells are presumptive myoblasts located between the basal lamina and cell membrane of skeletal muscle fibers. They are normally quiescent, but a muscle damage, via the release of a mitogenic factor, activates and re-enter them the replicative phase of the cell cycle. Satellite cells can form completely new fibers in the event of cell death or can help repair a focal injury that does not destroy the whole fiber. The state of a satellite cell largely relies on the interplay among three growth factors: fibroblast growth factor (FGF), insulin-like growth factor I (IGF- I), and TGF-β. In the early stages of regeneration, FGF and IGF-I in the presence of TGF-β, which inhibits differentiation, stimulate cell proliferation [247 - 253] (Fig. **31**).

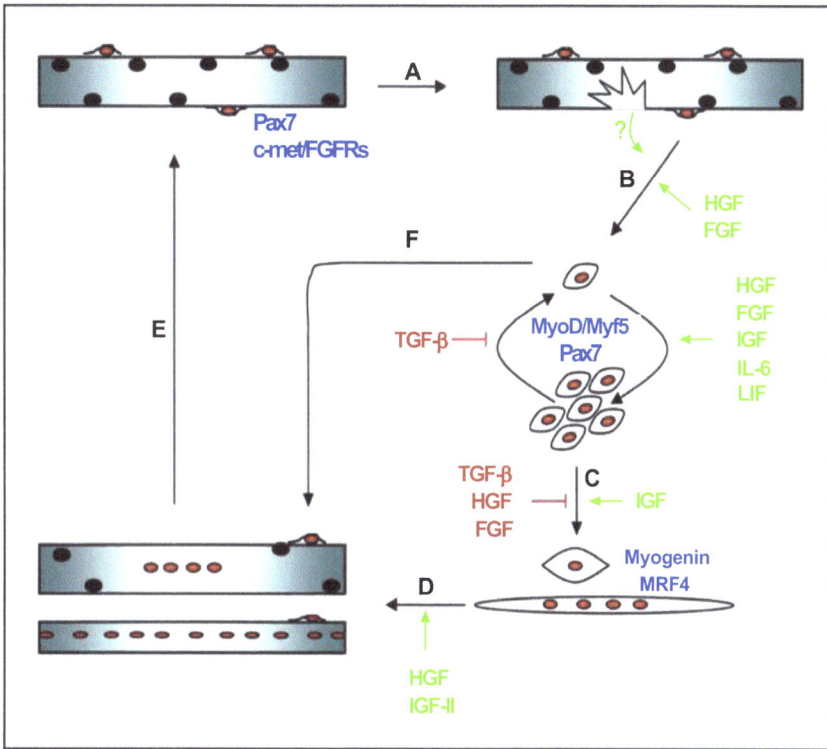

Fig. (31). From: Chargé SB, Rudnicki MA. Cellular and molecular regulation of muscle regeneration. Physiol Rev 2004; 84(1): 209-38.

The figure describes in sequence the regeneration process of the skeleton muscle. The damage active satellite quiescent cells (A) allowing the increase of myogenic cells (B) that can proliferate; the proliferative phase follows the stage of differentiation (C) and the fusion of myoblasts and myofibrils. Process ends with the complete repair (E).

It is in this stage that therapeutic US may have its greatest effect. In animal studies showed a positive effect of the US in muscle regeneration. The use of US 3 Hz with an intensity of 1.5 W/cm^2 on the gastrocnemius muscle lesion of rats resulted in a significant increase in proliferation of satellite cells demonstrated by immunohistochemistry [254]. Karnes and Burton examined the effect of US on the repair of muscle injured through repeated eccentric contractions.

The rats were anesthetized and subsequently each foot was secured to a motorized footplate with surgical tape, which determines the movement of the ankle with a constant interval of 110°. Furthermore, an electric stimulation was applied to the peroneal nerve during ankle plantarflexion. The bilateral lesion of extensor digitorum longus muscles has been obtained through the eccentric exercise by a flexion-extension injury device. The rats were divided into 4 groups: three groups received 5 minute of continuous 1.0 MHz ultrasound at 0.5W/cm^2 to either the left or right hind limb, immediately after injury and continued, respectively, daily for 3, 5, or 7 days. A fifth group of animals is the control group; their limbs were injured but they did not receive any treatment. Results of this study indicate that 7 daily treatments of continuous therapeutic US significantly improves maximum force production of muscles that have been injured by repeated eccentric contraction, compared with injured but untreated controls [255]. Matheus *et al.* analysed the mechanical properties of rats gastrocnemius muscles subjected to acute impact injury and treated with therapeutic US at frequency of 1 and 3 MHz. The treatment consisted of a single five-minute session per day, for six consecutive days. The injured muscles demonstrated a significant reduction in all analysed properties: reduction of 24% for stretching, to a maximal limit (*i.e.*. a stretching value from the starting point up to the point of rupture), of 44% for load, at a proportionality limit (*i.e.*, the maximal load value registered during the test), and of 45% for stiffness (*i.e.*, the elastic resistance to an applied force) [256].

The effect of the US has been evaluated on chick embryo cells [257] demonstrating that when the US are used in pulsed mode and at a low intensity are able to induce cell proliferation, however, when it used with low intensity with continuous wave induces muscle differentiation. It determines the cell death if used in high-intensity pulsed mode. These effects have been highlighted on cell cultures grown for 24 hours and exposed to treatment: four culture plate are exposed to US with different parameters, as described, and a control culture plate not exposed to treatment (Table **4**).

Table 4. Protocols for US wave treatments.

Mode	Intensity (W/cm^2)	Duration (minutes)
Pulsed	0.5	5
Pulsed	1.0	10
Continuous	0.5	5

From: Abrunhosa VM, Mermelstein CS, Costa ML, Costa-Felix RPB. Biological response *in vitro* of skeletal muscle cells treated with different intensity continuous and pulsed ultrasound fields Journal of Physics: Conference Series 279 2011; 012022.

It was observed that low-intensity pulsed US wave induces cell proliferation, whereas low-intensity continuous US wave induces muscle differentiation (Fig. **32**).

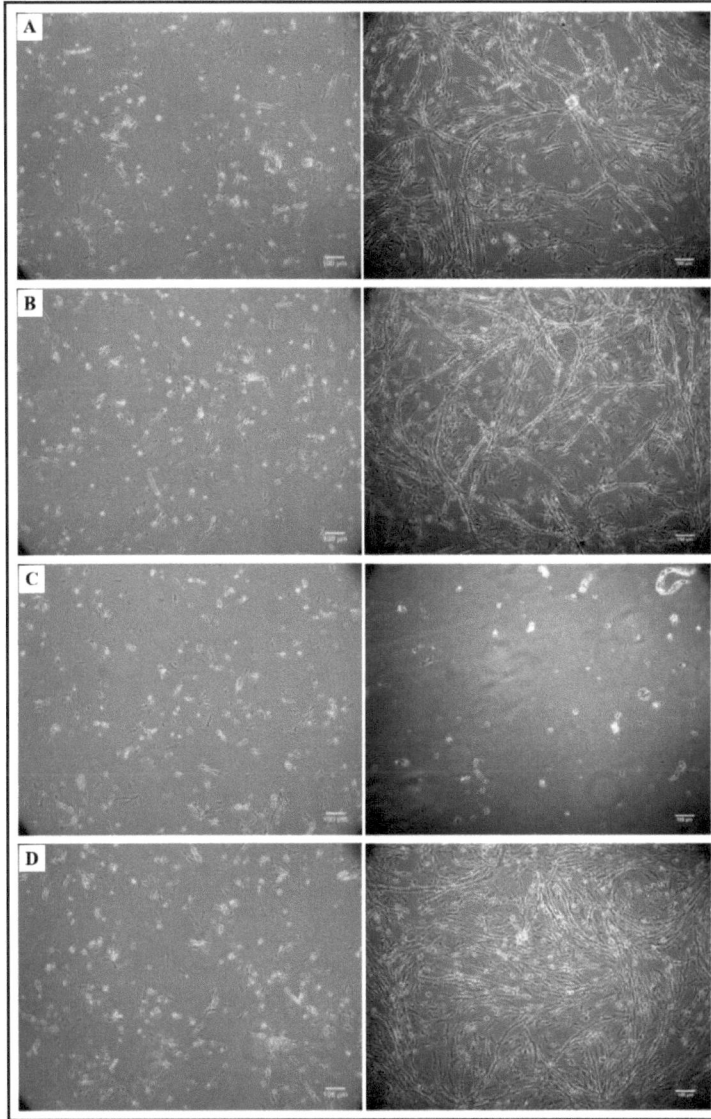

Fig. (32). **A**. Control cell culture grown for 24 hours (left), and after 72 hours (right). **B**. Cell culture treated with continuous US treatment (0.5 W/cm^2 intensity) during 5 minutes (left), and after 48 hours of US treatment (right). **C**. Cell culture treated with pulsed US treatment (1.0 W/cm^2 intensity) during 10 minutes (left), and after 48 hours of US treatment (right). **D**. Cell culture treated with pulsed US (0.5 W/cm^2 intensity) during 5 minutes (left), and after 48 hours of US treatment (right). From: Abrunhosa VM, Mermelstein CS, Costa ML, Costa-Felix RPB. Biological response *in vitro* of skeletal muscle cells treated with different intensity continuous and pulsed ultrasound fields Journal of Physics: Conference Series 279 2011; 012022.

The review of the scientific literature shows that there are no guidelines and/or standardized protocols in order to define the mode of application of the US, experimental recommendations reported to perform a treatment for 5 to 10 minutes and from 1 to 3 treatments per day, clinical treatments are performed almost exclusively once a day. The possibility exists that clinical treatment protocols commonly employed for US are not sufficient for therapeutic efficacy. Robertson and Baker [56] in a systematic review showed, in two methodologically acceptable studies, the clinical efficacy of the pulsed US (1: 4), with treatment times of 15 minutes, resulting in densities of 60 and 150 J energy/cm^2, respectively [258, 259]. *Vice versa*, the remaining 5 studies lacking effectiveness employed pulsed US and of 2 to 10 minutes exposure times, resulting in overall energy density of 2 to 40 J/cm^2 [89, 90, 92, 94, 95]. The frequency resonance hypothesis may suggest that different ultrasonic frequencies (1 MHz, 3 MHz, 45 kHz, and other) may require different durations of exposure (time), different energy densities (J/cm^2), or both, to reach therapeutic efficacy. In our experience, the best application of the US for therapy of muscle injury is with us to pulsed frequency 38 kHz 3 times per week for at least 2 weeks.

Carpal Tunnel Syndrome

The carpal tunnel syndrome (CTS) is the most common compression neuropathy of the upper limbs. It is a symptomatic neuropathy caused by compression of the median nerve at the wrist, characterized from the pathophysiological point of view by an increased pressure within the carpal tunnel and a consensual loss of function of the median nerve at this level [260, 261]. The typical symptoms and signs of CTS can be classified into three stages: a first stage (irritative phase), with a sensation of swelling and numbness of the hand (but sometimes irradiated to the forearm and shoulder) which causes night-time awakenings and a sensation of limb stiffness usually persisting at morning awakening. A second stage (deficit phase), with the paraesthesia persisting in the daytime, especially following the execution of repetitive movements of the fingers or hand, and intermittent motor deficits (difficulty in handling objects, which often fall down); a third stage (hypotrophic/atrophic phase), with appearance of hypotrophy or atrophy of the thenar eminence and possible attenuation of the sensory symptoms.

Conservative treatment approaches seem to offer clear advantages over surgical treatment of the CTS. Recent studies have confirmed short-term effects of steroid injections into the carpal tunnel, with modest or complete pain relief in up to 92% of the patients, although long-term recurrence rates seem to be variable.

Proposed mechanisms for potential benefit of US for patients with carpal tunnel syndrome include the anti-inflammatory and tissue-stimulating effects of this intervention. Experiments on the stimulation of nerve regeneration and on nerve conduction by US treatment and findings of an anti-inflammatory effect of such treatment support the concept that US treatment might facilitate recovery from nerve compression [262, 263]. However, Yildiz highlighted other research which suggests that US does not have an anti-inflammatory effect but rather accelerates the process of formation and resolution of pressure in the carpal tunnel canal [264]. Szumski summarized the effects of US on nervous tissue as follows: it selectively heats peripheral nerves; may alter or block impulse conduction; and may increase membrane permeability and tissue metabolism [196]. The author pointed out that any of the above-mentioned mechanisms may be due to the thermal effect of US and may cause pain relief. Pulsed US produced significantly greater improvement in subjective complaints, handgrip and finger pinch strength, and electromyographic variables (motor distal latency and sensory nerve antidromic conduction velocity) than sham US treatment. These benefits were sustained at 6-month follow-up. US was applied for 20 sessions at 1 MHz frequency, 1.0 W/cm^2 intensity, pulsed mode 1:4, for 15 minutes per session. Another randomized, placebo-controlled trial found clinical improvements in both US- and diclofenac-treated patients with mild to moderate carpal tunnel syndrome. Continuous US with an intensity of 0.5 W/cm^2 was applied to the palmar carpal tunnel for 10 minutes 5 days a week for 4 weeks. Only the US-treated group had electrophysiological changes (increased sensory nerve action potential amplitude), but the implications of these results are uncertain. Using pulsed US at 1 MHz, Ebenbichler *et al.* reported a significant effect of US on improvement of the symptoms after 7 weeks of treatment and at 6 months of follow-up [258]. Using continuous US at 3 MHz (a mean symptom duration of 84 months) for 10 treatments with a frequency of 5-min session five times a week, Oztas *et al.* showed a statistically significant improvement in pain, night pain and electromyographic characteristics [265]. Aygül *et al.* demonstrated the efficacy of phonophoresis with dexamethasone sodium phosphate in CTS demonstrating a significant improvement of motor and sensory conduction of the median nerve at electromyography [266]. Six trials observe therapeutic US effects as part of a complex rehabilitation protocols with another non-surgical intervention [267 - 272]. A systematic review of concluded that there was moderate evidence that US is more effective than placebo after 7 weeks of treatment and at 6 months of follow-up, but that no evidence of such an effect was noted if treatment was limited to 2 weeks [273].

Continuous US generally has not been recommended for the treatment of CTS because of the risk of adverse impact on nerve conduction velocity by overheating. More author reported a improvement of symptoms of CTS after the applications of US treatment, but their responses were not identical. We suggested that US effects on motor nerve conduction velocity may depend on intensity and duration, and could be a result of both thermal and non-thermal effects of insonation. Nowadays, there is insufficient evidence to support the use of therapeutic US as a treatment with greater efficacy compared to other non-surgical interventions for CTS (such as splinting, corticosteroid injections, and oral drugs), or to support the greater benefit of one type of therapeutic US regimen over another. Other studies are necessary to demonstrate the efficacy and safety of therapeutic US for CTS.

Dermal Ulcers And Complex Wounds

Complex wounds are an important source of morbidity to patients and generate high costs to hospitals and community health care organizations. Chronic wounds is a problem in modern society, and represent significant medical, economic and social costs: they are a physical and psychological disease, and they are responsible for considerable health care expenditure and long-term morbidity. Chronic or non-healing ulcers are characterized by defective remodelling of the ECM, a failure to re-epithelialize, and prolonged inflammation. Even under optimal conditions, the healing process can lead to fibrosis or scars, which can cause multiple disabilities. Chronic wounds are defined as wounds which have failed to proceed through an orderly and timely reparative process to produce anatomic and functional integrity over a period of 3 months [274 - 276].

The phenomenon of mechano-transduction, or the converting mechanical energy into cellular biological processes, is one of the most important molecular response related to cell regeneration and repair [277]. The use of negative pressure therapy, for example, through the application of a porous film and a semi-occlusive dressing connected to an aspiration system, for the treatment of surgical wounds and ulcers, has shown a good efficacy. This methodology acts through micro-deformations which stretch the cells generating micro-mechanical stress biologically expressed with increased cell proliferation [278].

Some authors suggest that the non-thermal effects of US aid the wound healing by inducing vasodilation of arterioles [279 - 281] and activation of adhesion molecules involved in the immune response [282, 283], as above-mentioned. Dyson and Suckling found that the addition of US treatment to conventional wound care procedures resulted in significantly greater reduction in the area of lower extremity varicose ulcers [117]. US was applied pulsed at 20% duty cycle, 1.0 W/cm^2 intensity, 3 MHz frequency, for 5 to 10 minutes to the intact skin around the border of 13 lower extremity varicose ulcers 3 times a week for 4 weeks. Sham US was applied, in a double-blind manner, to 12 other ulcers to serve as a control. At 28 days, the treated ulcers were approximately 30% reduced in size, whereas the sham-treated ulcers were not significantly smaller than their initial size. McDiarmid *et al.* show that infected pressure ulcers healed significantly more quickly with the application of US than with sham treatment, whereas clean wounds did not [284]. US was applied pulsed at a 20% duty cycle,

0.8 W/cm^2 intensity, 3 MHz frequency, for 5 to 10 minutes 3 times a week. Byl *et al.* conducted controlled, single-blinded, post-test experimental study to compare the differences in wound breaking strength and collagen deposition in pigs [213, 214]. The authors surgically induced incisions in 48 pigs and for 5 to 10 days US was applied with either high-dose or low-dose US. High-dose US parameters were 1.5 W/cm^2, continuous mode, 1 MHz for 5 minutes and low-dose parameters were 0.5 W/cm^2, pulsed mode, 20% duty cycle, 1 MHz for 5 minutes. Findings from the study revealed that US was beneficial in wound healing and stated that physical therapists can utilize high-dose US for about 1 week to enhance collagen deposition and wound strength. Low-dose US was suggested for treatment for 2 weeks or more. However, other studies failed to demonstrate improved healing of pressure [95] or venous ulcers with US [285, 286]. 1-MHz US was used in the first two of these studies, and it is possible that this lower frequency may have altered the effectiveness of the intervention. In the third study, 3 MHz pulsed US was used, but the addition of 0.1% chlorhexidine, a cytotoxic agent, to cleanse some of the wounds may have obscured the benefits of the US. Thus, recent reviews of randomized controlled trials on the treatment of venous ulcers and pressure ulcers with therapeutic US concluded that there is no good evidence of a benefit of US therapy in dermal ulcers, and additional well-controlled studies are needed to ascertain the effectiveness of this intervention [287, 288].

US can be applied to a dermal ulcer by applying transmission gel to the intact skin around the wound perimeter and treating only over this area the wound can be treated directly by covering it with a US coupling sheet or by placing it and the US transducer in water. In June 2004, a non-contact US device was approved by the Food and Drug Administration (FDA) for wounds. Non-contact US therapy also showed to enhance angiogenesis and collagen deposition in a diabetic mouse model. In May 2005, this device was approved for use in wound healing. The device applies 40 kHz frequency, 0.1 W/cm^2 to 0.5 W/cm^2 intensity US when held 5 to 15 mm from the wound. The device uses a saline mist as a coupling medium to deliver ultrasonic energy to the tissue. It is held perpendicular to the wound, and multiple vertical and horizontal passes are made over the wound during treatment [289] (Fig. **33**).

A randomized controlled trial by a different group of researchers found that 63% of patients treated with the standard of care plus non-contact US achieved greater than 50% wound healing at 12 weeks, whereas 29% of those treated with the standard of care alone achieved the same results [290]. The patients in this study all had non-healing leg and foot ulcers associated with chronic critical limb ischemia. Maan *et al.* [291] showed that non-contact, low-frequency US therapy with frequency of 3 sessions for week, significantly accelerated wound healing, reducing the number of days related to wound closure, in the controls that received standard dressing change. The study was performed on diabetic mice: the application of non-contact low-frequency US has highlighted the increase of collagen deposition and thickness of the dermis associated with an increase of fibroblast proliferation. Probably the primary stimulus is the production of VEGF, that determines the proliferation of endothelial cells and consequently angiogenesis, which is a critical step in tissue repair processes. The stimulation of stromal cells is of particular interest since it has been shown that this phenomenon is absent in diabetics, with decreased ability to recruit circulating progenitor necessary for wound healing [292, 293].

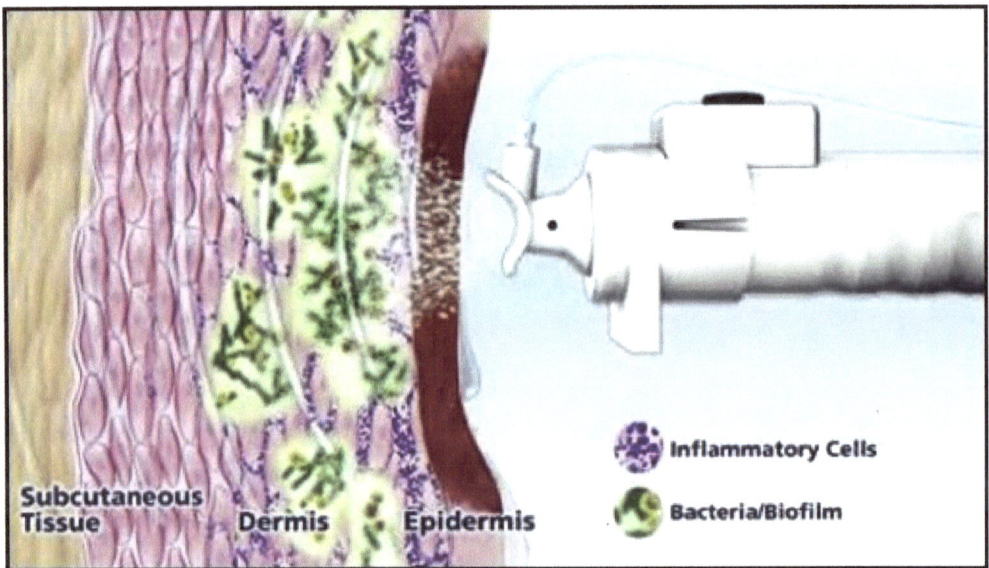

Fig. (33). Non-contact US device. From: https://s-media cachak0.pinimg.com.

In addition, a further advantage in the use of non-contact low-frequency US is related to the effective in reducing the biofilm of wound infection [294], the study showed during the latter two-thirds of the healing process that the reduction of lesion area is associated with a reduction of infections. Therefore, the use of the US can be a "neoadjuvant approach" before skin grafting interventions or through free flap tissue transfer, for definitive treatment. The non-contact mode is a less invasive approach, more sterile, unlike the negative pressure is more widely accepted by the patient with an improvement in the quality of life [295, 296].

Overall, the studies indicate that US can accelerate the healing of dermal ulcer and complex wound and facilitate development of stronger repair tissue. The treatment parameters found to be most effective were 0.5 to 0.8 W/cm^2 intensity, pulsed 20% for 3 to 5 minutes, 3 to 5 times a week.

Skin And Adipose Tissue: Aesthetic Applications

Aesthetic medicine and cosmetology have been developing dynamically in recent years.

US used for aesthetic purposes (body contouring) can be divided into two different categories: US of very low frequency (kHz), and focused US with very high intensity aimed to ablate the adipose tissue by heating (HIFU).

US applications without surgical intervention have been investigated to deliver energy through the skin. Ultrasonic energy may be delivered to the tissue in non-focused or focused wave form. In non-focused US delivery, skin and subcutaneous fat are exposed to approximately the same energy extent; in contrast, focused US can be concentrated in a defined subcutaneous focal area to produce lysis of adipocyte and no or minimal damage to surrounding tissues [149] (Fig. **34**).

Using appropriate devices, designed to work at frequencies that do not permit the development in depth of the US waves (typically around 3 MHz), the application of US in the aesthetic field is generally related to the treatment of wrinkles and localized fat deposits. The aesthetic applications are the following:

- application of cosmetic agents: US would facilitate the absorption of active substances on the face and body such as oils, fat soluble vitamins, products liposomes, emulsions and water-soluble agents: the effect would be the increasing of cells permeability, decreasing the functional skin barrier and increasing the channels activity of the active ingredients (sonophoresis);
- treatment for drying and/or polishing surface wrinkles: US, thanks to its thermal effects, heats the tissues and promotes biochemical and metabolic processes;
- eliminate or reduce localized fat deposits: US performs an action of the treated area of the fat mobilization, promoting fat metabolism and its removal.

Treatment for drying and/or polishing surface wrinkles. The transfer of mechanical energy through the vibration also occurs through massage with an average of 3 vibrations per second reaching three-million vibrations per second. The manual therapy and massage is always used for detaching the tissues, modulate the tone and elasticity of the skin. Similarly the US are able to transfer vibratory energy, by modulating the elasticity of the tissues through the action on collagen and extracellular matrix components, increasing the temperature also stimulate the flow of blood to the area, bringing with it more oxygen and nutrients for healing. A further aspect to consider is associated with washout of waste substances and toxins. The synergistic and combined effects make it possible to improve the quality of fabrics, improve the healing process, or the phenomena associated with skin aging. The use of US in skin generates different processes that have physiological and therapeutic effects. The mechanical effects generate a micromassage, cavitation increased permeability of the cells, improvements in the release of toxins and separation of collagen fibers. Thermal effects occur due to the mechanical effect, raising the temperature of the tissues and causing an increased metabolism, vasodilation and changes in the pattern of collagen. The thermal effect promotes healing, cell regeneration and tissue extensibility and relaxation [297]. The further effect of the US is to expand the intracellular spaces of skin superficial layer. By applying ultrasound and then a topical drug or cosmetic, it facilitates the conveyance of the product more effectively. To amplify the effect of sonoporation. Furthermore, it can perform a pre-treatment with microdermabrasion or the removal of the outer layer of the epidermis which further facilitates the absorption of topical [298].

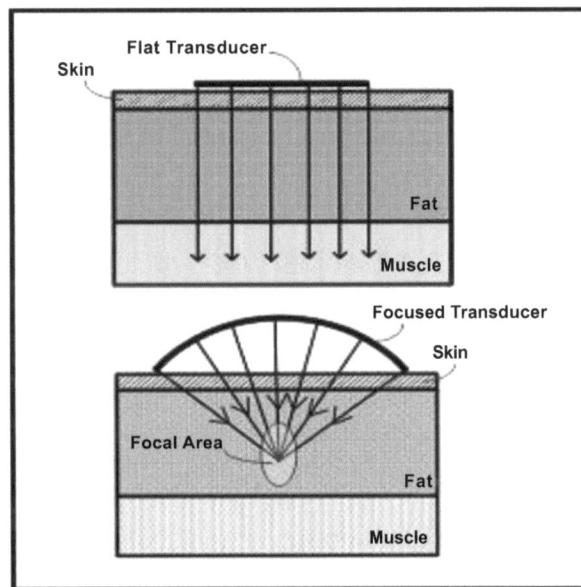

Fig. (34). Illustrations of the US beam extension when energy is emitted from a flat (above) or focused (below) transducer. From: Brown SA, Greenbaum L, Shtukmaster S, Zadok Y, Ben-Ezra S, Kushkuley L. Characterization of nonthermal focused ultrasound for noninvasive selective fat cell disruption (lysis): technical and preclinical assessment. Plast Reconstr Surg 2009; 124(1): 92-101.

Eliminate or reduce localized fat deposits. One of the most common uses of US in aesthetics is to treat the edemato-fibro-sclerotic panniculitis and the localised adiposity. Both conditions indicate an altered state of the subcutaneous tissue rich of adipocytes: *de facto*, the edemato-fibro-sclerotic panniculitis is more related to the microcirculation condition, systemic hormonal metabolism, dietary habits and lifestyle, whereas the localized adiposity is the result of a transformed deposit of fat tissue due to a localized lipodystrophy. The presence of such modifications represent a cosmetic and functional disorder which has been mostly reported in the Caucasian and female populations (85% of the lipodystrophy cases of the lower extremities affect women and 15% men). To treat both conditions, US is delivered to enhance action of a lymphatic drainage massage. On adipose tissue cavitation effect causes the fragmentation and subsequent leakage of the lipid matrix that reach the interstitial fluid. Emulsification of the lipid favours its metabolic assimilation. Through the generation of compression and depression cycles at appropriate frequency, US causes cavitation phenomena at the fat/water interface, adipocyte rupture and triglyceride release. US can be concentrated in a defined subcutaneous area to produce selective lipolysis and clinically relevant reduction of the volume of subcutaneous fat pad while avoiding any damage to surrounding tissues [149] (Fig. **35**).

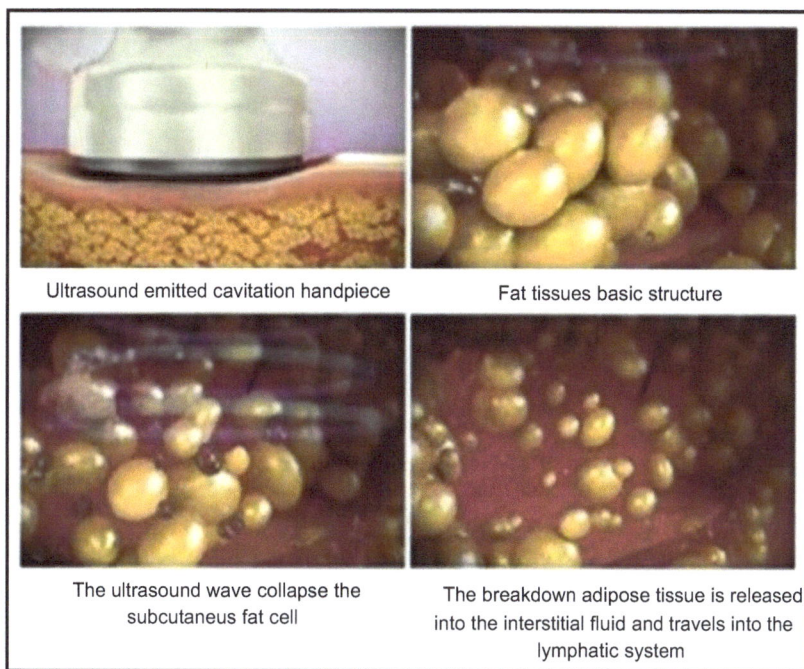

Ultrasound emitted cavitation handpiece

Fat tissues basic structure

The ultrasound wave collapse the subcutaneus fat cell

The breakdown adipose tissue is released into the interstitial fluid and travels into the lymphatic system

Fig. (35). Cavitation process and lipolysis. Modified from: http://www.prettislim.com/ u-lipo/ how-does-u-lipo-works.

US are delivered through a head that is in direct contact with skin, with a gel which help transmit the US waves. Treatment may last from 20 a 60 minutes depending on the areas to be treated and the particular case (Fig. **36**).

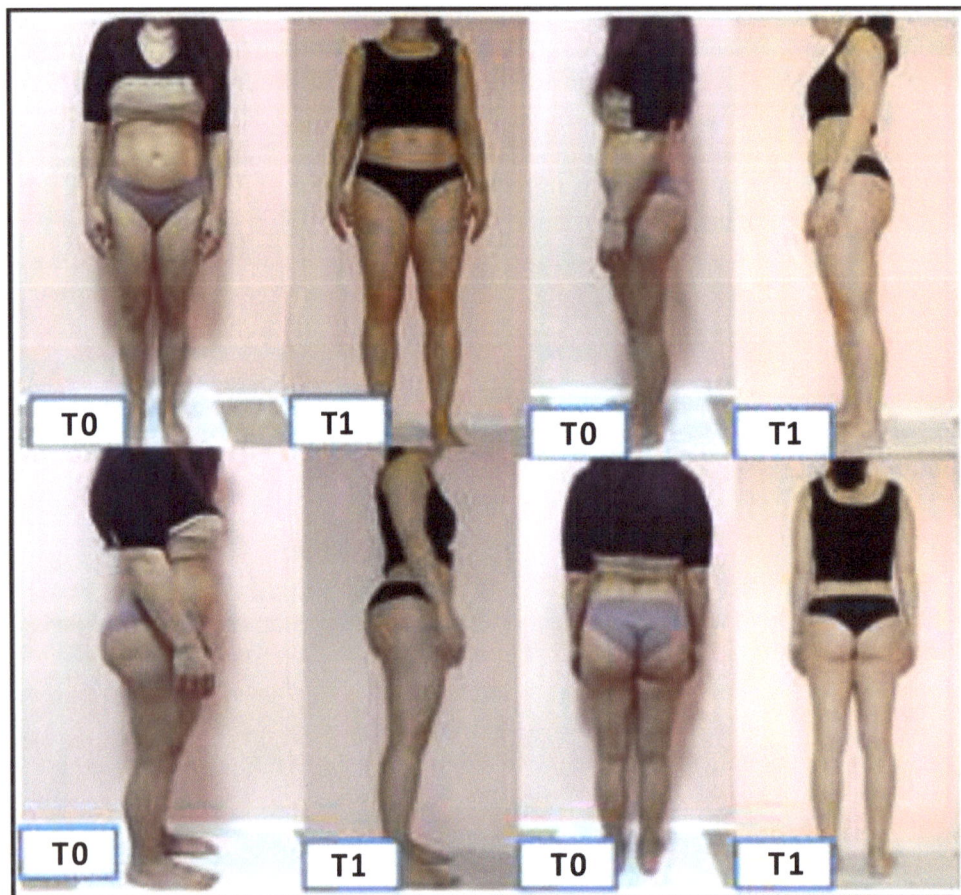

Fig. (36). Reduction of weight, edemato-fibro-sclerotic panniculitis, and localised adiposity after a 4-week therapy (2 session per week). Two clinical cases are presented in the figure: at the top of the panel - a 24 year old subject with lower limb edema; in the lower panel a 35 year old girl subject edematous-fibro-sclerotic panniculitis, before and after treatment.

University Center of Physical and Rehabilitation Medicine, "Gabriele d'Annunzio" University, Chieti-Pescara (Italy).

Over the 1980s, the US-assisted liposuction (UAL) was introduced. The technique consists of the use of the US simultaneously to an aspiration of the traditional type. The UAL provides a surgical incision and the subcutaneous application, directly into the adipose tissue to be treated, of an emitter of US hand piece with frequency of about 20 kHz, which for size is comparable to a normal from suction cannula. This surgical approach, although effective, has many drawbacks for patients related to the hospitalization, general anaesthesia, post-surgery pain, presence of bruising and swelling in the treated area, as well as other risks related to surgical procedures; possible complications are skin burns and irregularities, and damage of blood vessels, nerves and muscles [299, 300].

Phonophoresis

Transcutaneous drug delivery (*pharmaphoresis*) has a number of advantages over oral drug administration. It provides a higher initial drug concentration at the delivery site, without gastric irritation and first-pass metabolism by the liver. It also allows delivery to a larger area than is readily achieved by injection, avoiding the pain, trauma, and infection risk associated with injection [301]. Among various techniques of transcutaneous drug administration, *phonophoresis* consists in delivery of molecules through a medium (usually a conductive gel) by US, whereas *iontophoresis* consists in the delivery of ions by an applied electric field [302, 303]. Although the exact mechanism is not known, drug absorption may involve a disruption of the stratum corneum lipid allowing the drug to pass through the skin [304].

The first report on the use of US to enhance drug delivery across the skin was published in 1954 [305]. This was followed by a series of studies performed by Griffin *et al.* to evaluate the location and depth of hydrocortisone delivery and the effects of varying US parameters on hydrocortisone phonophoresis [306 - 309]. The authors of these first studies proposed that US enhanced drug delivery by exerting pressure on the drug to drive it through the skin. However, because US exerts only a few force, it is now thought that US increases transdermal drug penetration by increasing the permeability of the stratum corneum through both thermal and non-thermal mechanisms.

It has been proposed that US alters the skin porous pathways by enlarging the radius of cutaneous pore and creating more pores or making them less winding. When the permeability of the stratum corneum is increased, a drug will diffuse across it because of the difference in concentration on either side of the skin. Once a drug diffuses across the stratum corneum, it is initially more concentrated at the delivery site and is then distributed throughout the body via the blood circulation; therefore, physicians should be aware that drugs delivered by phonophoresis become systemic, and the contraindications for systemic delivery of these drugs also apply to this mode of delivery [310 - 312] (Fig. **37**).

Two procedures are used with the US: the application of the drug and immediately the ultrasound application or drug and/or the product is applied on the skin and left to act for time necessary for the absorption and subsequently US is applied. Nowadays, the latter approach is preferred [313 - 315].

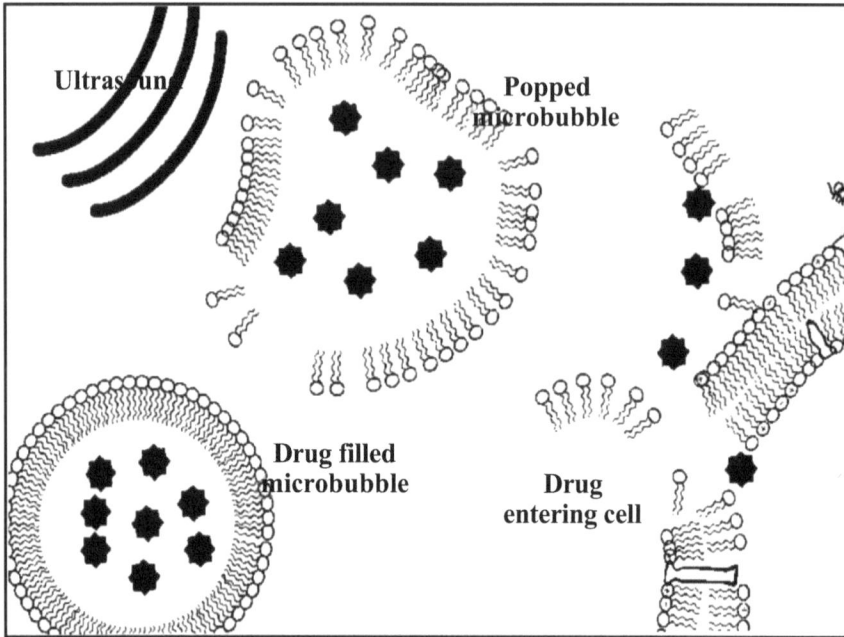

Fig. (37). Mechanism of phonophoresis. From: Unger EC, Hersh E, Vannan M, Matsunaga TO, McCreery T. Local drug and gene delivery through micro bubbles. Prog Cardiovasc Dis 2001; 44(1): 45-54.

The fundamental parameters which determine the variation of the phonophoresis action are: energy levels, the entity of cavitation, the coupling efficiency between the translator and substance conveyed, skin hydration, type of drug or product applied [316]. Energy levels are attenuated as the US waves are transmitted through the tissues due to either absorption of the energy by the tissues or by dispersion and scattering of the waves. Most of the recent research on phonophoresis uses low-frequency US, of 100 kHz or lower frequency. Ultrasound for therapeutic purposes, are used in physical and rehabilitation medicine with a range between 0.75 and 3 MHz: lower frequencies penetrate most deeply (3-5 cm) and are preferred in subjects with a high percentage of body fat, while higher frequencies are absorbed from superficial tissues (1-2 cm). Delivery of US can be either thermal and continuous (producing more thermal heating; intensity of 1.0 to 1.5 W/cm^2 for 5-7 minutes) or non-thermal and pulsed (producing less heating; 0.8 to 1.5 W/cm^2 with a duty cycle of 20-60% for 5-7 minutes). Another variable affecting dosage is the energy of application; 0.1 to 0.3 W/cm^2 is regarded as low intensity, 0.4 to 1.5 W/cm^2 is medium intensity and 1.6 to 3 W/cm^2 is high intensity; treatment times generally range from 5 to 10 minutes. US, also produces mechanical effects as microstreming and cavitation of cells, or in any case non-thermal effects as reduction of the membrane potential, alterations of lipid structure, with increasing cell permeability and ionic conductance [317, 318]. Cavitation refers to the formation and collapse of small air bubbles formed in a two liquid to a pressure change induced in the tissue fluid from the passage of ultrasound. Cavitation can be stable (when ultrasound of high intensity and low frequency passing through a liquid, produces small bubbles that swing rhythmically in size) or unstable (when high-frequency ultrasound that generated bubbles grow and collapse abruptly). For micro streaming it means the formation of vortices in small volumes of cytoplasmic and interstitial fluid, this improves the dissolution of the drug particles in the suspension and alter the cell membrane structure by setting the permeability to sodium and calcium ions. The micro streaming effect also relates to the metabolic activity of the cell (protein synthesis) generating a fibroblastic activation, a change of bloodstream and interstitial fluid movement. The good conveyance of the drug depends on the acoustic impedance of the crossed tissues, amount of protein in the tissues, tissue hydration and the frequency and intensity of the US. The product must not have a granular texture and it must have a low viscosity for manageability of application and handling of the transducer head movement, in common clinical practice specific gel formulations are used. The use of oil and emulsions can dissipate the US waves and it, also, determines a localized overheating. Obviously, it must not be interposed air that does not allow the transmission of the waves [319].

Numerous drugs have been administered using phonophoresis. In rehabilitation, phonophoresis is used to convey drugs such as corticosteroids and NSAIDs to treat diseases affecting the musculoskeletal system. Osteoarthritis can be treated with ketoprofen using an applicator 5 cm in diameter, with a frequency of 1 MHz, with a power of 1.5 W/cm^2 for 8 min, piroxicam in continuous mode, power, 1.0W/cm^2 obtaining excellent results for pain, diclofenac gel for myofascial syndrome, indomethacin for temporomandibular joint pain [320 - 322]. A number of research explored the use of phonophoresis to deliver insulin [323, 324], vaccines, and other drugs that can be given only by injection, and that are not typically administered by rehabilitation professionals. Although animal studies have been promising, this approach to drug delivery is hampered by difficulties with precise dose control. US is also being explored as a method for monitoring blood glucose levels [325]. Rehabilitation professionals use phonophoresis primarily for local delivery of corticosteroids and NSAIDs to treat tissue inflammation associated with conditions such as tendinitis or bursitis.

Sonotransfection

Gene transfection is a process consisting in introduction of DNA into eukaryotic cells; the introduced DNA is then integrated into chromosomes. The currents transfection methods uses physical, chemical or viral techniques. The US-mediated gene transfection is a method that uses as viral or chemical carriers for sonotransfection with demonstrated efficacy for gene therapy in particular for cancer treatment. The *in vitro* procedure uses several US exposure (sonication) setups [326], but although high transfection rates attained in some conditions replicating similar levels of transfection *in vivo* is been difficult; *in vivo* simulated setups offer hope for a more consistent outcome *in vivo*. To confirm and increase the data on the effectiveness of sonotransfection many studies are still ongoing. Very interesting are studies that plan to transfer therapeutic genes with micro bubbles directly inside the target cell by avoiding exposure to the cells and/or nearby tissues [327] (Fig. **38**).

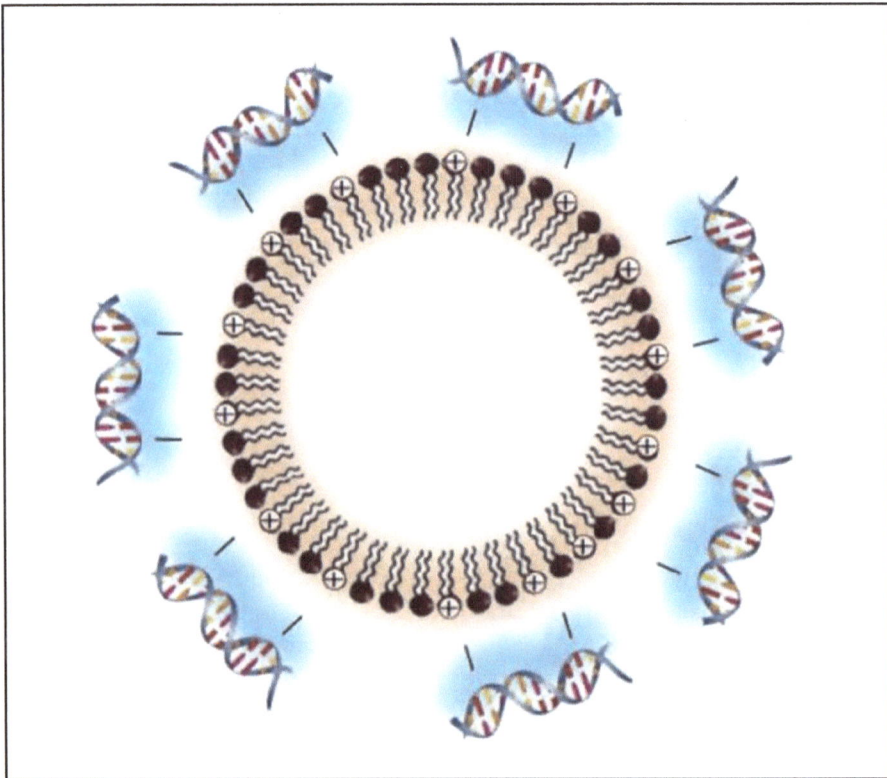

Fig. (38). Micro bubble for gene delivery. The gaseous core is coated by a monolayer of phospholipid containing cationic lipid imparting a net positive charge to the microbubble. DNA, as a polyanion, is adsorbed electrostatically to the exterior surface of the micro bubble.

Several studies have shown that the efficiency is considerably increased with the addition of contrast agents [120, 328 - 332] consisting of gas micro bubbles encapsulated, also often used in imaging as they are able to reflect the acoustic wave. The main properties of these means is to emphasize the effects of ultrasonic field on the sample for which, by adding them in the cell culture medium, reduced intensity US are required to generate cavitation.

Dosimetry

The absorption evaluation and study of the biological effects of US are linked to the development of a dosimetry that characterizes the physical agent and its potential interaction with the biological material and which requires the presence of three factors:

- quantification of one or more measurable values that define the output from the source;
- determining the effect on biological material energy propagated in various ways (by reflection, refraction, and others);
- determination of the cause-effect relationship between the previous quantities.

The history of other types of energies shows that it is, increasingly, difficult to define the concept of dose. For example, in the field of ionizing radiation dosimetry describes the amount of absorbed dose (energy imparted to the site of interest per unit mass) but over this to explain many biological effects it is necessary to introduce the concepts of cumulative dose, dose equivalent, the threshold dose. Similarly, in photobiology it refers to ultraviolet radiation as energy per unit area and in the field of electromagnetic radiation using the specific absorption rate and the absorbed power density.

As for US, dosimetry is much less developed and is still an open question. Dosimetric parameters for therapeutic US have been determined through experimental observations of bio-effects due to exposure: the most used parameters are the sound pressure and intensity. However, it should be stressed the importance of reaching a definition of the concept of «dose» for therapeutic applications of the US, which may be obtained by means of theoretical techniques, numerical simulation of the propagation of the US beam in tissues and biological samples, and experimental techniques. This objective requires a thorough knowledge of the characteristics of the US beam which is fundamental both in the study of the biological effects of the US and in the assessment of possible health risks linked to medical treatments. For this purpose appropriate dummies may be designed and produced, for example consisting in sandwich tissue-equivalent elements paired with thermocouples or thermal cameras to measure the local temperature, even by placing a consolidated database to evaluate the dosimetric models through studies *in vitro* and *in vivo* [333 - 335].

Clinical trials and adverse event reports have highlighted some risks related to the ultrasonic technology, including damage to non-target tissue and skin burns. Clinical trials for the uterine fibroid device found that 8 patients suffered temporary internal nerve damage from far-field heat, though all but one of these cases was resolved within 3 days. Patient movement can also result in ablation of the incorrect tissue, which occurred in two adverse event cases reported to FDA. Patients suffered from bowel perforation by the US treatment; the event was attributed to user error, since the operator should have adjusted the treatment plan after the patient moved. Clinical trial reports also cite skin irritation and burning at the site of application; 5 patients in the uterine fibroid pivotal trial experienced first- or second-degree skin burns, and 1 patient in the bone metastases pivotal trial experienced a 3 cm third-degree burn [336, 337].

Several biophysical mechanisms at the basis of biological effects of the US have been identified, which in turn may constitute the intended effect of the treatment or a side effect. For each mechanism may be more relevant a particular characteristic of the US wave: certainly the intensity plays a significant role in the case of the thermal effects; as for the non-thermal effects, other physical parameters may be more significant, such as the negative peak pressure (rarefaction) in the case of mechanical effects related to cavitation. The international standard of the International Electrotechnical Commission introduced a parameter to define an exposure or security index. It takes the properties of the tissues crossed by the US wave and technical properties of the devices into account (the "mechanical index"), as well as the so-called "thermal index", that evaluates the thermal effect through assessment of the temperature of the US source, the heat propagation mechanisms in each tissue, and the exposure time. The two indices are widely used in case of high-frequency US applications as security indicators of exposure; a recent study indicates that the direct application of these indices to the low frequencies (sonophoresis, body contouring, and others) needs of an accurate investigation, whereby while the thermal index can be used directly the mechanical index seems become less reliably.

It should be underlined the importance, especially as regards the emerging medical applications of the US (HIFU, aesthetic medicine, and others), to determine accurate methods for predicting the dose (or in any case the most significant physical quantities), and to develop specific procedures to characterize the transducers and monitor the performance of the devices. In particular, with regard to the HIFU, the ability to generate high temperature inside tissues makes it necessary guarantee that the treatment is provided in an appropriate manner and in the correct site. In fact, for this application, in particular, open problems remain relative to the measurement of physical quantities, which relate, for example, the most appropriate methods for the measurement of power in a highly focused ultrasonic field. Also for aesthetic medicine, a physical characterization of the US beam and its propagation in biological tissues is necessary to ensure the effectiveness and safety of treatments [104, 338].

Adverse Effects And Contraindications

Although US has rarely been reported to produce adverse effects [336, 337], a variety of adverse effects can occur if US is applied incorrectly, or when contraindicated. The most common adverse effect is a burn, which may occur when high- intensity, continuous US is applied, particularly if a stationary application technique is used [339].

There is general agreement in the literature regarding contraindications and precautions for the clinical application of therapeutic US. Precautions are recommended in application of US on specific organs (over the eyes, since cavitation in the ocular fluids may damage it, and in the area of the male or female reproductive organs, since US may affect gametogenesis) and in the following conditions:

- *cancer*. Although no research data are available on the effects of US cancer in humans. a study indicated that the application of continuous US at 1.0 W/cm^2, 1 MHz, for 5 minutes for 10 treatments over a period of 2 weeks to mice with subcutaneous malignant tumors significantly increase the rate of tumor growth compared with those of untreated controls, and treated animals also developed more lymph node metastases [340]. Hence, it is recommended not to apply US on malignant tumors in humans. Caution should be also used when treating a patient who has a history of a (malignant) tumor, because it can be difficult to ascertain whether any small tumors remain;
- *thrombophlebitis*. Because US may dislodge or cause partial disintegration of a thrombus, which could result in obstruction of the circulation to vital organs, US should not be applied over or near an area where a thrombus is or may be present;
- *pacemaker*. Because US may heat a pacemaker or interfere with its electrical circuitry, it should not be applied in the area of a pacemaker;
- *pregnancy*. Maternal hyperthermia has been associated with fetal abnormalities, including growth retardation, microphthalmia, microcephaly, anencephaly, neural tube defects, and myelodysplasia. A report also documents a case of microcephaly, sacral agenesia, and developmental delay in a child whose mother was treated 18 times with low-intensity pulsed US for a left psoas bursitis between days 6 and 29 of pregnancy [341, 342]. It is therefore recommended not to apply US at any level in areas where it may reach a developing fetus.

CONFLICT OF INTEREST

The author (editor) declares no conflict of interest, financial or otherwise.

ACKNOWLEDGEMENTS

Declared none.

REFERENCES

[1]   Wong RA, Schumann B, Townsend R, Phelps CA. A survey of therapeutic ultrasound use by physical therapists who are orthopaedic certified specialists. Phys Ther 2007; 87(8): 986-94.
[http://dx.doi.org/10.2522/ptj.20050392] [PMID: 17553923]

[2]   Humphrey VF. Ultrasound and matter physical interactions. Prog Biophys Mol Biol 2007; 93(1-3): 195-211.
[http://dx.doi.org/10.1016/j.pbiomolbio.2006.07.024] [PMID: 17079004]

[3]   Leighton TG. What is ultrasound? Prog Biophys Mol Biol 2007; 93(1-3): 3-83.
[http://dx.doi.org/10.1016/j.pbiomolbio.2006.07.026] [PMID: 17045633]

[4]   Pierce AD. Acoustics: an introduction to its physical principles and applications. New York: McGraw-Hill 1981.

[5]   Alvarenga AV, Costa-Félix RP. Metrological aspects on therapeutic ultrasound parameters: effective radiating area and non-uniformity ration. Phys Procedia 2010; 3(1): 643-9.
[http://dx.doi.org/10.1016/j.phpro.2010.01.081]

[6]   Williams AR. Production and transmission of ultrasound. Physiotherapy 1987; 73: 113-6.

[7]   Hekkenberg RT, Reibold R, Zeqiri B. Development of standard measurement methods for essential properties of ultrasound therapy equipment. Ultrasound Med Biol 1994; 20(1): 83-98.
[http://dx.doi.org/10.1016/0301-5629(94)90020-5] [PMID: 8197630]

[8]   Curie J, Curie P. Développement, par pression, de l'électricité polaire dans les cristaux hémièdres à faces inclinées. Comptes Rendus de l'Académie des Sciences 1880; 91: 294-5.

[9]   Curie J, Curie P. Phénomènes électriques des cristaux hémièdres à faces inclinées. J Phys Theor Appl 1882; 1(1): 245-51.
[http://dx.doi.org/10.1051/jphystap:018820010024500]

[10]   Chapelon JY, Cathignol D, Cain C, *et al.* New piezoelectric transducers for therapeutic ultrasound. Ultrasound Med Biol 2000; 26(1): 153-9.
[http://dx.doi.org/10.1016/S0301-5629(99)00120-9] [PMID: 10687803]

[11]   Manbachi A, Cobbold RS. Development and application of piezoelectric materials for ultrasound generation and detection. Ultrasound 2011; 19(4): 187-96.
[http://dx.doi.org/10.1258/ult.2011.011027]

[12]   Genovese M. Ultrasound transducers. J Diagn Med Sonogr 2016; 32(1): 48-53.
[http://dx.doi.org/10.1177/8756479315618207]

[13]   Damjanovic D. Ferroelectric, dielectric and piezoelectric properties of ferroelectric thin films and ceramics. Rep Prog Phys 1998; 61(9): 1267.
[http://dx.doi.org/10.1088/0034-4885/61/9/002]

[14]   Khodayari A, Pruvost S, Sebald G, Guyomar D, Mohammadi S. Nonlinear pyroelectric energy harvesting from relaxor single crystals. IEEE Trans Ultrason Ferroelectr Freq Control 2009; 56(4): 693-9.
[http://dx.doi.org/10.1109/TUFFC.2009.1092] [PMID: 19406698]

[15]   Pye SD, Milford C. The performance of ultrasound physiotherapy machines in Lothian Region, Scotland, 1992. Ultrasound Med Biol 1994; 20(4): 347-59.
[http://dx.doi.org/10.1016/0301-5629(94)90003-5] [PMID: 8085291]

[16]   Dalmont JP. Acoustic impedance measurement, part I: a review. J Sound Vibrat 2001; 243(3): 427-39.
[http://dx.doi.org/10.1006/jsvi.2000.3428]

[17]   Zagzebski JA. Essentials of ultrasound physics. St. Louis, MO: Mosby – Year Book 1996.

[18]   Kinsler LE, Frey AR, Coppens AB, Sanders JV. Fundamentals of acoustics. 4th ed., New York: John Wiley & Sons 1982.

[19]   ter Haar GR, Bamber JC, Hill CR. Physical Principles of Medical Ultrasonics. 2nd ed., Chichester: John Wiley & Sons 2004.

[20]   Chivers RC, Hill CR. Ultrasonic Attenuation in Human Tissue. Ultrasound Med Biol 1975; 2(1): 25-9.
[http://dx.doi.org/10.1016/0301-5629(75)90038-1] [PMID: 1216368]

[21]   Dunn F, Edmonds PD, Fry WJ. Absorption and dispersion of ultrasound in biological media. In: Schwan HP, Ed. Biological Engineering. New York: McGraw-Hill 1969; pp. 205-332.

[22]   Dyson M. Mechanisms involved in therapeutic ultrasound. Physiotherapy 1987; 73: 116-20.

[23]   Gann N. Ultrasound: current concepts. Clin Manage 1991; 11: 64-9.

[24]   Ziskin MC, McDiarmid T, Michlovitz SL. Therapeutic ultrasound. In: Michlovitz S, Ed. Thermal agents in rehabilitation. Philadelphia: FA Davis Company 1990.

[25]   OBrien WD Jr. Ultrasound-biophysics mechanisms. Prog Biophys Mol Biol 2007; 93(1-3): 212-55.
[http://dx.doi.org/10.1016/j.pbiomolbio.2006.07.010] [PMID: 16934858]

[26]   Hunt JW. Applications of microwave, ultrasound, and radiofrequency heating. Natl Cancer Inst Monogr 1982; 61: 447-56.
[PMID: 7177189]

[27]   Langevin P. French Patent No. 505,703. Filed September 17, 1917. Issued August 5, 1920.

[28]   Wood RW, Loomis AL. The physical and biological effects of high-frequency sound waves of great intensity. Phil Mag S 7 1927; 4(22): 417-36.
[http://dx.doi.org/10.1080/14786440908564348]

[29]   Harvey EN. Biological aspects of ultrasonic waves: a general survey. Biol Bull 1930; 59: 306-25.
[http://dx.doi.org/10.2307/1536819]

[30]   Kremkau FW. Ultrasonic treatment of experimental animal tumours. Br J Cancer Suppl 1982; 5: 226-32.
[PMID: 6279136]

[31]   Lyng H, Monge OR, Bøhler PJ, Rofstad EK. Relationships between thermal dose and heat-induced tissue and vascular damage after thermoradiotherapy of locally advanced breast carcinoma. Int J Hyperthermia 1991; 7(3): 403-15.
[http://dx.doi.org/10.3109/02656739109005006] [PMID: 1919137]

[32]   Lynn JG, Zwemer RL, Chick AJ, Miller AE. A new method for the generation and use of focused ultrasound in experimental biology. J Gen Physiol 1942; 26(2): 179-93.
[http://dx.doi.org/10.1085/jgp.26.2.179] [PMID: 19873337]

[33]   Fry WJ, Fry RB. Determination of absolute sound levels and acoustic absorption coefficients by thermocouple probes – experiment. J Acoust Soc Am 1954; 26(3): 311-7.
[http://dx.doi.org/10.1121/1.1907333]

[34]   Sjöberg A, Stahle J, Johnson S, Sahl R. Treatment of Menieres disease by ultrasonic irradiation. Acta Otolaryngol 1963; 56(2-6): 171-5.
[http://dx.doi.org/10.3109/00016486309127401] [PMID: 13977816]

[35]   Sjöberg A, Stahle J, Johnson S, Sahl R. Treatment of Menieres disease by ultrasonic irradiation. Physical, experimental and clinical studies. Acta Otolaryngol Suppl 1963; 179: 1-86.
[PMID: 13977815]

[36]   Breazeale MA, Dunn F. Comparison of methods for absolute calibration of ultrasonic fields. J Acoust Soc Am 1974; 55(3): 671-2.
[http://dx.doi.org/10.1121/1.1914581]

[37]   Apfel RE. Acoustic cavitation prediction. J Acoust Soc Am 1981; 69(6): 1624-33.
[http://dx.doi.org/10.1121/1.385939]

[38]   Apfel RE. Acoustic cavitation. In: Edmonds PD, Ed. Methods in Experimental Physics: Ultrasonics. New York: Academic Press 1981; Vol. 19: pp. 356-411.

[39]   Apfel RE. Acoustic cavitation: a possible consequence of biomedical uses of ultrasound. Br J Cancer Suppl 1982; 5 (Suppl. 5): 140-6.
[PMID: 6950749]

[40]   Appel RE. Possibility of microcavitation from diagnostic ultrasound. IEEE Trans Ultrason Ferroelectr Freq Control 1986; 33(2): 139-42.
[http://dx.doi.org/10.1109/T-UFFC.1986.26805] [PMID: 18291762]

[41]   Holland CK, Apfel RE. An improved theory for the prediction of microcavitation thresholds. IEEE Trans Ultrason Ferroelectr Freq Control 1989; 36(2): 204-8.
[http://dx.doi.org/10.1109/58.19152] [PMID: 18284969]

[42]   Holland CK, Apfel RE. Thresholds for transient cavitation produced by pulsed ultrasound in a controlled nuclei environment. J Acoust Soc Am 1990; 88(5): 2059-69.
[http://dx.doi.org/10.1121/1.400102] [PMID: 2269722]

[43]   Apfel RE, Holland CK. Gauging the likelihood of cavitation from short-pulse, low-duty cycle diagnostic ultrasound. Ultrasound Med Biol 1991; 17(2): 179-85.
[http://dx.doi.org/10.1016/0301-5629(91)90125-G] [PMID: 2053214]

[44]   Flynn HG. Generation of transient cavities in liquids by microsecond pulses of ultrasound. J Acoust Soc Am 1982; 72(6): 1926-32.
[http://dx.doi.org/10.1121/1.388622]

[45]   Flynn HG, Church CC. Erratum: transient pulsations of small gas bubbles in water [J. Acoust. Soc. Am. 84, 985998 (1988)] [corrected and republished]. J Acoust Soc Am 1988; 84(5): 1863-76.
[Erratum in: J Acoust Soc Am 1988; 84(5): 1863-76].
[http://dx.doi.org/10.1121/1.397253] [PMID: 3209777]

[46]   ter Haar G, Dyson M, Oakley EM. The use of ultrasound by physiotherapists in Britain, 1985. Ultrasound Med Biol 1987; 13(10): 659-63.
[http://dx.doi.org/10.1016/0301-5629(87)90064-0] [PMID: 3686730]

[47]   Dunn F, Frizzell LA. Bioeffects of ultrasound. In: Lehmann JF, Ed. Therapeutic Heat and Cold. Baltimore: Williams and Wilkins 1982; vol. 9: pp. 386-403.

[48]   Baker KG, Robertson VJ, Duck FA. A review of therapeutic ultrasound: biophysical effects. Phys Ther 2001; 81(7): 1351-8.
[PMID: 11444998]

[49]   ter Haar G. Therapeutic applications of ultrasound. Prog Biophys Mol Biol 2007; 93(1-3): 111-29.
[http://dx.doi.org/10.1016/j.pbiomolbio.2006.07.005] [PMID: 16930682]

[50]   Watson T. Ultrasound in contemporary physiotherapy practice. Ultrasonics 2008; 48(4): 321-9.
[http://dx.doi.org/10.1016/j.ultras.2008.02.004] [PMID: 18466945]

[51]   Kuitert JH. Ultrasonic energy as an adjunct in the management of radiculitis and similar referred pain.
Am J Phys Med 1954; 33(1): 61-5.
[PMID: 13124482]

[52]   Coleman DJ, Lizzi FL, Driller J, *et al.* Therapeutic ultrasound in the treatment of glaucoma. I.
Experimental model. Ophthalmology 1985; 92(3): 339-46.
[http://dx.doi.org/10.1016/S0161-6420(85)34029-0] [PMID: 3991121]

[53]   Quan KM, Shiran M, Watmough DJ. Applicators for generating ultrasound-induced hyperthermia in
neoplastic tumours and for use in ultrasound physiotherapy. Phys Med Biol 1989; 34(11): 1719-31.
[http://dx.doi.org/10.1088/0031-9155/34/11/019] [PMID: 2587630]

[54]   Foster RS, Bihrle R, Sanghvi NT, Fry FJ, Donohue JP. High-intensity focused ultrasound in the
treatment of prostatic disease. Eur Urol 1993; 23 (Suppl. 1): 29-33.
[PMID: 7685694]

[55]   Schatzl G, Madersbacher S, Djavan B, Lang T, Marberger M. Two-year results of transurethral
resection of the prostate versus four less invasive treatment options. Eur Urol 2000; 37(6): 695-701.
[http://dx.doi.org/10.1159/000020220] [PMID: 10828670]

[56]   Robertson VJ, Baker KG. A review of therapeutic ultrasound: effectiveness studies. Phys Ther 2001;
81(7): 1339-50.
[PMID: 11444997]

[57]   Johns LD, Straub SJ, Howard SM. Analysis of effective radiating area, power, intensity, and field
characteristics of ultrasound transducers. Arch Phys Med Rehabil 2007; 88(1): 124-9.
[http://dx.doi.org/10.1016/j.apmr.2006.09.016] [PMID: 17207688]

[58]   Denegar CR, Saliba E, Saliba S. Therapeutic Modalities for Musculoskeletal Injuries. 4th ed. Human
Kinetics 2016; pp. 12-3.

[59]   Johns LD, Straub SJ, Howard SM. Variability in effective radiating area and output power of new
ultrasound transducers at 3 MHz. J Athl Train 2007; 42(1): 22-8.
[PMID: 17597939]

[60]   Straub SJ, Johns LD, Howard SM. Variability in effective radiating area at 1 MHz affects ultrasound
treatment intensity. Phys Ther 2008; 88(1): 50-7.
[http://dx.doi.org/10.2522/ptj.20060358] [PMID: 17940107]

[61]   Gutiérrez MI, Vera A, Leija L. Methods for characterization of physiotherapy ultrasonic transducers.
In: Campolo D, Ed. New Developments in Biomedical Engineering. InTech 2010; 28: pp. 517-42.
[http://dx.doi.org/10.5772/7600]

[62]   OBrien WD Jr, Frizzell LA, Weigel RM, Zachary JF. Ultrasound-induced lung hemorrhage is not
caused by inertial cavitation. J Acoust Soc Am 2000; 108(3 Pt 1): 1290-7.
[http://dx.doi.org/10.1121/1.1287706] [PMID: 11008829]

[63]   OBrien WD Jr, Simpson DG, Frizzell LA, Zachary JF. Superthreshold behavior and threshold
estimates of ultrasound-induced lung hemorrhage in adult rats: role of beamwidth. IEEE Trans
Ultrason Ferroelectr Freq Control 2001; 48(6): 1695-705.
[http://dx.doi.org/10.1109/58.971723] [PMID: 11800133]

[64]   OBrien WD Jr, Abbott JG, Stratmeyer ME, *et al.* Acoustic output upper limits proposition: should
upper limits be retained? J Ultrasound Med 2002; 21(12): 1335-41.
[http://dx.doi.org/10.7863/jum.2002.21.12.1335] [PMID: 12494975]

[65]   OBrien WD Jr, Simpson DG, Ho MH, Miller RJ, Frizzell LA, Zachary JF. Superthreshold behavior and threshold estimation of ultrasound-induced lung hemorrhage in pigs: role of age dependency. IEEE Trans Ultrason Ferroelectr Freq Control 2003; 50(2): 153-69.
[http://dx.doi.org/10.1109/TUFFC.2003.1182119] [PMID: 12625588]

[66]   OBrien WD Jr, Simpson DG, Frizzell LA, Zachary JF. Threshold estimates and superthreshold behavior of ultrasound-induced lung hemorrhage in adult rats: role of pulse duration. Ultrasound Med Biol 2003; 29(11): 1625-34.
[http://dx.doi.org/10.1016/j.ultrasmedbio.2003.08.002] [PMID: 14654157]

[67]   OBrien WD Jr, Simpson DG, Frizzell LA, Zachary JF. Threshold estimates and superthreshold behavior of ultrasound-induced lung hemorrhage in adult rats: role of pulse duration. J Ultrasound Med 2006; 25(7): 873-82.
[http://dx.doi.org/10.7863/jum.2006.25.7.873] [PMID: 16798898]

[68]   Barnett SB, ter Haar GR, Ziskin MC, Nyborg WL, Maeda K, Bang J. Current status of research on biophysical effects of ultrasound. Ultrasound Med Biol 1994; 20(3): 205-18.
[http://dx.doi.org/10.1016/0301-5629(94)90060-4] [PMID: 8059482]

[69]   Coleman AJ, Choi MJ, Saunders JE. Detection of acoustic emission from cavitation in tissue during clinical extracorporeal lithotripsy. Ultrasound Med Biol 1996; 22(8): 1079-87.
[http://dx.doi.org/10.1016/S0301-5629(96)00118-4] [PMID: 9004432]

[70]   Graff KF. A history of ultrasonics. In: Mason WP, Thurston RN, Eds. Physical Acoustics. New York: Academic Press 1981; 15(1): pp. 1-97.
[http://dx.doi.org/10.1016/B978-0-12-477915-0.50006-3]

[71]   Kitchen SS, Partridge CJ. A review of therapeutic ultrasound. Physiotherapy 1990; 76: 593-600.

[72]   Duck FA. Radiation pressure and acoustic streaming. In: Duck FA, Baker AC, Starritt HC, Eds. Ultrasound in Medicine. Bristol: Institute of Physics Publishing 1998; 3: pp. 39-56.
[http://dx.doi.org/10.1887/0750305932/b673c3]

[73]   Draper DO, Sunderland S, Kirkendall DT, Ricard M. A comparison of temperature rise in human calf muscles following applications of underwater and topical gel ultrasound. J Orthop Sports Phys Ther 1993; 17(5): 247-51.
[http://dx.doi.org/10.2519/jospt.1993.17.5.247] [PMID: 8343782]

[74]   Draper DO, Schulthies S, Sorvisto P, Hautala AM. Temperature changes in deep muscles of humans during ice and ultrasound therapies: an *in vivo* study. J Orthop Sports Phys Ther 1995; 21(3): 153-7.
[http://dx.doi.org/10.2519/jospt.1995.21.3.153] [PMID: 7742841]

[75]   Draper DO, Castel JC, Castel D. Rate of temperature increase in human muscle during 1 MHz and 3 MHz continuous ultrasound. J Orthop Sports Phys Ther 1995; 22(4): 142-50.
[http://dx.doi.org/10.2519/jospt.1995.22.4.142] [PMID: 8535471]

[76]   Ashton DF, Draper DO, Myrer JW. Temperature rise in human muscle during ultrasound treatments using flex-all as a coupling agent. J Athl Train 1998; 33(2): 136-40.
[PMID: 16558500]

[77]   Chan AK, Myrer JW, Measom GJ, Draper DO. Temperature changes in human patellar tendon in response to therapeutic ultrasound. J Athl Train 1998; 33(2): 130-5.
[PMID: 16558499]

[78]   Lehmann JF, McMillan JA, Brunner GD, Blumberg JB. Comparative study of the efficiency of short-wave, microwave and ultrasonic diathermy in heating the hip joint. Arch Phys Med Rehabil 1959; 40: 510-2.
[PMID: 14415376]

[79]   ter Haar GR, Hopewell JW. Ultrasonic heating of mammalian tissues *in vivo*. Br J Cancer Suppl 1982; 5: 65-7.
[PMID: 6950777]

[80]   Lehmann JF, de Lateur BJ. Therapeutic heat. In: Lehmann JF, Ed. Therapeutic Heat and Cold. 4th ed. Baltimore: Williams and Wilkins 1990; pp. 417-581.

[81]   Vander AJ, Luciano D, Sherman J. Human Physiology: The Mechanisms of Body Function. 8th ed., Boston: McGraw-Hill Higher Education 2001.

[82]   Abraham P, Leftheriotis G, Desvaux B, Saumet M, Saumet JL. Diameter and blood velocity changes in the saphenous vein during thermal stress. Eur J Appl Physiol Occup Physiol 1994; 69(4): 305-8.
[http://dx.doi.org/10.1007/BF00392035] [PMID: 7851365]

[83]   Wyper DJ, McNiven DR. Effects of some physiotherapeutic agents on skeletal muscle blood flow. Physiotherapy 1976; 62(3): 83-5.
[PMID: 1265149]

[84]   Robinson SE, Buono MJ. Effect of continuous-wave ultrasound on blood flow in skeletal muscle. Phys Ther 1995; 75(2): 145-9.
[http://dx.doi.org/10.1093/ptj/75.2.145] [PMID: 7846134]

[85]   Bickford RH, Duff RS. Influence of ultrasonic irradiation on temperature and blood flow in human skeletal muscle. Circ Res 1953; 1(6): 534-8.
[http://dx.doi.org/10.1161/01.RES.1.6.534] [PMID: 13106924]

[86]   Paul WD, Imig CJ. Temperature and blood flow studies after ultrasonic irradiation. Am J Phys Med 1955; 34(2): 370-5.
[PMID: 14361716]

[87]   Akyürekli D, Gerig LH, Raaphorst GP. Changes in muscle blood flow distribution during hyperthermia. Int J Hyperthermia 1997; 13(5): 481-96.
[http://dx.doi.org/10.3109/02656739709023547] [PMID: 9354933]

[88]   Low J, Reed A. Electrotherapy Explained: Principles and Practice. Oxford: Butterworth-Heinemann 1994.

[89]   Hashish I, Harvey W, Harris M. Anti-inflammatory effects of ultrasound therapy: evidence for a major placebo effect. Br J Rheumatol 1986; 25(1): 77-81.
[http://dx.doi.org/10.1093/rheumatology/25.1.77] [PMID: 2417648]

[90]   Hashish I, Hai HK, Harvey W, Feinmann C, Harris M. Reduction of postoperative pain and swelling by ultrasound treatment: a placebo effect. Pain 1988; 33(3): 303-11.
[http://dx.doi.org/10.1016/0304-3959(88)90289-8] [PMID: 3419838]

[91]   Lundeberg T, Abrahamsson P, Haker E. A comparative study of continuous ultrasound, placebo ultrasound and rest in epicondylalgia. Scand J Rehabil Med 1988; 20(3): 99-101.
[PMID: 3187466]

[92]   Grant A, Sleep J, McIntosh J, Ashurst H. Ultrasound and pulsed electromagnetic energy treatment for perineal trauma. A randomized placebo-controlled trial. Br J Obstet Gynaecol 1989; 96(4): 434-9.
[http://dx.doi.org/10.1111/j.1471-0528.1989.tb02419.x] [PMID: 2665802]

[93]   Munting E. Ultrasonic therapy for painful shoulders. Physiotherapy 1978; 64(6): 180-1.
[PMID: 674402]

[94]   Nykänen M. Pulsed ultrasound treatment of the painful shoulder a randomized, double-blind, placebo-controlled study. Scand J Rehabil Med 1995; 27(2): 105-8.
[PMID: 7569819]

[95]   ter Riet G, Kessels AG, Knipschild P. A randomized clinical trial of ultrasound in the treatment of pressure ulcers. Phys Ther 1996; 76(12): 1301-11.
[http://dx.doi.org/10.1093/ptj/76.12.1301] [PMID: 8959999]

[96]   Rigby BJ. The effect of mechanical extension upon the thermal stability of collagen. Biochim Biophys Acta 1964; 79: 634-6.
[PMID: 14179468]

[97]   Lehmann JF, Masock AJ, Warren CG, Koblanski JN. Effect of therapeutic temperatures on tendon extensibility. Arch Phys Med Rehabil 1970; 51(8): 481-7.
[PMID: 5448112]

[98]   Reed B, Ashikaga T. The effects of heating with ultrasound on knee joint displacement. J Orthop Sports Phys Ther 1997; 26(3): 131-7.
[http://dx.doi.org/10.2519/jospt.1997.26.3.131] [PMID: 9276853]

[99]   Reed BV, Ashikaga T, Fleming BC, Zimny NJ. Effects of ultrasound and stretch on knee ligament extensibility. J Orthop Sports Phys Ther 2000; 30(6): 341-7.
[http://dx.doi.org/10.2519/jospt.2000.30.6.341] [PMID: 10871146]

[100] Sarvazyan AP, Rudenko OV, Nyborg WL. Biomedical applications of radiation force of ultrasound: historical roots and physical basis. Ultrasound Med Biol 2010; 36(9): 1379-94.
[http://dx.doi.org/10.1016/j.ultrasmedbio.2010.05.015] [PMID: 20800165]

[101] Church CC. Spontaneous homogeneous nucleation, inertial cavitation and the safety of diagnostic ultrasound. Ultrasound Med Biol 2002; 28(10): 1349-64.
[http://dx.doi.org/10.1016/S0301-5629(02)00579-3] [PMID: 12467862]

[102] Bremond N, Arora M, Ohl CD, Lohse D. Controlled multibubble surface cavitation. Phys Rev Lett 2006; 96(22): 224501.
[http://dx.doi.org/10.1103/PhysRevLett.96.224501] [PMID: 16803310]

[103] Coleman AJ, Saunders JE, Crum LA, Dyson M. Acoustic cavitation generated by an extracorporeal shockwave lithotripter. Ultrasound Med Biol 1987; 13(2): 69-76.
[http://dx.doi.org/10.1016/0301-5629(87)90076-7] [PMID: 3590362]

[104] Hodnett M, Zeqiri B. A strategy for the development and standardisation of measurement methods for high power/cavitating ultrasonic fields: review of high power field measurement techniques. Ultrason Sonochem 1997; 4(4): 273-88.
[http://dx.doi.org/10.1016/S1350-4177(97)00042-4] [PMID: 11233809]

[105] Shi WT, Forsberg F, Tornes A, Ostensen J, Goldberg BB. Destruction of contrast microbubbles and the association with inertial cavitation. Ultrasound Med Biol 2000; 26(6): 1009-19.
[http://dx.doi.org/10.1016/S0301-5629(00)00223-4] [PMID: 10996701]

[106] Ince NH, Tezcanli G, Belen RK, Apikyan İG. Ultrasound as a catalyzer of aqueous reaction systems: the state of the art and environmental applications. Appl Catal B 2011; 29: 167-76.
[http://dx.doi.org/10.1016/S0926-3373(00)00224-1]

[107] Dahlem O, Demaiffe V, Halloin V, Reisse J. Direct sonication system suitable for medium scale sonochemical reactors. AIChE J 1998; 44(12): 2724-30.
[http://dx.doi.org/10.1002/aic.690441213]

[108] Reisse J. Introduction to sonochemistry. Proceedings of the 15th International Congress on Acoustics. Trondheim, Norway. 1995; pp. 409-12.

[109] Paliwal S, Mitragotri S. Ultrasound-induced cavitation: applications in drug and gene delivery. Expert Opin Drug Deliv 2006; 3(6): 713-26.
[http://dx.doi.org/10.1517/17425247.3.6.713] [PMID: 17076594]

[110] Wu CC, Roberts PH. A model of sonoluminescence. Proc R Soc Lond, A Contain Pap Math Phys Character 1924; 1994(445): 323-49.

[111] Moss WC, Clarke DB, White WJ, Young DA. Hydrodynamic simulations of bubble collapse and picosecond sonoluminescence. Phys Fluids 1994; 6(9): 2979-85.
[http://dx.doi.org/10.1063/1.868124]

[112] Lepoint T, De Pauw D, Lepoint-Mullie F, Goldman M, Goldman A. Sonoluminescence: an alternative "electrohydrodynamic" hypothesis. J Acoust Soc Am 1997; 101(4): 2012.
[http://dx.doi.org/10.1121/1.418242]

[113] Yasui K. Influence of ultrasonic frequency on multibubble sonoluminescence. J Acoust Soc Am 2002; 112(4): 1405-13.
[http://dx.doi.org/10.1121/1.1502898] [PMID: 12398448]

[114] Lepoint T, Mullie F. What exactly is cavitation chemistry? Ultrason Sonochem 1994; 1(1): S13-22.
[http://dx.doi.org/10.1016/1350-4177(94)90020-5]

[115] Hickling R. Transient, high-pressure solidification associated with cavitation in water. Phys Rev Lett 1994; 73(21): 2853-6.
[http://dx.doi.org/10.1103/PhysRevLett.73.2853] [PMID: 10057212]

[116] Margulis MA. Fundamental problems of sonochemistry and cavitation. Ultrason Sonochem 1994; 1(2): S87-90.
[http://dx.doi.org/10.1016/1350-4177(94)90003-5]

[117] Dyson M, Suckling J. Stimulation of tissue repair by ultrasound: a survey of the mechanisms involved. Physiotherapy 1978; 64(4): 105-8.
[PMID: 349580]

[118] Dinno MA, Dyson M, Young SR, Mortimer AJ, Hart J, Crum LA. The significance of membrane changes in the safe and effective use of therapeutic and diagnostic ultrasound. Phys Med Biol 1989; 34(11): 1543-52.
[http://dx.doi.org/10.1088/0031-9155/34/11/003] [PMID: 2685832]

[119] Champion JV, Langton CM, Meeten GH, Sherman NE. Near-field ultrasonic measurement apparatus for fluids. Meas Sci Technol 1990; 1(8): 786-92.
[http://dx.doi.org/10.1088/0957-0233/1/8/020]

[120] Miller DL, Quddus J. Sonoporation of monolayer cells by diagnostic ultrasound activation of contrast-agent gas bodies. Ultrasound Med Biol 2000; 26(4): 661-7.
[http://dx.doi.org/10.1016/S0301-5629(99)00170-2] [PMID: 10856630]

[121] Fuciarelli AF, Sisk EC, Thomas RM, Miller DL. Induction of base damage in DNA solutions by ultrasonic cavitation. Free Radic Biol Med 1995; 18(2): 231-8.
[http://dx.doi.org/10.1016/0891-5849(94)00119-5] [PMID: 7744306]

[122] Riesz P, Kondo T. Free radical formation induced by ultrasound and its biological implications. Free Radic Biol Med 1992; 13(3): 247-70.
[http://dx.doi.org/10.1016/0891-5849(92)90021-8] [PMID: 1324205]

[123] Huang YM, Zhao J, Yu X, Zhong W, Sun SQ. Effects of free radicals on the molecular fluidity and structure of the RBC membrane. Biorheology 1995; 32(2-3): 321.
[http://dx.doi.org/10.1016/0006-355X(95)92287-K]

[124] Huang Y, Liu D, Sun S. Mechanism of free radicals on the molecular fluidity and chemical structure of the red cell membrane damage. Clin Hemorheol Microcirc 2000; 23(2-4): 287-90.
[PMID: 11321453]

[125] Pozzi D, Fattibene P, Viscomi D, *et al.* Use of EPR and FTIR to detect biological effects of ultrasound and microbubbles on a fibroblast cell line. Eur Biophys J 2011; 40(10): 1115-20.
[http://dx.doi.org/10.1007/s00249-011-0738-8] [PMID: 21866359]

[126] Ohhashi Y, Kihara M, Naiki H, Goto Y. Ultrasonication-induced amyloid fibril formation of β_2-microglobulin. J Biol Chem 2005; 280(38): 32843-8.
[http://dx.doi.org/10.1074/jbc.M506501200] [PMID: 16046408]

[127] Marchioni C, Riccardi E, Spinelli S, *et al.* Structural changes induced in proteins by therapeutic ultrasounds. Ultrasonics 2009; 49(6-7): 569-76.
[http://dx.doi.org/10.1016/j.ultras.2009.02.003] [PMID: 19278707]

[128] Krasovitski B, Kimmel E. Shear stress induced by a gas bubble pulsating in an ultrasonic field near a wall. IEEE Trans Ultrason Ferroelectr Freq Control 2004; 51(8): 973-9.
[http://dx.doi.org/10.1109/TUFFC.2004.1324401] [PMID: 15344403]

[129] Koshiyama K, Kodama T, Yano T, Fujikawa S. Structural change in lipid bilayers and water penetration induced by shock waves: molecular dynamics simulations. Biophys J 2006; 91(6): 2198-205.
[http://dx.doi.org/10.1529/biophysj.105.077677] [PMID: 16798798]

[130] Selman GG, Jurand A. An electron microscope study of the endoplasmic reticulum in newt notochord cells after disturbance with ultrasonic treatment and subsequent regeneration. J Cell Biol 1964; 20: 175-83.
[http://dx.doi.org/10.1083/jcb.20.1.175] [PMID: 14105208]

[131] Frenkel V, Kimmel E, Iger Y. Ultrasound-induced intercellular space widening in fish epidermis. Ultrasound Med Biol 2000; 26(3): 473-80.
[http://dx.doi.org/10.1016/S0301-5629(99)00164-7] [PMID: 10773379]

[132] Lewin PA, Bjørnø L. Acoustically induced shear stresses in the vicinity of microbubbles in tissue. J Acoust Soc Am 1982; 71(3): 728-34.
[http://dx.doi.org/10.1121/1.387549]

[133] Church CC. The effect of an elastic solid surface layer on the radial pulsations of gas bubbles. J Acoust Soc Am 1995; 97(3): 1510-21.
[http://dx.doi.org/10.1121/1.412091]

[134] Huang H, Kamm RD, Lee RT. Cell mechanics and mechanotransduction: pathways, probes, and physiology. Am J Physiol Cell Physiol 2004; 287(1): C1-C11.
[http://dx.doi.org/10.1152/ajpcell.00559.2003] [PMID: 15189819]

[135] Lelièvre S, Weaver VM, Bissell MJ. Extracellular matrix signaling from the cellular membrane skeleton to the nuclear skeleton: a model of gene regulation. Recent Prog Horm Res 1996; 51: 417-32.
[PMID: 8701089]

[136] Ruwhof C, van der Laarse A. Mechanical stress-induced cardiac hypertrophy: mechanisms and signal transduction pathways. Cardiovasc Res 2000; 47(1): 23-37.
[http://dx.doi.org/10.1016/S0008-6363(00)00076-6] [PMID: 10869527]

[137] Basson MD. Paradigms for mechanical signal transduction in the intestinal epithelium. Category: molecular, cell, and developmental biology. Digestion 2003; 68(4): 217-25.
[http://dx.doi.org/10.1159/000076385] [PMID: 14739529]

[138] Kishikawa H, Miura S, Yoshida H, *et al.* Transmural pressure induces IL-6 secretion by intestinal epithelial cells. Clin Exp Immunol 2002; 129(1): 86-91.
[http://dx.doi.org/10.1046/j.1365-2249.2002.01895.x] [PMID: 12100026]

[139] Suslick KS. Sonochemistry. Science 1990; 247(4949): 1439-45.
[http://dx.doi.org/10.1126/science.247.4949.1439] [PMID: 17791211]

[140] Mason TJ. Introduction. In: Mason TJ, Ed. Chemistry with Ultrasound. Amsterdam: Elsevier Science 1990; pp. 1-26.

[141] Mason TJ. Sonochemistry: the uses of ultrasound in chemistry. Cambridge: Royal Society of Chemistry 1990.

[142] Mason TJ. Practical Sonochemistry: User's Guide to Applications in Chemistry and Chemical Engineering. Ellis Horwood Ltd 1991.

[143] Mason TJ, Lorimer JP. Applied Sonochemistry: Uses of Power Ultrasound in Chemistry and Processing. Wiley-VCH Verlag 2002.
[http://dx.doi.org/10.1002/352760054X]

[144] Brujan EA, Ikeda T, Matsumoto Y. Jet formation and shock wave emission during collapse of ultrasound-induced cavitation bubbles and their role in the therapeutic applications of high-intensity focused ultrasound. Phys Med Biol 2005; 50(20): 4797-809.
[http://dx.doi.org/10.1088/0031-9155/50/20/004] [PMID: 16204873]

[145] Feril LB Jr, Kondo T. Major factors involved in the inhibition of ultrasound-induced free radical production and cell killing by pre-sonication incubation or by high cell density. Ultrason Sonochem 2005; 12(5): 353-7.
[http://dx.doi.org/10.1016/j.ultsonch.2004.05.004] [PMID: 15590309]

[146] Krasovitski B, Frenkel V, Shoham S, Kimmel E. Intramembrane cavitation as a unifying mechanism for ultrasound-induced bioeffects. Proc Natl Acad Sci USA 2011; 108(8): 3258-63.
[http://dx.doi.org/10.1073/pnas.1015771108] [PMID: 21300891]

[147] Buldakov MA, Hassan MA, Zhao QL, *et al.* Influence of changing pulse repetition frequency on chemical and biological effects induced by low-intensity ultrasound *in vitro*. Ultrason Sonochem 2009; 16(3): 392-7.
[http://dx.doi.org/10.1016/j.ultsonch.2008.10.006] [PMID: 19022698]

[148] Forrest G, Rosen K. Ultrasound: effectiveness of treatments given under water. Arch Phys Med Rehabil 1989; 70(1): 28-9.
[PMID: 2916914]

[149] Brown SA, Greenbaum L, Shtukmaster S, Zadok Y, Ben-Ezra S, Kushkuley L. Characterization of nonthermal focused ultrasound for noninvasive selective fat cell disruption (lysis): technical and preclinical assessment. Plast Reconstr Surg 2009; 124(1): 92-101.
[http://dx.doi.org/10.1097/PRS.0b013e31819c59c7] [PMID: 19346998]

[150] Bélanger AY. Ultrasound. In: Bélanger AY, Ed. Evidence-Based Guide to Therapeutic Physical Agents. Philadelphia: Lippincott Williams & Wilkins 2003.

[151] Ahmadi F, McLoughlin IV, Chauhan S, ter-Haar G. Bio-effects and safety of low-intensity, low-frequency ultrasonic exposure. Prog Biophys Mol Biol 2012; 108(3): 119-38.
[http://dx.doi.org/10.1016/j.pbiomolbio.2012.01.004] [PMID: 22402278]

[152] Binder A, Hodge G, Greenwood AM, Hazleman BL, Page Thomas DP. Is therapeutic ultrasound effective in treating soft tissue lesions? Br Med J (Clin Res Ed) 1985; 290(6467): 512-4.
[http://dx.doi.org/10.1136/bmj.290.6467.512] [PMID: 3918652]

[153] DVaz AP, Ostor AJ, Speed CA, *et al.* Pulsed low-intensity ultrasound therapy for chronic lateral epicondylitis: a randomized controlled trial. Rheumatology (Oxford) 2006; 45(5): 566-70.
[http://dx.doi.org/10.1093/rheumatology/kei210] [PMID: 16303817]

[154] Padilla F, Puts R, Vico L, Guignandon A, Raum K. Stimulation of Bone Repair with Ultrasound. Adv Exp Med Biol 2016; 880(21): 385-427.
[http://dx.doi.org/10.1007/978-3-319-22536-4_21] [PMID: 26486349]

[155] Duarte LR. The stimulation of bone growth by ultrasound. Arch Orthop Trauma Surg 1983; 101(3): 153-9.
[http://dx.doi.org/10.1007/BF00436764] [PMID: 6870502]

[156] Pilla AA, Mont MA, Nasser PR, *et al.* Non-invasive low-intensity pulsed ultrasound accelerates bone healing in the rabbit. J Orthop Trauma 1990; 4(3): 246-53.
[http://dx.doi.org/10.1097/00005131-199004030-00002] [PMID: 2231120]

[157] Warden SJ, Fuchs RK, Kessler CK, Avin KG, Cardinal RE, Stewart RL. Ultrasound produced by a conventional therapeutic ultrasound unit accelerates fracture repair. Phys Ther 2006; 86(8): 1118-27.
[PMID: 16879045]

[158] Busse JW, Bhandari M, Kulkarni AV, Tunks E. The effect of low-intensity pulsed ultrasound therapy on time to fracture healing: a meta-analysis. CMAJ 2002; 166(4): 437-41.
[PMID: 11873920]

[159] Heckman JD, Ryaby JP, McCabe J, Frey JJ, Kilcoyne RF. Acceleration of tibial fracture-healing by non-invasive, low-intensity pulsed ultrasound. J Bone Joint Surg Am 1994; 76(1): 26-34.
[http://dx.doi.org/10.2106/00004623-199401000-00004] [PMID: 8288661]

[160] Kristiansen TK, Ryaby JP, McCabe J, Frey JJ, Roe LR. Accelerated healing of distal radial fractures with the use of specific, low-intensity ultrasound. A multicenter, prospective, randomized, double-blind, placebo-controlled study. J Bone Joint Surg Am 1997; 79(7): 961-73.
[http://dx.doi.org/10.2106/00004623-199707000-00002] [PMID: 9234872]

[161] Mayr E, Rudzki MM, Rudzki M, Borchardt B, Häusser H, Rüter A. Beschleunigt niedrig intensiver, gepulster Ultraschall die Heilung von Skaphoidfrakturen? Handchir Mikrochir Plast Chir 2000; 32(2): 115-22.
[http://dx.doi.org/10.1055/s-2000-19253] [PMID: 10857066]

[162] Cook SD, Ryaby JP, McCabe J, Frey JJ, Heckman JD, Kristiansen TK. Acceleration of tibia and distal radius fracture healing in patients who smoke. Clin Orthop Relat Res 1997; (337): 198-207.
[http://dx.doi.org/10.1097/00003086-199704000-00022] [PMID: 9137191]

[163] Emami A, Petrén-Mallmin M, Larsson S. No effect of low-intensity ultrasound on healing time of intramedullary fixed tibial fractures. J Orthop Trauma 1999; 13(4): 252-7.
[http://dx.doi.org/10.1097/00005131-199905000-00005] [PMID: 10342350]

[164] Emami A, Larsson A, Petrén-Mallmin M, Larsson S. Serum bone markers after intramedullary fixed tibial fractures. Clin Orthop Relat Res 1999; (368): 220-9.
[PMID: 10613172]

[165] Warden SJ, Bennell KL, McMeeken JM, Wark JD. Acceleration of fresh fracture repair using the sonic accelerated fracture healing system (SAFHS): a review. Calcif Tissue Int 2000; 66(2): 157-63.
[http://dx.doi.org/10.1007/s002230010031] [PMID: 10652965]

[166] Hadjiargyrou M, McLeod K, Ryaby JP, Rubin C. Enhancement of fracture healing by low intensity ultrasound. Clin Orthop Relat Res 1998; (355): (Suppl.)S216-29.
[http://dx.doi.org/10.1097/00003086-199810001-00022] [PMID: 9917641]

[167] Pounder NM, Harrison AJ. Low intensity pulsed ultrasound for fracture healing: a review of the clinical evidence and the associated biological mechanism of action. Ultrasonics 2008; 48(4): 330-8.
[http://dx.doi.org/10.1016/j.ultras.2008.02.005] [PMID: 18486959]

[168] Einhorn TA. The cell and molecular biology of fracture healing. Clin Orthop Relat Res 1998; (355): (Suppl.)S7-S21.
[http://dx.doi.org/10.1097/00003086-199810001-00003] [PMID: 9917622]

[169] Claes L, Willie B. The enhancement of bone regeneration by ultrasound. Prog Biophys Mol Biol 2007; 93(1-3): 384-98.
[http://dx.doi.org/10.1016/j.pbiomolbio.2006.07.021] [PMID: 16934857]

[170] Tai K, Pelled G, Sheyn D, *et al.* Nanobiomechanics of repair bone regenerated by genetically modified mesenchymal stem cells. Tissue Eng Part A 2008; 14(10): 1709-20.
[http://dx.doi.org/10.1089/ten.tea.2007.0241] [PMID: 18620480]

[171] Sun JS, Hong RC, Chang WH, Chen LT, Lin FH, Liu HC. *In vitro* effects of low-intensity ultrasound stimulation on the bone cells. J Biomed Mater Res 2001; 57(3): 449-56.
[http://dx.doi.org/10.1002/1097-4636(20011205)57:3<449::AID-JBM1188>3.0.CO;2-0]   [PMID: 11523040]

[172] Snow CJ, Johnson KA. Effects of therapeutic ultrasound on acute inflammation. Physiotherapy 1987; 73(3): 116-20.

[173] Martinez de Albornoz P, Khanna A, Longo UG, Forriol F, Maffulli N. The evidence of low-intensity pulsed ultrasound for *in vitro*, animal and human fracture healing. Br Med Bull 2011; 100: 39-57.
[http://dx.doi.org/10.1093/bmb/ldr006] [PMID: 21429948]

[174]   Maxwell L, Collecutt T, Gledhill M, Sharma S, Edgar S, Gavin JB. The augmentation of leucocyte adhesion to endothelium by therapeutic ultrasound. Ultrasound Med Biol 1994; 20(4): 383-90.
[http://dx.doi.org/10.1016/0301-5629(94)90007-8] [PMID: 8085295]

[175]   Dyson M, Luke DA. Induction of mast cell degranulation in skin by ultrasound. IEEE Trans Ultrason Ferroelectr Freq Control 1986; 33(2): 194-201.
[http://dx.doi.org/10.1109/T-UFFC.1986.26814] [PMID: 18291771]

[176]   Young SR, Dyson M. Macrophage responsiveness to therapeutic ultrasound. Ultrasound Med Biol 1990; 16(8): 809-16.
[http://dx.doi.org/10.1016/0301-5629(90)90045-E] [PMID: 2095011]

[177]   Rappolee DA, Werb Z. Macrophage-derived growth factors. Curr Top Microbiol Immunol 1992; 181: 87-140.
[http://dx.doi.org/10.1007/978-3-642-77377-8_4] [PMID: 1424786]

[178]   Reher P, Doan N, Bradnock B, Meghji S, Harris M. Effect of ultrasound on the production of IL-8, basic FGF and VEGF. Cytokine 1999; 11(6): 416-23.
[http://dx.doi.org/10.1006/cyto.1998.0444] [PMID: 10346981]

[179]   Wu CC. Exposure to low intensity ultrasound stimulates aggrecan gene expression by cultured chondrocytes. Trans Orthop Res Soc 1996; 21: 622.

[180]   Yang KH, Parvizi J, Wang SJ, *et al.* Exposure to low-intensity ultrasound increases aggrecan gene expression in a rat femur fracture model. J Orthop Res 1996; 14(5): 802-9.
[http://dx.doi.org/10.1002/jor.1100140518] [PMID: 8893775]

[181]   Parvizi J, Parpura V, Greenleaf JF, Bolander ME. Calcium signaling is required for ultrasound-stimulated aggrecan synthesis by rat chondrocytes. J Orthop Res 2002; 20(1): 51-7.
[http://dx.doi.org/10.1016/S0736-0266(01)00069-9] [PMID: 11853090]

[182]   Parvizi J, Parpura V, Kinnick RR, Greenleaf JF, Bolander ME. Low intensity ultrasound increases intracellular concentrations of calcium in chondrocytes. Trans Orthop Res Soc 1997; 22: 465.

[183]   Mortimer AJ, Dyson M. The effect of therapeutic ultrasound on calcium uptake in fibroblasts. Ultrasound Med Biol 1988; 14(6): 499-506.
[http://dx.doi.org/10.1016/0301-5629(88)90111-1] [PMID: 3227573]

[184]   Elmer WA, Fleischer AC. Enhancement of DNA synthesis in neonatal mouse tibial epiphyses after exposure to therapeutic ultrasound. J Clin Ultrasound 1974; 2(3): 191-5.
[http://dx.doi.org/10.1002/jcu.1870020307] [PMID: 4220238]

[185]   Wiltink A, Nijweide PJ, Oosterbaan WA, Hekkenberg RT, Helders PJ. Effect of therapeutic ultrasound on endochondral ossification. Ultrasound Med Biol 1995; 21(1): 121-7.
[http://dx.doi.org/10.1016/0301-5629(94)00092-1] [PMID: 7754572]

[186]   Nolte PA, Klein-Nulend J, Albers GH, *et al.* Low-intensity ultrasound stimulates endochondral ossification *in vitro*. J Orthop Res 2001; 19(2): 301-7.
[http://dx.doi.org/10.1016/S0736-0266(00)00027-9] [PMID: 11347705]

[187]   Rutten S, Nolte PA, Guit GL, Bouman DE, Albers GH. Use of low-intensity pulsed ultrasound for posttraumatic nonunions of the tibia: a review of patients treated in the Netherlands. J Trauma 2007; 62(4): 902-8.
[http://dx.doi.org/10.1097/01.ta.0000238663.33796.fb] [PMID: 17426546]

[188]   Romano CL, Romano D, Logoluso N. Low-intensity pulsed ultrasound for the treatment of bone delayed union or nonunion: a review. Ultrasound Med Biol 2009; 35(4): 529-36.
[http://dx.doi.org/10.1016/j.ultrasmedbio.2008.09.029] [PMID: 19097683]

[189] Bashardoust Tajali S, Houghton P, MacDermid JC, Grewal R. Effects of low-intensity pulsed ultrasound therapy on fracture healing: a systematic review and meta-analysis. Am J Phys Med Rehabil 2012; 91(4): 349-67.
[http://dx.doi.org/10.1097/PHM.0b013e31822419ba] [PMID: 21904188]

[190] Snyder BM, Conley J, Koval KJ. Does low-intensity pulsed ultrasound reduce time to fracture healing? A meta-analysis. Am J Orthop 2012; 41(2): E12-9.
[PMID: 22482096]

[191] Francis CW, Önundarson PT, Carstensen EL, *et al.* Enhancement of fibrinolysis *in vitro* by ultrasound. J Clin Invest 1992; 90(5): 2063-8.
[http://dx.doi.org/10.1172/JCI116088] [PMID: 1430229]

[192] Blinc A, Francis CW, Trudnowski JL, Carstensen EL. Characterization of ultrasound-potentiated fibrinolysis *in vitro*. Blood 1993; 81(10): 2636-43.
[PMID: 8490172]

[193] Young SR, Dyson M. The effect of therapeutic ultrasound on angiogenesis. Ultrasound Med Biol 1990; 16(3): 261-9.
[http://dx.doi.org/10.1016/0301-5629(90)90005-W] [PMID: 1694604]

[194] Carvalho PdeT, Silva IS, Reis FA, *et al.* Histological study of tendon healing in malnourished Wistar rats treated with ultrasound therapy. Acta Cir Bras 2006; 21 (Suppl. 4): 13-7.
[http://dx.doi.org/10.1590/S0102-86502006001000004] [PMID: 17293959]

[195] Fyfe MC, Chahl LA. The effect of ultrasound on experimental oedema in rats. Ultrasound Med Biol 1980; 6(2): 107-11.
[http://dx.doi.org/10.1016/0301-5629(80)90038-1] [PMID: 7404841]

[196] Szumski AJ. Mechanisms of pain relief as a result of therapeutic application of ultrasound. Phys Ther Rev 1960; 40: 116-9.
[PMID: 13836468]

[197] Culav EM, Clark CH, Merrilees MJ. Connective tissues: matrix composition and its relevance to physical therapy. Phys Ther 1999; 79(3): 308-19.
[PMID: 10078774]

[198] Aparecida de Aro A, Vidal B de C, Pimentel ER. Biochemical and anisotropical properties of tendons. Micron 2012; 43(2-3): 205-14.
[http://dx.doi.org/10.1016/j.micron.2011.07.015] [PMID: 21890364]

[199] Ingber DE, Dike L, Hansen L, *et al.* Cellular tensegrity: exploring how mechanical changes in the cytoskeleton regulate cell growth, migration, and tissue pattern during morphogenesis. Int Rev Cytol 1994; 150: 173-224.
[http://dx.doi.org/10.1016/S0074-7696(08)61542-9] [PMID: 8169080]

[200] Sachs F. Mechanical transduction by membrane ion channels: a mini review. Mol Cell Biochem 1991; 104(1-2): 57-60.
[http://dx.doi.org/10.1007/BF00229804] [PMID: 1717821]

[201] Webster DF, Harvey W, Dyson M, Pond JB. The role of ultrasound-induced cavitation in the *in vitro* stimulation of collagen synthesis in human fibroblasts. Ultrasonics 1980; 18(1): 33-7.
[http://dx.doi.org/10.1016/0041-624X(80)90050-5] [PMID: 7350723]

[202] Doan N, Reher P, Meghji S, Harris M. *in vitro* effects of therapeutic ultrasound on cell proliferation, protein synthesis, and cytokine production by human fibroblasts, osteoblasts, and monocytes. J Oral Maxillofac Surg 1999; 57(4): 409-19.
[http://dx.doi.org/10.1016/S0278-2391(99)90281-1] [PMID: 10199493]

[203] Chiquet M. Regulation of extracellular matrix gene expression by mechanical stress. Matrix Biol 1999; 18(5): 417-26.
[http://dx.doi.org/10.1016/S0945-053X(99)00039-6] [PMID: 10601729]

[204] Kobayashi Y, Sakai D, Iwashina T, Iwabuchi S, Mochida J. Low-intensity pulsed ultrasound stimulates cell proliferation, proteoglycan synthesis and expression of growth factor-related genes in human nucleus pulposus cell line. Eur Cell Mater 2009; 17: 15-22.
[http://dx.doi.org/10.22203/eCM.v017a02] [PMID: 19598131]

[205] Riser BL, Cortes P, Heilig C, *et al.* Cyclic stretching force selectively up-regulates transforming growth factor-beta isoforms in cultured rat mesangial cells. Am J Pathol 1996; 148(6): 1915-23.
[PMID: 8669477]

[206] Hori Y, Katoh T, Hirakata M, *et al.* Anti-latent TGF-beta binding protein-1 antibody or synthetic oligopeptides inhibit extracellular matrix expression induced by stretch in cultured rat mesangial cells. Kidney Int 1998; 53(6): 1616-25.
[http://dx.doi.org/10.1046/j.1523-1755.1998.00908.x] [PMID: 9607192]

[207] Gutierrez JA, Perr HA. Mechanical stretch modulates TGF-beta1 and alpha1(I) collagen expression in fetal human intestinal smooth muscle cells. Am J Physiol 1999; 277(5 Pt 1): G1074-80.
[PMID: 10564114]

[208] Lee AA, Delhaas T, McCulloch AD, Villarreal FJ. Differential responses of adult cardiac fibroblasts to *in vitro* biaxial strain patterns. J Mol Cell Cardiol 1999; 31(10): 1833-43.
[http://dx.doi.org/10.1006/jmcc.1999.1017] [PMID: 10525421]

[209] Lindahl GE, Chambers RC, Papakrivopoulou J, *et al.* Activation of fibroblast procollagen alpha 1(I) transcription by mechanical strain is transforming growth factor-beta-dependent and involves increased binding of CCAAT-binding factor (CBF/NF-Y) at the proximal promoter. J Biol Chem 2002; 277(8): 6153-61.
[http://dx.doi.org/10.1074/jbc.M108966200] [PMID: 11748224]

[210] Chambers RC, Laurent GJ. Collagens. In: Crystal RD, West JB, Weibel ER, Barnes PJ, Eds. The Lung: Scientific Foundations. Philadelphia: Lippincott-Raven 1997; pp. 709-27.

[211] Webster DF, Harvey W, Dyson M, Pond JB. The role of ultrasound-induced cavitation in the 'in vitro' stimulation of collagen synthesis in human fibroblasts. Ultrasonics. 1980; 18: pp. (1)33-7.

[212] Frieder S, Weisberg J, Fleming B, Stanek A. A pilot study: the therapeutic effect of ultrasound following partial rupture of Achilles tendons in male rats. J Orthop Sports Phys Ther 1988; 10(2): 39-46.
[http://dx.doi.org/10.2519/jospt.1988.10.2.39] [PMID: 18796976]

[213] Byl NN, McKenzie AL, West JM, Whitney JD, Hunt TK, Scheuenstuhl HA. Low-dose ultrasound effects on wound healing: a controlled study with Yucatan pigs. Arch Phys Med Rehabil 1992; 73(7): 656-64.
[PMID: 1622322]

[214] Byl NN, McKenzie A, Wong T, West J, Hunt TK. Incisional wound healing: a controlled study of low and high dose ultrasound. J Orthop Sports Phys Ther 1993; 18(5): 619-28.
[http://dx.doi.org/10.2519/jospt.1993.18.5.619] [PMID: 8268965]

[215] Pocock BJZ. The effect of therapeutic ultrasound on the mechanical properties of surgical incisions in Wistar rats BSc thesis. London: University of London 1994.

[216] Leung MC, Ng GY, Yip KK. Effect of ultrasound on acute inflammation of transected medial collateral ligaments. Arch Phys Med Rehabil 2004; 85(6): 963-6.
[http://dx.doi.org/10.1016/j.apmr.2003.07.018] [PMID: 15179651]

[217] da Cunha A, Parizotto NA, Vidal B de C. The effect of therapeutic ultrasound on repair of the Achilles tendon (*tendo calcaneus*) of the rat. Ultrasound Med Biol 2001; 27(12): 1691-6.
[http://dx.doi.org/10.1016/S0301-5629(01)00477-X] [PMID: 11839414]

[218] Frasson NF, Taciro C, Parizotto NA. Análise nanoestrutural da ação do ultra-som terapêutico sobre o processo de regeneração do tendão de ratos. Fisioter Pesqui 2009; 16(3): 198-204.
[http://dx.doi.org/10.1590/S1809-29502009000300002]

[219] Jackson BA, Schwane JA, Starcher BC. Effect of ultrasound therapy on the repair of Achilles tendon injuries in rats. Med Sci Sports Exerc 1991; 23(2): 171-6.
[http://dx.doi.org/10.1249/00005768-199102000-00005] [PMID: 2017013]

[220] Ng GY, Ng CO, See EK. Comparison of therapeutic ultrasound and exercises for augmenting tendon healing in rats. Ultrasound Med Biol 2004; 30(11): 1539-43.
[http://dx.doi.org/10.1016/j.ultrasmedbio.2004.08.030] [PMID: 15588965]

[221] Yeung CK, Guo X, Ng YF. Pulsed ultrasound treatment accelerates the repair of Achilles tendon rupture in rats. J Orthop Res 2006; 24(2): 193-201.
[http://dx.doi.org/10.1002/jor.20020] [PMID: 16435348]

[222] Sparrow KJ, Finucane SD, Owen JR, Wayne JS. The effects of low-intensity ultrasound on medial collateral ligament healing in the rabbit model. Am J Sports Med 2005; 33(7): 1048-56.
[http://dx.doi.org/10.1177/0363546504267356] [PMID: 15888724]

[223] Warden SJ, Avin KG, Beck EM, DeWolf ME, Hagemeier MA, Martin KM. Low-intensity pulsed ultrasound accelerates and a nonsteroidal anti-inflammatory drug delays knee ligament healing. Am J Sports Med 2006; 34(7): 1094-102.
[http://dx.doi.org/10.1177/0363546505286139] [PMID: 16476921]

[224] Jeremias Júnior SL, Camanho GL, Bassit AC, Forgas A, Ingham SJ, Abdalla RJ. Low-intensity pulsed ultrasound accelerates healing in rat calcaneus tendon injuries. J Orthop Sports Phys Ther 2011; 41(7): 526-31.
[http://dx.doi.org/10.2519/jospt.2011.3468] [PMID: 21335926]

[225] Kerr CL, Gregory DW, Chan KK, Watmough DJ, Wheatley DN. Ultrasound-induced damage of veins in pig ears, as revealed by scanning electron microscopy. Ultrasound Med Biol 1989; 15(1): 45-52.
[http://dx.doi.org/10.1016/0301-5629(89)90131-2] [PMID: 2922880]

[226] De Deyne PG, Kirsch-Volders M. *In vitro* effects of therapeutic ultrasound on the nucleus of human fibroblasts. Phys Ther 1995; 75(7): 629-34.
[http://dx.doi.org/10.1093/ptj/75.7.629] [PMID: 7604082]

[227] Wessling KC, DeVane DA, Hylton CR. Effects of static stretch versus static stretch and ultrasound combined on triceps surae muscle extensibility in healthy women. Phys Ther 1987; 67(5): 674-9.
[http://dx.doi.org/10.1093/ptj/67.5.674] [PMID: 3575424]

[228] Usuba M, Miyanaga Y, Miyakawa S, Maeshima T, Shirasaki Y. Effect of heat in increasing the range of knee motion after the development of a joint contracture: an experiment with an animal model. Arch Phys Med Rehabil 2006; 87(2): 247-53.
[http://dx.doi.org/10.1016/j.apmr.2005.10.015] [PMID: 16442980]

[229] Cameron MH. Physical Agents in Rehabilitation – From Research to Practice. 4th ed., St. Louis, MO: Elsevier Inc. 2013.

[230] Chargé SB, Rudnicki MA. Cellular and molecular regulation of muscle regeneration. Physiol Rev 2004; 84(1): 209-38.
[http://dx.doi.org/10.1152/physrev.00019.2003] [PMID: 14715915]

[231] Schmalbruch H, Lewis DM. Dynamics of nuclei of muscle fibers and connective tissue cells in normal and denervated rat muscles. Muscle Nerve 2000; 23(4): 617-26.
[http://dx.doi.org/10.1002/(SICI)1097-4598(200004)23:4<617::AID-MUS22>3.0.CO;2-Y] [PMID: 10716774]

[232] Kasemkijwattana C, Menetrey J, Somogyl G, *et al.* Development of approaches to improve the healing following muscle contusion. Cell Transplant 1998; 7(6): 585-98.
[http://dx.doi.org/10.1016/S0963-6897(98)00037-2] [PMID: 9853587]

[233] Menetrey J, Kasemkijwattana C, Fu FH, Moreland MS, Huard J. Suturing versus immobilization of a muscle laceration. A morphological and functional study in a mouse model. Am J Sports Med 1999; 27(2): 222-9.
[PMID: 10102105]

[234] Taylor DC, Dalton JD Jr, Seaber AV, Garrett WE Jr. Experimental muscle strain injury. Early functional and structural deficits and the increased risk for reinjury. Am J Sports Med 1993; 21(2): 190-4.
[http://dx.doi.org/10.1177/036354659302100205] [PMID: 8465911]

[235] Nicholson GA, Gardner-Medwin D, Pennington RJ, Walton JN. Carrier detection in Duchenne muscular dystrophy: Assessment of the effect of age on detection-rate with serum-creatine-kinae-activity. Lancet 1979; 1(8118): 692-4.
[http://dx.doi.org/10.1016/S0140-6736(79)91147-4] [PMID: 85935]

[236] Coulton GR, Morgan JE, Partridge TA, Sloper JC. The mdx mouse skeletal muscle myopathy: I. A histological, morphometric and biochemical investigation. Neuropathol Appl Neurobiol 1988; 14(1): 53-70.
[http://dx.doi.org/10.1111/j.1365-2990.1988.tb00866.x] [PMID: 2967442]

[237] Sorichter S, Mair J, Koller A, *et al.* Creatine kinase, myosin heavy chains and magnetic resonance imaging after eccentric exercise. J Sports Sci 2001; 19(9): 687-91.
[http://dx.doi.org/10.1080/02640410152475810] [PMID: 11522144]

[238] Chetverikova EP, Pashovkin TN, Rosanova NA, Sarvazyan AP, Williams AR. Interaction of therapeutic ultrasound with purified enzymes *in vitro*. Ultrasonics 1985; 23(4): 183-8.
[http://dx.doi.org/10.1016/0041-624X(85)90028-9] [PMID: 4012893]

[239] Johns LD. Nonthermal effects of therapeutic ultrasound: the frequency resonance hypothesis. J Athl Train 2002; 37(3): 293-9.
[PMID: 16558674]

[240] Orimo S, Hiyamuta E, Arahata K, Sugita H. Analysis of inflammatory cells and complement C3 in bupivacaine-induced myonecrosis. Muscle Nerve 1991; 14(6): 515-20.
[http://dx.doi.org/10.1002/mus.880140605] [PMID: 1852158]

[241] Fielding RA, Manfredi TJ, Ding W, Fiatarone MA, Evans WJ, Cannon JG. Acute phase response in exercise. III. Neutrophil and IL-1 beta accumulation in skeletal muscle. Am J Physiol 1993; 265(1 Pt 2): R166-72.
[PMID: 8342683]

[242] Robertson TA, Maley MA, Grounds MD, Papadimitriou JM. The role of macrophages in skeletal muscle regeneration with particular reference to chemotaxis. Exp Cell Res 1993; 207(2): 321-31.
[http://dx.doi.org/10.1006/excr.1993.1199] [PMID: 8344384]

[243] Tidball JG. Inflammatory cell response to acute muscle injury. Med Sci Sports Exerc 1995; 27(7): 1022-32.
[http://dx.doi.org/10.1249/00005768-199507000-00011] [PMID: 7564969]

[244] Lescaudron L, Peltékian E, Fontaine-Pérus J, *et al.* Blood borne macrophages are essential for the triggering of muscle regeneration following muscle transplant. Neuromuscul Disord 1999; 9(2): 72-80.
[http://dx.doi.org/10.1016/S0960-8966(98)00111-4] [PMID: 10220861]

[245] Merly F, Lescaudron L, Rouaud T, Crossin F, Gardahaut MF. Macrophages enhance muscle satellite cell proliferation and delay their differentiation. Muscle Nerve 1999; 22(6): 724-32.
[http://dx.doi.org/10.1002/(SICI)1097-4598(199906)22:6<724::AID-MUS9>3.0.CO;2-O] [PMID: 10366226]

[246] Wigmore PM, Evans DJ. Molecular and cellular mechanisms involved in the generation of fiber diversity during myogenesis. Int Rev Cytol 2002; 216: 175-232.
[http://dx.doi.org/10.1016/S0074-7696(02)16006-2] [PMID: 12049208]

[247] Mauro A. Satellite cell of skeletal muscle fibers. J Biophys Biochem Cytol 1961; 9: 493-5.
[http://dx.doi.org/10.1083/jcb.9.2.493] [PMID: 13768451]

[248] Campion DR. The muscle satellite cell: a review. Int Rev Cytol 1984; 87: 225-51.
[http://dx.doi.org/10.1016/S0074-7696(08)62444-4] [PMID: 6370890]

[249] Allen RE, Rankin LL. Regulation of satellite cells during skeletal muscle growth and development. Proc Soc Exp Biol Med 1990; 194(2): 81-6.
[http://dx.doi.org/10.3181/00379727-194-43060] [PMID: 2190237]

[250] Zammit PS. The muscle satellite cell: the story of a cell on the edge! In: Schiaffino S, Partridge P, Eds. Skeletal Muscle Repair and Regeneration. Berlin: Springer 2008; 3: pp. 45-64.

[251] Boonen KJ, Post MJ. The muscle stem cell niche: regulation of satellite cells during regeneration. Tissue Eng Part B Rev 2008; 14(4): 419-31.
[http://dx.doi.org/10.1089/ten.teb.2008.0045] [PMID: 18817477]

[252] Berdeaux R, Stewart R. cAMP signaling in skeletal muscle adaptation: hypertrophy, metabolism, and regeneration. Am J Physiol Endocrinol Metab 2012; 303(1): E1-E17.
[http://dx.doi.org/10.1152/ajpendo.00555.2011] [PMID: 22354781]

[253] Yin H, Price F, Rudnicki MA. Satellite cells and the muscle stem cell niche. Physiol Rev 2013; 93(1): 23-67.
[http://dx.doi.org/10.1152/physrev.00043.2011] [PMID: 23303905]

[254] Rantanen J, Thorsson O, Wollmer P, Hurme T, Kalimo H. Effects of therapeutic ultrasound on the regeneration of skeletal myofibers after experimental muscle injury. Am J Sports Med 1999; 27(1): 54-9.
[PMID: 9934419]

[255] Karnes JL, Burton HW. Continuous therapeutic ultrasound accelerates repair of contraction-induced skeletal muscle damage in rats. Arch Phys Med Rehabil 2002; 83(1): 1-4.
[http://dx.doi.org/10.1053/apmr.2002.26254] [PMID: 11782824]

[256] Matheus JP, Oliveira FB, Gomide LB, Milani JG, Volpon JB, Shimano AC. Effects of therapeutic ultrasound on the mechanical properties of skeletal muscles. Rev Bras Fisioter 2008; 12(3): 241-7.
[http://dx.doi.org/10.1590/S1413-35552008000300013]

[257] Abrunhosa VM, Mermelstein CS, Costa ML, Costa-Felix RP. Biological response *in vitro* of skeletal muscle cells treated with different intensity continuous and pulsed ultrasound fields. J Phys Conf Ser 2011; 279: 012022.
[http://dx.doi.org/10.1088/1742-6596/279/1/012022]

[258] Ebenbichler GR, Resch KL, Nicolakis P, *et al.* Ultrasound treatment for treating the carpal tunnel syndrome: randomised sham controlled trial. BMJ 1998; 316(7133): 731-5.
[http://dx.doi.org/10.1136/bmj.316.7133.731] [PMID: 9529407]

[259] Ebenbichler GR, Erdogmus CB, Resch KL, *et al.* Ultrasound therapy for calcific tendinitis of the shoulder. N Engl J Med 1999; 340(20): 1533-8.
[http://dx.doi.org/10.1056/NEJM199905203402002] [PMID: 10332014]

[260] Kerwin G, Williams CS, Seiler JG III. The pathophysiology of carpal tunnel syndrome. Hand Clin 1996; 12(2): 243-51.
[PMID: 8724576]

[261] Werner RA, Andary M. Carpal tunnel syndrome: pathophysiology and clinical neurophysiology. Clin Neurophysiol 2002; 113(9): 1373-81.
[http://dx.doi.org/10.1016/S1388-2457(02)00169-4] [PMID: 12169318]

[262] Rozmaryn LM, Dovelle S, Rothman ER, Gorman K, Olvey KM, Bartko JJ. Nerve and tendon gliding exercises and the conservative management of carpal tunnel syndrome. J Hand Ther 1998; 11(3): 171-9.
[http://dx.doi.org/10.1016/S0894-1130(98)80035-5] [PMID: 9730093]

[263] Nathan PA, Keniston RC, Myers LD, Meadows KD, Lockwood RS. Natural history of median nerve sensory conduction in industry: relationship to symptoms and carpal tunnel syndrome in 558 hands over 11 years. Muscle Nerve 1998; 21(6): 711-21.
[http://dx.doi.org/10.1002/(SICI)1097-4598(199806)21:6<711::AID-MUS2>3.0.CO;2-A] [PMID: 9585324]

[264] Yildiz N, Atalay NS, Gungen GO, Sanal E, Akkaya N, Topuz O. Comparison of ultrasound and ketoprofen phonophoresis in the treatment of carpal tunnel syndrome. J Back Musculoskeletal Rehabil 2011; 24(1): 39-47.
[http://dx.doi.org/10.3233/BMR-2011-0273] [PMID: 21248399]

[265] Oztas O, Turan B, Bora I, Karakaya MK. Ultrasound therapy effect in carpal tunnel syndrome. Arch Phys Med Rehabil 1998; 79(12): 1540-4.
[http://dx.doi.org/10.1016/S0003-9993(98)90416-6] [PMID: 9862296]

[266] Aygül R, Ulvi H, Karatay S, Deniz O, Varoglu AO. Determination of sensitive electrophysiologic parameters at follow-up of different steroid treatments of carpal tunnel syndrome. J Clin Neurophysiol 2005; 22(3): 222-30.
[PMID: 15933496]

[267] Gerritsen AA, de Vet HC, Scholten RJ, Bertelsmann FW, de Krom MC, Bouter LM. Splinting vs surgery in the treatment of carpal tunnel syndrome: a randomized controlled trial. JAMA 2002; 288(10): 1245-51.
[http://dx.doi.org/10.1001/jama.288.10.1245] [PMID: 12215131]

[268] Piravej K, Boonhong J. Effect of ultrasound thermotherapy in mild to moderate carpal tunnel syndrome. J Med Assoc Thai 2004; 87 (Suppl. 2): S100-6.
[PMID: 16083171]

[269] Baysal O, Altay Z, Ozcan C, Ertem K, Yologlu S, Kayhan A. Comparison of three conservative treatment protocols in carpal tunnel syndrome. Int J Clin Pract 2006; 60(7): 820-8.
[http://dx.doi.org/10.1111/j.1742-1241.2006.00867.x] [PMID: 16704676]

[270] Ekim A, Colak E. Ultrasound treatment in carpal tunnel syndrome: a placebo controlled study. Turkish Journal of Physical Medicine and Rehabilitation 2008.

[271] Dincer U, Cakar E, Kiralp MZ, Kilac H, Dursun H. The effectiveness of conservative treatments of carpal tunnel syndrome: splinting, ultrasound, and low-level laser therapies. Photomed Laser Surg 2009; 27(1): 119-25.
[http://dx.doi.org/10.1089/pho.2008.2211] [PMID: 19196106]

[272] Duymaz T, Sindel D, Kesiktas N, Muslumanoglu L. Efficacy of some combined conservative methods in the treatment of carpal tunnel syndrome: a randomized controlled clinical and electrophysiological trial. Turk J Rheum 2012; 27: 1.
[http://dx.doi.org/10.5606/tjr.2012.005]

[273] Carlson H, Colbert A, Frydl J, Arnall E, Elliot M, Carlson N. Current options for nonsurgical management of carpal tunnel syndrome. Int J Clin Rheumatol 2010; 5(1): 129-42.
[http://dx.doi.org/10.2217/ijr.09.63] [PMID: 20490348]

[274] Hasan A, Murata H, Falabella A, *et al.* Dermal fibroblasts from venous ulcers are unresponsive to the action of transforming growth factor-β 1. J Dermatol Sci 1997; 16(1): 59-66.
[http://dx.doi.org/10.1016/S0923-1811(97)00622-1] [PMID: 9438909]

[275] Agren MS, Steenfos HH, Dabelsteen S, Hansen JB, Dabelsteen E. Proliferation and mitogenic response to PDGF-BB of fibroblasts isolated from chronic venous leg ulcers is ulcer-age dependent. J Invest Dermatol 1999; 112(4): 463-9.
[PMID: 10201530]

[276] Cook H, Davies KJ, Harding KG, Thomas DW. Defective extracellular matrix reorganization by chronic wound fibroblasts is associated with alterations in TIMP-1, TIMP-2, and MMP-2 activity. J Invest Dermatol 2000; 115(2): 225-33.
[http://dx.doi.org/10.1046/j.1523-1747.2000.00044.x] [PMID: 10951240]

[277] Zhang H, Landmann F, Zahreddine H, Rodriguez D, Koch M, Labouesse M. A tension-induced mechanotransduction pathway promotes epithelial morphogenesis. Nature 2011; 471(7336): 99-103.
[http://dx.doi.org/10.1038/nature09765] [PMID: 21368832]

[278] Lancerotto L, Bayer LR, Orgill DP. Mechanisms of action of microdeformational wound therapy. Semin Cell Dev Biol 2012; 23(9): 987-92.
[http://dx.doi.org/10.1016/j.semcdb.2012.09.009] [PMID: 23036531]

[279] Chokshi SK, Rongione AJ, Freeman I, Gal D, Gunwald AM, Alliger W. Ultrasonic energy produces endothelium dependent vasomotor-relaxation *in vitro*. Circulation 1989; 80 (Suppl. 2): 565.

[280] Fischell TA, Abbas MA, Grant GW, Siegel RJ. Ultrasonic energy. Effects on vascular function and integrity. Circulation 1991; 84(4): 1783-95.
[http://dx.doi.org/10.1161/01.CIR.84.4.1783] [PMID: 1914114]

[281] Steffen W, Cumberland D, Gaines P, *et al.* Catheter-delivered high intensity, low frequency ultrasound induces vasodilation *in vivo*. Eur Heart J 1994; 15(3): 369-76.
[http://dx.doi.org/10.1093/oxfordjournals.eurheartj.a060505] [PMID: 8013511]

[282] Pardi R, Inverardi L, Bender JR. Regulatory mechanisms in leukocyte adhesion: flexible receptors for sophisticated travelers. Immunol Today 1992; 13(6): 224-30.
[http://dx.doi.org/10.1016/0167-5699(92)90159-5] [PMID: 1304726]

[283] Rustad KC, Wong VW, Gurtner GC. The role of focal adhesion complexes in fibroblast mechanotransduction during scar formation. Differentiation 2013; 86(3): 87-91.
[http://dx.doi.org/10.1016/j.diff.2013.02.003] [PMID: 23623400]

[284] McDiarmid T, Burns PN, Lewith GT, *et al.* Ultrasound and the treatment of pressure sores. Physiotherapy 1985; 71: 66-70.

[285] Lundeberg T, Nordström F, Brodda-Jansen G, Eriksson SV, Kjartansson J, Samuelson UE. Pulsed ultrasound does not improve healing of venous ulcers. Scand J Rehabil Med 1990; 22(4): 195-7.
[PMID: 2263919]

[286] Eriksson SV, Lundeberg T, Malm M. A placebo controlled trial of ultrasound therapy in chronic leg ulceration. Scand J Rehabil Med 1991; 23(4): 211-3.
[PMID: 1785031]

[287] Baba-Akbari Sari A, Flemming K, Cullum NA, Wollina U. Therapeutic ultrasound for pressure ulcers. Cochrane Database Syst Rev 2006; (3): CD001275.
[PMID: 16855964]

[288] Cullum NA, Al-Kurdi D, Bell-Syer SE. Therapeutic ultrasound for venous leg ulcers. Cochrane Database Syst Rev 2010; (6): CD001180.
[PMID: 20556749]

[289] Ennis WJ, Valdes W, Gainer M, Meneses P. Evaluation of clinical effectiveness of MIST ultrasound therapy for the healing of chronic wounds. Adv Skin Wound Care 2006; 19(8): 437-46.
[http://dx.doi.org/10.1097/00129334-200610000-00011] [PMID: 17008814]

[290] Kavros SJ, Miller JL, Hanna SW. Treatment of ischemic wounds with noncontact, low-frequency ultrasound: the Mayo clinic experience, 20042006. Adv Skin Wound Care 2007; 20(4): 221-6.
[http://dx.doi.org/10.1097/01.ASW.0000266660.88900.38] [PMID: 17415030]

[291] Maan ZN, Januszyk M, Rennert RC, *et al*. Noncontact, low-frequency ultrasound therapy enhances neovascularization and wound healing in diabetic mice. Plast Reconstr Surg 2014; 134(3): 402e-11e.
[http://dx.doi.org/10.1097/PRS.0000000000000467] [PMID: 25158717]

[292] Connolly DT. Vascular permeability factor: a unique regulator of blood vessel function. J Cell Biochem 1991; 47(3): 219-23.
[http://dx.doi.org/10.1002/jcb.240470306] [PMID: 1791186]

[293] Gallagher KA, Liu ZJ, Xiao M, *et al*. Diabetic impairments in NO-mediated endothelial progenitor cell mobilization and homing are reversed by hyperoxia and SDF-1 alpha. J Clin Invest 2007; 117(5): 1249-59.
[http://dx.doi.org/10.1172/JCI29710] [PMID: 17476357]

[294] Seth AK, Nguyen KT, Geringer MR, *et al*. Noncontact, low-frequency ultrasound as an effective therapy against *Pseudomonas aeruginosa*-infected biofilm wounds. Wound Repair Regen 2013; 21(2): 266-74.
[http://dx.doi.org/10.1111/wrr.12000] [PMID: 23421692]

[295] Isaac AL, Armstrong DG. Negative pressure wound therapy and other new therapies for diabetic foot ulceration: the current state of play. Med Clin North Am 2013; 97(5): 899-909.
[http://dx.doi.org/10.1016/j.mcna.2013.03.015] [PMID: 23992900]

[296] Upton D, Stephens D, Andrews A. Patients experiences of negative pressure wound therapy for the treatment of wounds: a review. J Wound Care 2013; 22(1): 34-9.
[http://dx.doi.org/10.12968/jowc.2013.22.1.34] [PMID: 23299356]

[297] Paul MD. An overview of cosmetic medicine and surgery: past, present, and future. Clin Plast Surg 2011; 38(3): 329-334, v.
[http://dx.doi.org/10.1016/j.cps.2011.02.004] [PMID: 21824533]

[298] Mulholland RS, Paul MD, Chalfoun C. Noninvasive body contouring with radiofrequency, ultrasound, cryolipolysis, and low-level laser therapy. Clin Plast Surg 2011; 38(3): 503-520, vii-iii.
[http://dx.doi.org/10.1016/j.cps.2011.05.002] [PMID: 21824546]

[299] Rawlings AV. Cellulite and its treatment. Int J Cosmet Sci 2006; 28(3): 175-90.
[http://dx.doi.org/10.1111/j.1467-2494.2006.00318.x] [PMID: 18489274]

[300] Ascher B. Safety and efficacy of UltraShape Contour I treatments to improve the appearance of body contours: multiple treatments in shorter intervals. Aesthet Surg J 2010; 30(2): 217-24.
[http://dx.doi.org/10.1177/1090820X09360692] [PMID: 20442099]

[301] McNeill SC, Potts RO, Francoeur ML. Local enhanced topical delivery (LETD) of drugs: does it truly exist? Pharm Res 1992; 9(11): 1422-7.
[http://dx.doi.org/10.1023/A:1015854728278] [PMID: 1475228]

[302] Burnette RR. Transdermal Drug Delivery: Developmental Issues and Research Initiatives, Drugs and the Pharmaceutical Sciences. New York: Marcel Dekker 1989; Vol. 35, pp. 247-92.

[303] Srinivasan V, Higuchi WI. A model for iontophoresis incorporating the effect of convective solvent flow. Int J Pharm 1990; 60(2): 133-8.
[http://dx.doi.org/10.1016/0378-5173(90)90298-I]

[304] Mitragotri S, Edwards DA, Blankschtein D, Langer R. A mechanistic study of ultrasonically-enhanced transdermal drug delivery. J Pharm Sci 1995; 84(6): 697-706.
[http://dx.doi.org/10.1002/jps.2600840607] [PMID: 7562407]

[305] Fellinger K, Schmid J. Klinik und Therapie des chronischen Gelenkrheumatismus. Vienna: Maudrich 1954.

[306] Griffin JE, Touchstone JC. Ultrasonic movement of cortisol into pig tissues. I. Movement into skeletal muscle. Am J Phys Med 1963; 42: 77-85.
[http://dx.doi.org/10.1097/00002060-196304000-00001] [PMID: 13950393]

[307] Griffin JE, Touchstone JC, Liu AC. Ultrasonic movement of cortisol into pig tissues. II. Movement into paravertebral nerve. Am J Phys Med 1965; 44: 20-5.
[http://dx.doi.org/10.1097/00002060-196502000-00003] [PMID: 14261632]

[308] Griffin JE, Touchstone JC. Low-intensity phonophoresis of cortisol in swine. Phys Ther 1968; 48(12): 1336-44.
[PMID: 5704952]

[309] Griffin JE, Touchstone JC. Effects of ultrasonic frequency on phonophoresis of cortisol into swine tissues. Am J Phys Med 1972; 51(2): 62-78.
[PMID: 5021935]

[310] Tang H, Mitragotri S, Blankschtein D, Langer R. Theoretical description of transdermal transport of hydrophilic permeants: application to low-frequency sonophoresis. J Pharm Sci 2001; 90(5): 545-68.
[http://dx.doi.org/10.1002/1520-6017(200105)90:5<545::AID-JPS1012>3.0.CO;2-H] [PMID: 11288100]

[311] Tezel A, Sens A, Mitragotri S. Description of transdermal transport of hydrophilic solutes during low-frequency sonophoresis based on a modified porous pathway model. J Pharm Sci 2003; 92(2): 381-93.
[http://dx.doi.org/10.1002/jps.10299] [PMID: 12532387]

[312] Mitragotri S, Kost J. Low-frequency sonophoresis: a review. Adv Drug Deliv Rev 2004; 56(5): 589-601.
[http://dx.doi.org/10.1016/j.addr.2003.10.024] [PMID: 15019748]

[313] Smith NB. Applications of ultrasonic skin permeation in transdermal drug delivery. Expert Opin Drug Deliv 2008; 5(10): 1107-20.
[http://dx.doi.org/10.1517/17425247.5.10.1107] [PMID: 18817516]

[314] Bommannan D, Okuyama H, Stauffer P, Guy RH, Sonophoresis I. Sonophoresis. I. The use of high-frequency ultrasound to enhance transdermal drug delivery. Pharm Res 1992; 9(4): 559-64.
[http://dx.doi.org/10.1023/A:1015808917491] [PMID: 1495903]

[315] Bommannan D, Menon GK, Okuyama H, Elias PM, Guy RH, Sonophoresis II. Sonophoresis. II. Examination of the mechanism(s) of ultrasound-enhanced transdermal drug delivery. Pharm Res 1992; 9(8): 1043-7.
[http://dx.doi.org/10.1023/A:1015806528336] [PMID: 1409375]

[316] Tang H, Wang CC, Blankschtein D, Langer R. An investigation of the role of cavitation in low-frequency ultrasound-mediated transdermal drug transport. Pharm Res 2002; 19(8): 1160-9.
[http://dx.doi.org/10.1023/A:1019898109793] [PMID: 12240942]

[317] Stride E, Saffari N. Microbubble ultrasound contrast agents: a review. Proc Inst Mech Eng H 2003; 217(6): 429-47.
[http://dx.doi.org/10.1243/09544110360729072] [PMID: 14702981]

[318] Ma J, Xu CS, Gao F, Chen M, Li F, Du LF. Diagnostic and therapeutic research on ultrasound microbubble/nanobubble contrast agents (Review). Mol Med Rep 2015; 12(3): 4022-8. [Review].
[PMID: 26081968]

[319] Byl NN. The use of ultrasound as an enhancer for transcutaneous drug delivery: phonophoresis. Phys Ther 1995; 75(6): 539-53.
[http://dx.doi.org/10.1093/ptj/75.6.539] [PMID: 7770499]

[320] Bare AC, McAnaw MB, Pritchard AE, *et al.* Phonophoretic delivery of 10% hydrocortisone through the epidermis of humans as determined by serum cortisol concentrations. Phys Ther 1996; 76(7): 738-45.
[http://dx.doi.org/10.1093/ptj/76.7.738] [PMID: 8677278]

[321] Sarrafzadeh J, Ahmadi A, Yassin M. The effects of pressure release, phonophoresis of hydrocortisone, and ultrasound on upper trapezius latent myofascial trigger point. Arch Phys Med Rehabil 2012; 93(1): 72-7.
[http://dx.doi.org/10.1016/j.apmr.2011.08.001] [PMID: 21982324]

[322] Allen LV Jr. Basics of compounding: phonophoresis. Int J Pharm Compd 2002; 6(5): 362-5.
[PMID: 23979415]

[323] Tachibana K, Tachibana S. Transdermal delivery of insulin by ultrasonic vibration. J Pharm Pharmacol 1991; 43(4): 270-1.
[http://dx.doi.org/10.1111/j.2042-7158.1991.tb06681.x] [PMID: 1676740]

[324] Park EJ, Werner J, Smith NB. Ultrasound mediated transdermal insulin delivery in pigs using a lightweight transducer. Pharm Res 2007; 24(7): 1396-401.
[http://dx.doi.org/10.1007/s11095-007-9306-4] [PMID: 17443398]

[325] Chuang H, Taylor E, Davison TW. Clinical evaluation of a continuous minimally invasive glucose flux sensor placed over ultrasonically permeated skin. Diabetes Technol Ther 2004; 6(1): 21-30.
[http://dx.doi.org/10.1089/152091504322783378] [PMID: 15000766]

[326] Feril LB Jr. Ultrasound-mediated gene transfection. Methods Mol Biol 2009; 542: 179-94.
[http://dx.doi.org/10.1007/978-1-59745-561-9_10] [PMID: 19565903]

[327] Zarnitsyn VG, Prausnitz MR. Physical parameters influencing optimization of ultrasound-mediated DNA transfection. Ultrasound Med Biol 2004; 30(4): 527-38.
[http://dx.doi.org/10.1016/j.ultrasmedbio.2004.01.008] [PMID: 15121255]

[328] Deng CX, Sieling F, Pan H, Cui J. Ultrasound-induced cell membrane porosity. Ultrasound Med Biol 2004; 30(4): 519-26.
[http://dx.doi.org/10.1016/j.ultrasmedbio.2004.01.005] [PMID: 15121254]

[329] Zhigang W, Zhiyu L, Haitao R, *et al.* Ultrasound-mediated microbubble destruction enhances VEGF gene delivery to the infarcted myocardium in rats. Clin Imaging 2004; 28(6): 395-8.
[http://dx.doi.org/10.1016/j.clinimag.2004.04.003] [PMID: 15531137]

[330] Akowuah EF, Gray C, Lawrie A, *et al.* Ultrasound-mediated delivery of TIMP-3 plasmid DNA into saphenous vein leads to increased lumen size in a porcine interposition graft model. Gene Ther 2005; 12(14): 1154-7.
[http://dx.doi.org/10.1038/sj.gt.3302498] [PMID: 15829995]

[331] Kodama T, Tan PH, Offiah I, *et al.* Delivery of oligodeoxynucleotides into human saphenous veins and the adjunct effect of ultrasound and microbubbles. Ultrasound Med Biol 2005; 31(12): 1683-91.
[http://dx.doi.org/10.1016/j.ultrasmedbio.2005.08.002] [PMID: 16344130]

[332] Newman CM, Bettinger T. Gene therapy progress and prospects: ultrasound for gene transfer. Gene Ther 2007; 14(6): 465-75.
[http://dx.doi.org/10.1038/sj.gt.3302925] [PMID: 17339881]

[333] Miller MW, Brayman AA. Biological effect of ultrasound. The perceived safety of diagnostic ultrasound within the context of ultrasound biophysics: a personal perspective. Echocardiography 1997; 14(6 Pt 1): 615-28.
[http://dx.doi.org/10.1111/j.1540-8175.1997.tb00771.x] [PMID: 11175001]

[334] Barnett SB, Ter Haar GR, Ziskin MC, Rott HD, Duck FA, Maeda K. International recommendations and guidelines for the safe use of diagnostic ultrasound in medicine. Ultrasound Med Biol 2000; 26(3): 355-66.
[http://dx.doi.org/10.1016/S0301-5629(00)00204-0] [PMID: 10773365]

[335] Nyborg WL. Biological effects of ultrasound: development of safety guidelines. Part II: general review. Ultrasound Med Biol 2001; 27(3): 301-33.
[http://dx.doi.org/10.1016/S0301-5629(00)00333-1] [PMID: 11369117]

[336] Nyborg WL. Biological effects of ultrasound: development of safety guidelines. Part I: personal histories. Ultrasound Med Biol 2000; 26(6): 911-64.
[http://dx.doi.org/10.1016/S0301-5629(00)00243-X] [PMID: 10996695]

[337] ter Haar G, Shaw A, Pye S, *et al.* Guidance on reporting ultrasound exposure conditions for bio-effects studies. Ultrasound Med Biol 2011; 37(2): 177-83.
[http://dx.doi.org/10.1016/j.ultrasmedbio.2010.10.021] [PMID: 21257086]

[338] Shaw A, Hodnett M. Calibration and measurement issues for therapeutic ultrasound. Ultrasonics 2008; 48(4): 234-52.
[http://dx.doi.org/10.1016/j.ultras.2007.10.010] [PMID: 18234261]

[339] Batavia M. Contraindications for superficial heat and therapeutic ultrasound: do sources agree? Arch Phys Med Rehabil 2004; 85(6): 1006-12.
[http://dx.doi.org/10.1016/j.apmr.2003.08.092] [PMID: 15179658]

[340] Sicard-Rosenbaum L, Lord D, Danoff JV, Thom AK, Eckhaus MA. Effects of continuous therapeutic ultrasound on growth and metastasis of subcutaneous murine tumors. Phys Ther 1995; 75(1): 3-11.
[http://dx.doi.org/10.1093/ptj/75.1.3] [PMID: 7809195]

[341] Shiota K. Neural tube defects and maternal hyperthermia in early pregnancy: epidemiology in a human embryo population. Am J Med Genet 1982; 12(3): 281-8.
[http://dx.doi.org/10.1002/ajmg.1320120306] [PMID: 7114091]

[342] Kalter H, Warkany J. Medical progress. Congenital malformations: etiologic factors and their role in prevention (first of two parts). N Engl J Med 1983; 308(8): 424-31.
[http://dx.doi.org/10.1056/NEJM198302243080804] [PMID: 6337330]

CHAPTER 4

The Applied Mechanical Vibration as Extracorporeal Shock Wave

Maria Cristina D'Agostino[1], Simona Maria Carmignano[2,*] and **Andrea Saggini[3]**

[1] *Shock Waves Therapy and Research Centre, Humanitas Research Hospital, "Humanitas" University, Rozzano, Italy*

[2] *School of Specialty in Physical and Rehabilitation Medicine, "Gabriele d'Annunzio" University, Chieti-Pescara, Italy*

[3] *Dermatology Specialist, Anatomic Pathology, Department of Biomedicine and Prevention, University of Rome Tor Vergata, Rome, Italy*

Abstract: After its originary introduction as urological lithotripsy (still clinically applied), shock wave progressively gained a growing therapeutic importance in some different medical fields. Initially restricted in many musculo-skeletal disorders, in more recent years, thanks to a better knowledge about its mechanisms of actions (mainly antiflogistic, angiogenic and analgesic), this particular form of mechanical vibration nowadays represents a real innovative and unexpected therapeutic tool at the service of rehabilitation and regenerative medicine. The effectiveness, safety and ductility of shock wave therapy make it a unique and versatile strategy with further promising therapeutic perspectives in the near future.

Keywords : Focused and unfocused waves, Lithotripsy, Mechanical stimulation, Radial wave, Regenerative processes, Shock wave generators, Shock waves.

INTRODUCTION

Shock waves are a particular form of mechanical stimulation, whose first medical application was limited to the treatment (breaking up) of kidney stones (as extracorporeal shock wave lithotripsy). In the following years, it expanded to the musculo-skeletal field, mainly for the treatment of some tendon and bone diseases, and more recently some other important and revolutionary clinical applications in the field of regenerative medicine have been studied and introduced in clinical practice [1 - 3]. Nowadays, Extracorporeal Shock Waves

---

* **Corresponding authors Simona Maria Carmignano:** School of Specialty in Physical and Rehabilitation Medicine, "Gabriele d'Annunzio" University, Chieti-Pescara, Italy; Tel: 03908713555306; Fax: 03909713553224; E-mail: simona.carmignano@gmail.com

Raoul Saggini (Ed.)

Therapy (ESWT) represent a valid tool for a wide range of disorders, both in orthopedics and rehabilitative medicine (tendon pathologies, bone diseases, vascular bone pathologies), but also in dermatology and vulnology (chronic wounds, ulcers, scars) [4 - 19], neurology complications such us spasticity [20, 21], or some sexual disturbances (*induratio penis plastica* and erectile dysfunctions) [22 - 28], and cardiology (in relation to ischemic heart diseases) [29 - 32].

Based on its noninvasiveness, safety (as absence of main side effects) tolerability, repeatability, and efficacy (if properly applied), extracorporeal shock waves constitutes a unique therapeutic tool in a broad range of medical conditions, representing a very useful medical solution especially when other conservative or surgical treatments are ineffective or failing [33 - 35].

GENERAL CHARACTERISTICS OF SHOCK WAVES

Shock wave (SW) is a particular form of mechanical stimulation, firstly described, as physical entity, at the beginning of the 19th century; only two centuries later, during World War II, based on fortuitous findings, some researchers began to study their possible therapeutic application in humans (other than their technical usage), aimed to exploit their potential for breaking structures. In fact, besides some early experimental attempts for destroying brain tumors in 1960, the main interest was reserved to the fragmentation of kidney stones (urolithiasis), and, at the beginning of the nineties, in Munich, extracorporeal shock wave lithotripsy was applied for the first time [36].

Soon after, in 1991, still based on some occasional observations, it was discovered that, from a simple mechanical stimulation (shock waves), it is possible to induce some relevant medical effects, unexpected before that time, and related to a biological action. Valchanov and Michailov in 1991 described the successful treatment of bone healing disturbances by SW application (that is osteogenesis induction), as the first non-urological application [37]. This should be considered as a milestone in the evolution of SW therapy, that is the changeover from the "mechanical model" of extracorporeal shock wave lithotripsy to its application as "mechanotherapy" on living tissues in all extra urological fields, where mechanical stimulations are applied for therapeutic purposes, based on biological reactions, as described below [38].

Since 1991 until now, SWs rapidly spread as orthotripsy for many musculoskeletal disorders (mainly bone healing diseases and tendon disturbances), although still considered as a relatively "pioneristic therapy" until few years ago, especially as this technique was inherited from urological applications, where it acts as a pure mechanical force. Still having in mind the "mechanical" action of breaking renal stones, at the beginning of the musculoskeletal applications and for some years later, the main interest was addressed toward calcifications disruption. Finally, in the early years of the new millennium, due to the discovery of its regenerative potential, and the increasing number of scientific results published in literature, the efficacy of SW as a biological tool was made clear (not only a pure mechanical one). From a general point of view, it was necessary to wait for some years, since the emergence of their originary successful clinical applications, to know a great deal about the mechanisms of action of SW at the tissue and cellular level, in order to explain many clinical therapeutic results.

SWs are acoustic waves, characterized by a pick pressure rises from the ambient value to its maximum within very few nanoseconds. SWs can be distinguished from some other acoustic waves (as ultrasounds for examples), due to their shape, characterized by initial high peak-pressure amplitude, rapidly followed by a drop to a negative value within few microseconds [39 - 45].

In 1997, the physical characteristics of SWs, used in the therapeutic fields, were established by a Consensus Conference, relative to the parameters recognized by numerous SW Scientific Societies [40] (Fig. **1**):

• rapid rise in pressure (< 10 ns);
• high peak pressure (up to 100 MPa);
• short-time duration (< 1000 ns).

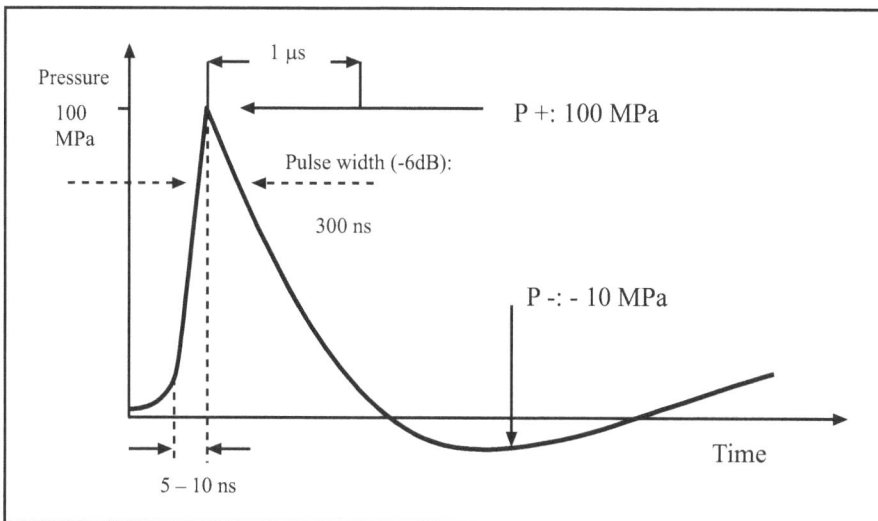

Fig. (1). ESWT: physical characteristics of wave. From: Ogden JA, Tóth-Kischkat A, Schultheiss R. Principles of shock wave therapy. Clin Orthop Relat Res 2001; (387): 8-17.

Both the negative and positive phase occur in a few seconds causing mechanical effects in transitional areas between tissues with different characteristics (acoustic impedance). The step of wave's deflection determines cavitation phenomenon with formation of bubbles gas that then subsequently implode at higher speed, thus generating a second front of shock waves or microjets of fluid (Fig. **2**).

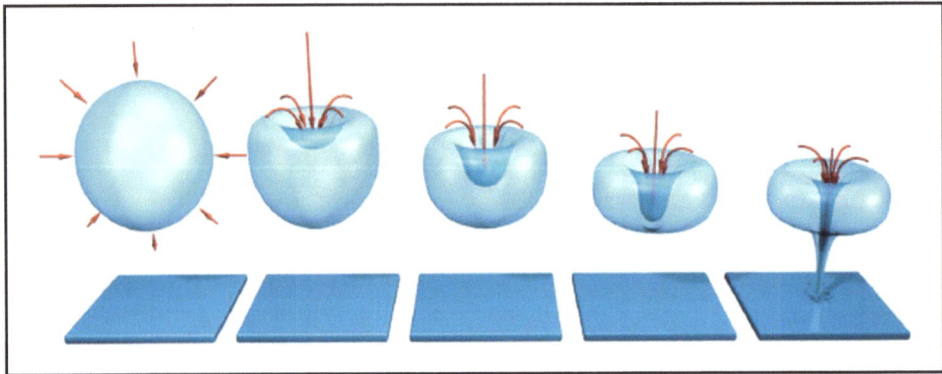

Fig. (2). Microjet formation by cavitation bubble collapse. From left to right: close to a boundary, the bubble cannot collapse symmetrically because the surrounding fluid cannot flow in symmetrically. Thus a torus is formed with a jet stream towards the boundary. From: Wess O, Ueberle F, Dührssen RN, *et al.* Working group technical developments – consensus report. In: Chaussy C, Eisenberger F, Jocham D, Wilbert D, Eds. High energy shock waves in medicine. Stuttgart, Thieme 1997; pp. 59-71.

These events are responsible, as the final result, for the direct (physical) and indirect (biological) effects of the shock waves on the treated tissues [39, 41, 43, 44].

Nowadays, in clinical practice, three different types of SW generators are available, equipped with different types of sources: electromagnetic, electrohydraulic and piezoelectric ones. In all these sources, SWs are produced due to a rapid increase in pressure (like a micro-explosion) into the water, and sooner, in order to obtain a therapeutic effect, they are concentrated or "focused" on the target (that is the pathological site of treatment). Focusing SW are realized by a parabolic lens, which directs the front of SWs, as soon as they originate from the source. Some technical characteristics of the different sources are described in more details below [42 - 44]:

- In the *electromagnetic generator,* the SW source is represented by a flat or a cylindrical coil (with multiple windings of copper wire) (depending on the model); at this level, a high energy transient electrical discharge induces a rapid expansion/contraction of the metal membrane of the flat coil or of the cylinder, thus generating SW.
- The source of the *electrohydraulic generator* is composed of two electrodes

(electrical terminals) located very close to each other in an aqueous environment, where a high energy transient electrical discharge passes (named "spark gap"). This causes a vapor bubble, that expands up to collapse sooner quickly, thus causing a wave of high pressure or SW (Fig. **3**).

- Differently, in the *piezoelectric generator*, the sources are composed of a set of piezoelectric crystals that instantly vibrate, as soon as a transient electrical discharge is produced. The rapid expansion and contraction of the piezoelectric crystals give rise to the SW front (Fig. **4**).

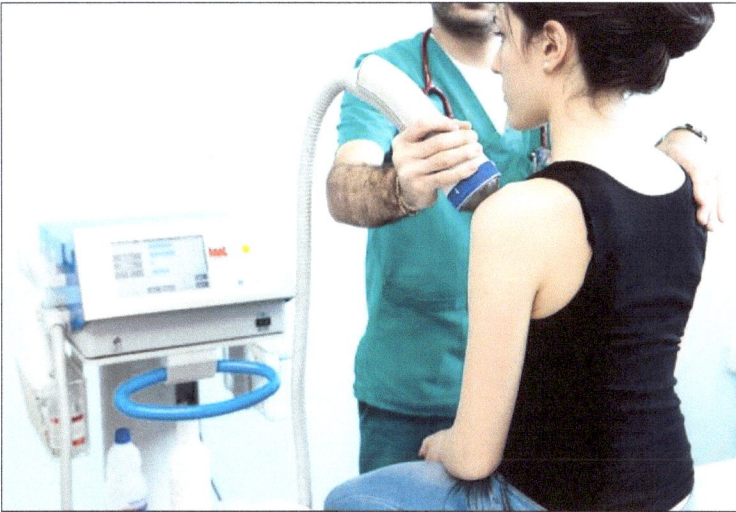

Fig. (3). Electrohydraulic generator of focused ESW, MTS Europe GmbH, Konstanz (Germany).

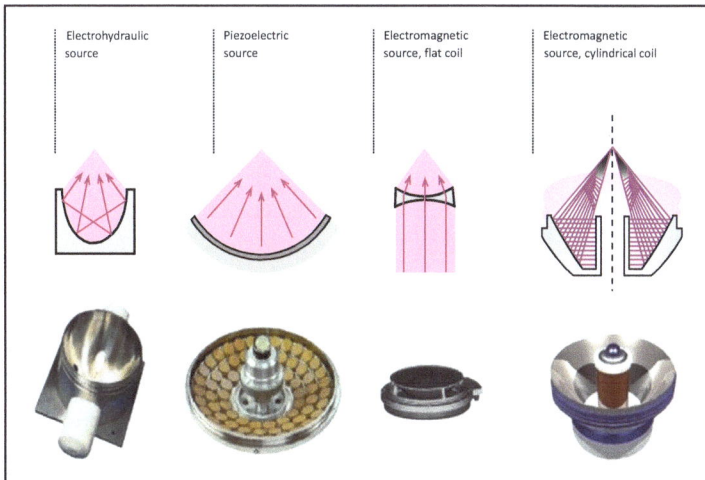

Fig. (4). Shock wave generators used in medicine. From: Wess O. Physics and technology of shock wave and pressure wave, International Society for Medical Shockwave Treatment Newsletter 2007.

From the technical point of view, some different types of lithotripters and sources will imply different treatment protocols, in relation to the number of impulses and the corresponding energy levels to be applied. On the basis of some standardized physical parameters, it is possible to describe the characteristics of different devices, trying, at least in part, to standardize and compare the different protocols with different focused SW source [42] (Fig. **5**).

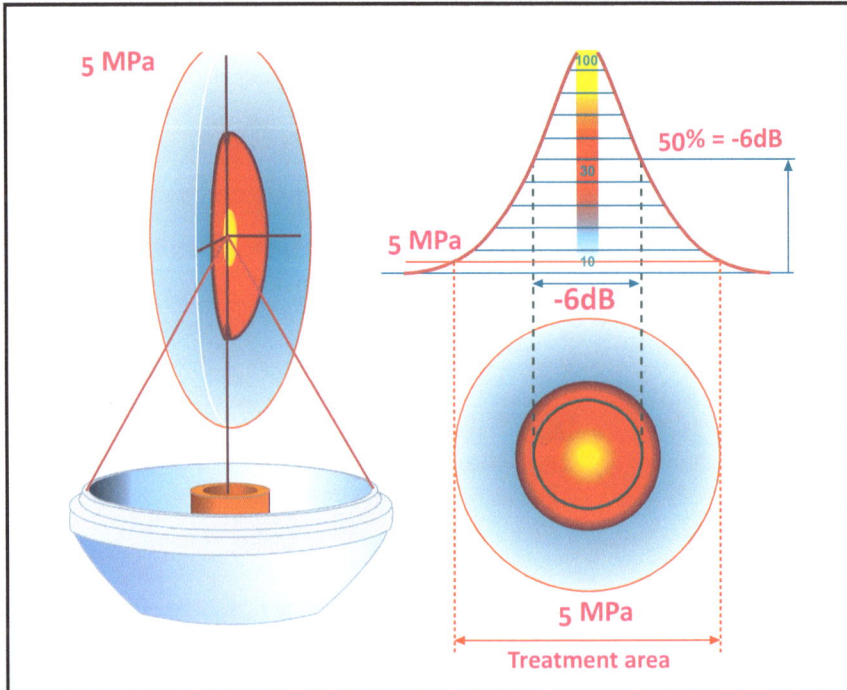

Fig. (5). Pressure distribution and focal zone. Typical focal zone (red) has an ellipsoid shape. Within the larger treatment zone (blue), therapeutic effects may still occur. From: Wess O. Physics and technology of shock wave and pressure wave, International Society for Medical Shockwave Treatment Newsletter 2007.

In more recent years, technological advances have supported the observations that SW could be effective also for tissue regeneration. To treat larger surfaces of tissue loss (as in ulcers, chronic or complicated wounds) some modified sources are needed, that although retaining the same physical characteristics (SW as such) are able to distribute the energy on a larger surface area. For this purpose, some focused SW generators were designed and marketed, being able to generate unfocused SW: the same biphasic wave assumes the form of a planar or unfocused wave during application. Obviously, for these devices the depth of penetration is lower, so that their therapeutic indication is limited to the more superficial lesions, like cutaneous ulcers and related disorders [2, 19]. Type of generator, energy flux density, frequency, number of pulses per square centimeter, number of treatment sessions, and time interval between each session are further parameters to be modulated and compared [44, 46].

Besides focused SW and its planar version, based on scientific works and clinical practice, since many years, another form of mechanical wave, *i.e:* the radial wave, is successfully applied for many musculoskeletal diseases, especially of the soft tissues (Fig. **6**). Radial wave is an acoustic wave (that is a mechanical stimulation) as well, but generated in a different way. In this case, the source (or applicator) is constituted by a barrel hand piece, where, by means of compressed air or a magnetic field, a metallic bullet is accelerated at a very high speed. The high kinetic energy generated in this way makes impacts against the tip of the applicator itself, directly applied on the skin. Energy is accumulated during run and transferred directly to the body surface in the affected area. The so-produced wave, after impact, continues to propagate in the body as a ball-shaped wave which propagates in a spherical way, thus deriving the descriptive term of "radial wave". The energy produced by the pressure wave is highest at the level of skin surface, but spreads and weakens as it penetrates deeper. In the radial shock wave, the focal point is not centered on the target zone as in the focused SW, but on the tip of the applicator. Due to the mechanism of production, radial SWs are not focused in depth, but have a radial transmission mode limited to the more superficial layers of the body, which is applied for treatment. From the physical point of view, although both of them are acoustic or mechanical waves, they differ in term of the shape of the waves themselves. Moreover, they share some clinical indications, but differ from some other ones (see Chapter 2) [41 - 44, 47].

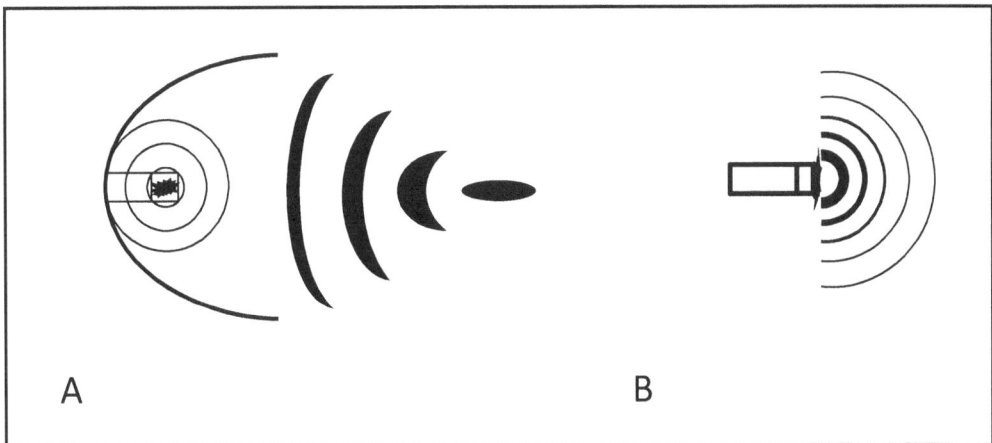

Fig. (6). A) Focused shockwave. **B)** Radial shockwave device. From: van der Worp H, van den Akker-Scheek I, van Schie H, Zwerver J. ESWT for tendinopathy: technology and clinical implications. Knee Surg Sports Traumatol Arthrosc 2013; 21(6): 1451-8.

Based on the tissue to be treated, (mainly soft tissues and bone), it can be appropriate to use a specific lithotripther rather than another one, relative to the different therapeutic requirements, especially the function of the energy to be applied while expecting a different biological effect. Low-medium energy level for treating tendon pathologies, or medium-high for bone [1, 2, 33] (Fig. 7).

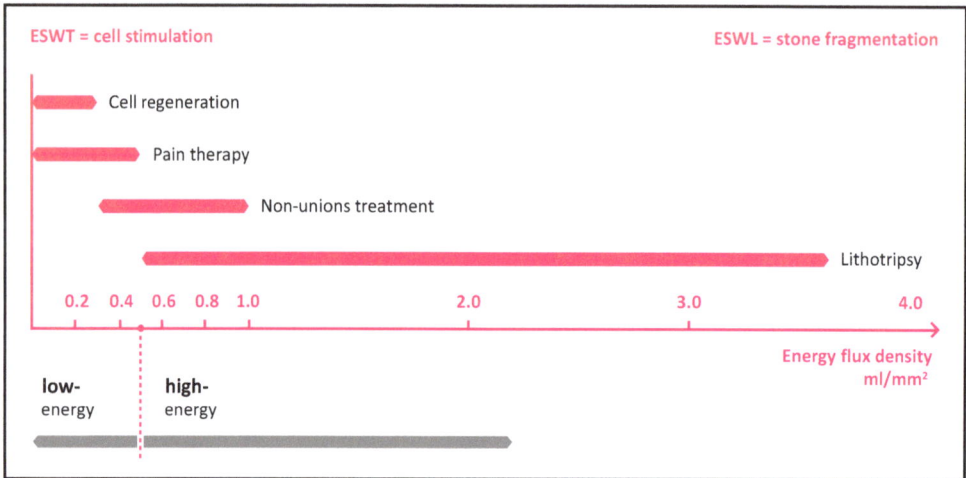

Fig. (7). Fields of application and relative energy levels of shock waves in medicine.

It is important to outline that, relative to the modalities of applying ESWT, international guidelines include all essential requirements for accurate application. If, for the treatments of bone disorders, it is important to target the anatomical area of pathology (better by fluoroscopic control), for those of tendons and related structures, this is not so primary. It could be, in any case, of great value to have a control "coupled" the system of generation of shock waves, in order to target SW precisely in the areas affected by degenerative processes, with/without calcifications, in this case the best instrumental method for targeting can be considered diagnostic ultrasound [48]. In spite of the type of device we use, if applied according to a good clinical practice, based on learning and training, from a general point of view, low-dose shock wave therapy without anaesthetic can be considered a safe and effective treatment [49 - 51]. Scientific literature or clinical experiences not report, systemic, or local complications [52].

MECHANISMS OF ACTION OF SHOCK WAVES

Nowadays, although partly unknown, there is a scientific evidence those SWs, on living tissues. Characterized with mechanical energy, do not produce some destructive or harmful effects, but properly make some biological actions on living tissues and cells, thus exerting a positive and regulatory influence. Thus, the pure mechanical stimuli (mechanical energy) can be considered as the "trigger" or a *primum movens* of the biological reactions, rather than the direct responsible of the ultimate effects of the stimulation. Although still partly unknown, basic science articles and clinical experiences point out that the main mechanisms of action for the SWs in extra urological fields can be summarized as follows [1, 2, 33, 53]:

- small unmyelinated nerve fibers reduction;
- substance P dilution;
- nitric oxide (NO) production;
- changes in cellular membrane permeability;
- possible antibacterial effect (still under study);
- growth factors secretion and some other biological mediators;
- proliferation, migration and differentiation of stem cells.

Based on these mechanisms of action at the tissue and cellular level, these general important clinical results can follow [2, 53]:

- antiflogistic and anti-edema effects;
- angiogenesis and tissue-specific regeneration (especially skin and bone);
- analgesic effect.

As mentioned above, not all details of the biological mechanisms induced by SW application are completely known, partly they are still under study.

From a general point of view, mechanotransduction is possible as most of the cells of the body, due to surface receptors and other transmission signals, can perceive and transmit the stimuli to the nucleus, thus activating it with the final result of producing growth factors and some other biochemical substances. In the specific field of SW, these different biochemical substances are able to influence the processes of different cell lineages, besides inducing the formation of new small blood vessels. Specific stem cells of each tissue along with endothelial cells and their precursors can be activated. Angiogenesis (either from "scratch" or "budding" from pre-existing small blood vessels) is one of the basic condition for supporting regenerative processes in the different affected tissues [53].

In the past, the action of the extracorporeal shock waves was only relative to the mechanical effect, namely to the possibility of being able to destroy the ectopic formations in the tissues, today the therapeutic approaches are motivated by the knowledge of the biological and molecular effects that can be achieved by modulating the specific usage parameters [38].

Nowadays it is possible to apply in clinical practice some mechanical stimulations, better known as "vibratory mechanotherapies", both for many disorders of bone and soft tissues as well.

According to a revisited definition by Huang C *et al:* of the term and based on the current knowledge in mechanobiology, mechanotherapies include «all therapeutic interventions that reduce and reverse injury to damaged tissues, or promote the homeostasis of healthy tissues by mechanical means at the molecular, cellular, or tissue level». In other words, they include all «active mechano-interventions, that aim to convert potentially destructive mechanical effects into constructive influences and target normal mechano-adaptation to promote recovery» [38].

Therefore, it is evident that, within the framework of the mechanotherapy, Extracorporeal Shock Waves Therapy (ESWT) has a revealing importance in relation to a number of biological and molecular actions already discovered and to those which are still under study [38].

Its importance, as mechanotherapy, is related to the possibility of positively influencing some cells metabolism and functionalities, so it is possible to improve repair and regenerative process. A number of recent studies, in fact, underline as its effect is manifested as ability to stimulate stem cells proliferation, migration and differentiation, thus obtaining tissue healing and regeneration. Moreover, other than stem cells and bone marrow – stromal cells, some different lines can be a sensible target of mechanotrasduction pathways following SW stimulation, including tenocytes, bone cells, endothelial cells, fibroblasts, some other ones, including all their direct precursors [1 - 3, 54 - 63].

The neoangiogenetic capacity, could be related to an initial inhibition of endothelial cells apoptosis and adhesion, described *in vitro* in the very early phase (first 3 hours), after SW stimulation. It has been postulated that, some early gene responses of endothelial cells to SW, as mechanotherapy, are similar to those induced by the laminar shear stress flow that is characterized by an anti-apoptotic effect as well. To elaborate, although at 3 hours after SW application, there is no neoangiogenic activity (observed as it will appear after 12 hours), there are already some "warning" or "preparatory" signals, like downregulation of cell cycle and adhesion genes, perhaps related to an oncoming detachment of endothelial junctions [57].

Moreover, increasing scientific evidences seem to describe that SW mechanotransduction pathways are not only dose-related but can also differ various cell types and stem cells in different stages of differentiation. As a possible consequence, each cell lineage seems to be responsive to SW stimulation; but, probably, it exists a different and specific pattern and range of optimal mechanical stimulation, being able to evoke some different biological responses, as much as the up regulation of TGF beta-1 (TGF-β1) and NO expression, other than suppression of the nuclear factor kB (NF-kB) activity and pro-inflammatory cytokines production [38, 54, 55, 64 - 66].

In very recent animal studies, aimed to evaluate the possible antifibrotic effect of SW application, used intramuscular injection of silicone, reduced formation of the dense fibrous envelope was described. Moreover, when applied in multiple SW treatments, it was possible to obtain active degradation of the fibrous capsule, due to synergistic modifications in pro- and anti-fibrotic proteins (TGF-β1 and matrix metalloproteinase 2, respectively), thus underlining a possible role of SW in reducing capsule formation and inducing fibrotic tissue resorption/remodeling as well [67, 68].

While describing the mechanisms of action of ESWT, based on similar experimental and clinical data, it hypothesize that this mechano-therapy would be able, not only to improve the healing events, but also to give rise to some regenerative processes; above all where fibrous tissue can be reduced at the source, or in any case, can be later remodeled (as in scar tissue).

These preliminary observations seem to foresee some further interesting applications in clinical practice, especially in cardiology, where some studies are already being conducted where regeneration of the original tissue, instead of scar tissue, is fundamental for heart vitality. On the other hand, many recent evidences would indicate that ESWT can ameliorate ventricular function in heart failure and ischemic diseases [69 - 71].

Moreover, recent studies in SW mechanobiology and basic science suggest that SW would influence the Toll-like receptor 3 (TLR3) pathway [69], suggesting its role in inducing tissue regeneration and remodeling as mechanotherapy, other than implying the role of this mechanotherapy as immunomodulator in wound healing, mainly through an anti-inflammatory pathway [30, 66, 72 - 74].

Surely, the most revolutionary evidence can be considered the data about the possible effect of SW on macrophages activities, in particular on the pro-resolving macrophages (or M2), that are able, at the crossroad between inflammation and regeneration, to induce resolution of the pathologic inflammatory processes at the tissue levels, thus increasing the possibility of a regenerative action [75].

Some studies showed how ESWT and the related mechanotransduction are effective in stimulating several endogenous growth factors such as epidermal growth factor, insulin-like growth factor 1, vascular endothelial growth factor

(VEGF) and NO production, inducing angiogenesis and promoting the healing of tendons, muscles, cartilage, bone and skin, fractures, ulcers and complex lesions.

Vulpiani *et al:*, [76, 77] described the clinical effectiveness of ESWT in Jumper's knee and in Achilles tendinopathy.

Saggini *et al:*, [78 - 80] showed the long-term effectiveness of ESWT in the rotator cuff syndrome and in jumper's knee.

Wang [81] highlighted the effect of increase in the performance of the knee after ACL reconstruction surgery, confirming the evidence of efficacy of this treatment in tendon and ligament diseases.

The efficacy of unfocused shock wave to improve "regenerative" processes was be demonstrated in a study by Saggini *et al:*, on retracting scars of the hand [82]. Selected patients were randomly divided into four groups (group A to D): group A (30 patients), consisting of individuals with (Group A-II, 15 patients) or without (Group A-I, 15 patients) surgery-induced complex regional pain syndrome (CRPS) of the hand; this group was administered treatment with unfocused ESWT alone, at a frequency of two sessions per week for 5 weeks; group B (15 patients with no evidence of CRPS) was treated with a combination of ESWT and manual myofascial therapy at a frequency of two sessions per week for 5 weeks; group C (15 patients with no evidence of CRPS) received ESWT treatment associated with manual myofascial therapy and local treatment with I-Coon system at a frequency of two sessions per week for 5 weeks; group D (10 patients with no evidence of CRPS) did not receive any treatment. Focal depth of shock waves was 49 mm with a total energy applied for each impulse of 0.13 mJ/mm^2; treatment frequency was 6 Hz and duration of each session was 1.5 min (500 pulses for session per 360 impulses/min), with a focus where the scar was hypertrophic and very painful. Scar assessment and evaluation were performed before the beginning of the treatment cycle (T0), after the fifth treatment session (T1) and after the second week, after the end of the 10th treatment session (T2). Scar height (cm), pigmentation, vascularization and pain were assessed using the modified Vancouver Scar Scale. Rating of subjective pain was performed using the Visual Analogue Scale (VAS); the VAS score is a simple tool commonly used for the evaluation of changes in pain intensity, with values ranging from 0 (no pain) to 10 (worst pain ever). Deficit in passive mobility because of scar-related contractures was evaluated using a range of motion (ROM) score ranging from a minimum of 0 to a maximum of 100. Biopsy specimens were taken from pathologic scars treated with unfocused ESWT at T0 and T2. A 3-mm, wedge-shaped incisional biopsy was collected from treated areas, perpendicular to clinically palpable scars, and sent for tissue processing and staining. Significant improvements were observed in group A (treated with shock waves): the most important change was detected in skin biopsies. Histopathological examination (Fig. **8**) revealed significant increase in dermal fibroblasts in each active treatment group (*i.e:*, groups A, B and C), as well as in neoangiogenetic response and type I collagen concentration; likewise, in each active treatment group, significant qualitative improvement in dermal collagen was observed, with a finer and more fibrillar appearance. Staining with picrosirius red indicated that treatment with ESWT resulted in a collagen fiber arrangement parallel to the skin surface and replacement of type III collagen with type I collagen (thus restoring the physiologic relationship between type I and III collagen).

Immunohistochemical comparison of pre- and post-ESWT treatment biopsies revealed that administration of a shock wave regimen resulted in a significant increase in infiltrating fXIIIa-positive fibrocytes, CD34 dermal expression and CD31-positive small vessels.

By contrast, no significant changes were observed in the control group (group D) by either hematoxylin-eosin, picrosirius red or immune-histochemical staining.

The results of this study seem to confirm that shock wave treatment is capable of inducing an increase in the number of activated fibroblasts, CD34-positive fibrocytes and fXIIIa-positive dendritic cells. This process is thought to lead to the deposition of new collagen, characterized by thinner collagen fascicles and parallel orientation to the dermo-epidermal junction. Additionally, shock wave therapy may be regarded as playing a significant role in increasing CD31-positive vessel density in the dermis of treated patients, allowing an improved tissue metabolism.

In healthy human skin, type I and III collagen have relatively substantial roles during collagen formation, comprising 80-85% and 10-15%, respectively. Newly developed scars undergo a maturation process, with type III collagen being gradually replaced by type I collagen to restore normal type I-to-III collagen ratio (which is approximately 5:1). Into repair process of skin as well as tissue tendon collagen is a fundamental element for the tone and elasticity. A variation of the characteristics and amount of collagen can result in a pathological repair process and pathological scarring. Collagen fibers within scar dermis show a reduced resistance potential, being only 70% in the normal skin. Our studies on skin and pathological scars demonstrated and confirmed the biostimulating effectiveness of ESWT on skin through modulation of the 3 phases of tissue repair (inflammatory, proliferative, remodeling). The principle effect is restoring the normal relationship between type I and III collagen. Therefore, the fibroblasts are the most mechanoresponsive cell type and play a key role in the remodeling of the extracellular matrix synthesizing and reorganizing the connective tissue components.

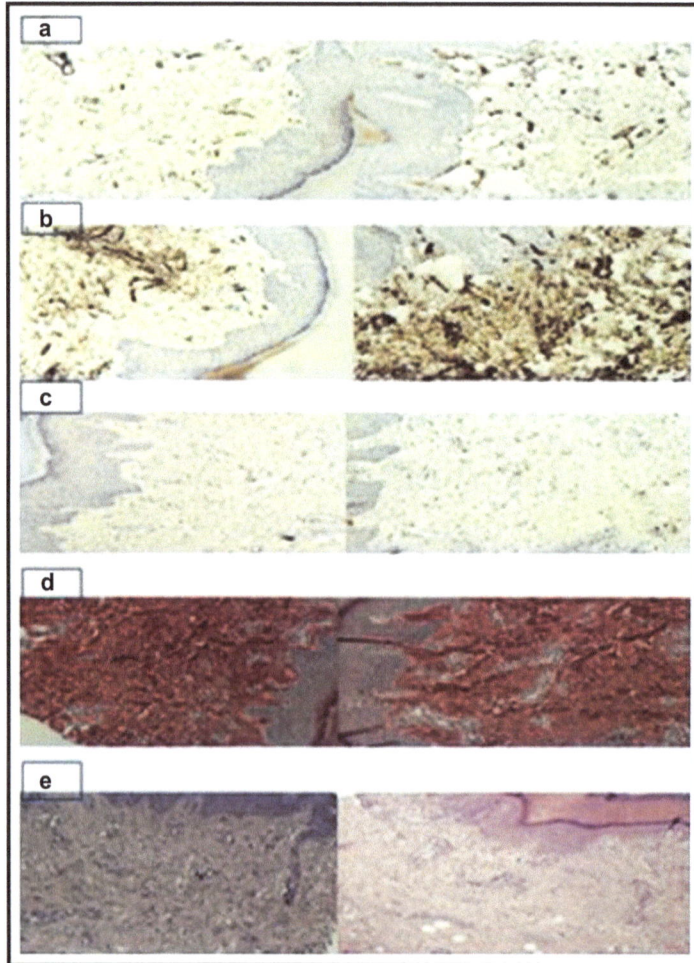

Fig. (8). Biopsy specimens taken from patients in the group treated with ESWT. (a) Immunohistochemical staining of fibroblasts and angiogenesis (right, before the treatment; left, after treatment) for FXIII reveals a significant increase in FXIII1 dendrocytes after treatment with ESWT. (b) Immunohistochemical staining for CD34 of fibroblasts, type I collagen and angiogenesis (right, before the treatment; left, after treatment) shows a significant increase in CD341dendrocytes and CD341vessels after treatment with ESWT. (c) Immunohistochemical staining for CD31 of angiogenesis (right, before the treatment; left, after treatment) demonstrates a significant increase in CD311 vessels after treatment with ESWT. (d) Picrosirius red (right, before the treatment; left, after treatment) staining reveals modified arrangement of collagen fibers after treatment with ESWT, parallel to the epidermis, and increased type I-to-III collagen ratio. (e) Hematoxylin-eosin (right, before the treatment; left, after treatment) highlights significant improvement in dermal collagen after treatment with ESWT, showing a thinner and more fibrillary collagen. From: Saggini R, Saggini A, Spagnoli AM, *et al:* Extracorporeal Shock Wave Therapy: An Emerging Treatment Modality for Retracting Scars of the Hands. Ultrasound Med Biol 2016; 42(1): 185-95.

Maffulli, in 2011 [83], described how changes in tendon structure in overload diseases (cit.) "are represented by: degeneration, disorganization and thickening of the collagen fibers, increase in degradation of collagen and interfibrillar glycosaminoglycans and, in particular, by altering of the normal relationship between type I and III collagen, as observed in the skin." Compatibly what has been observed in human skin, tissue regeneration is related to fibroblast infiltration and collagen remodeling, and based on the evidence of clinical efficacy of ESWT on the tendon, we can assume the existence of a similar reparative model *in vivo* in human tendon.

Mechanotransduction pathways and mechanobiology can also be advocated to describe and explain the analgesic effect of ESWT, more evident in the more precocious phases of application. Regarding this topic, recently Saggini *et al.*, described the effects of mechanotransduction on pain [84]; various hypotheses have been formulated, although one of the most reliable one is the theory of the "hyperstimulation analgesia". This theory states that a painful stimulation, as it can be in the case of SW, is soon transmitted to the central nervous system through the posterior column of the spinal cord, and it may activate the descending inhibitory system; it in turn blocks the transmission of nociceptive stimuli in the posterior column. Moreover, analgesia obtained can also improve the joint function as well. SW can also induce overstimulation of the nerve fibers, thus resulting in the increase of the painful stimulus and meanwhile intensifying the analgesic effect ("gate control" theory) [85].

Another biological explanation for the analgesic effect of SW application can be considered a possible degeneration of the nerve fibers originating from the small neurons immunoreactive to Activating Transcription Factor 3, a protein linked to the activation of genes related to protein coding pro-inflammatory, which seems to derive a relieved pain. Releasing of these bioactive substances (mainly substance P and calcitonin gene-related peptide) at the level of sensory nerve endings plays an important role in the maintenance of pain and chronic inflammation [86].

Chronic inflammation can contribute to increase the pain, for example in epicondylitis, chronic plantar fasciitis and tendinous disorders of the rotator cuff [87, 88]. A study revealed the contribution of substance P (as interleukin 1-alpha and TGF-β1) in the pathogenesis of tennis elbow, without any apparent infiltration of inflammatory cells [89].

From a general point of view, it likely that the mechanisms of action of SW in the treatment of musculoskeletal pain cannot be defined in a single pathogenetic mechanism, thus posing a demand for further studies. Nevertheless, all researches conducted on muscle pain during the last years, and the experience gained in ESWT clinical practice for musculoskeletal pain, confirm the important role of this "mechanotherapy" as a conservative treatment option, which can also be applied to some other diseases characterized by functional disorders and pain syndromes.

CLINICAL GUIDELINES

The different therapeutic indications for SW treatment are described in the guidelines by the Società Italiana Terapia con Onde D'urto (SITOD) and the International Society for Medical Shockwave Treatment (ISMST).

Regarding the SITOD guidelines, all the following indications are considered.

- Standard indications
  - Pseudoarthrosis or delayed bone healing
  - Stress fractures
    - Shoulder tendinopathies (with or without calcification/s)
  - Chronic enthesopathies (insertional tendinopathies)
  - Plantar fascitis (with or without heel spur)
  - Early aseptic osteonecrosis
  - Early dissecans osteochondritis (after closure of the metaphyseal plates)
  - Algoneurodystrophy (Sudeck's disease)
- Relative indications
  - Miofascial syndromes
  - Muscle injury without discontinuity
  - Skin ulcers
  - Spasticity

In SITOD guidelines, it is reported that one of the most important factors to be considered for obtaining the best results is to formulate a correct diagnosis, as well as to exclude from ESWT, all those patients who present the following contraindications:

- Local bone or soft tissue acute infection;
- Primary pernicious diseases;
- Growth plates in the focal point (if high energies are applied);
- Disorders of coagulation;
- Pregnancy;
- Pacemaker;
- Presence in the focal point of brain, spinal cord, main nerves, lung tissue (neurocranium, spinal column, ribs).

On March 2008, a Consensus Conference by ISMST stated that «scientific results (both experimental and clinical ones) are related to the different parameters of the SW sources, single and total energy applied, to the modalities of targeting, to the frequency of the applications and the aim of the treatment (calcium deposits dissolution, connective tissue angiogenesis and pain therapy)» and that all the clinical and therapeutic general principles of orthopedic medicine and rehabilitation have to be taken into account while applying ESWT. According to this Consensus Conference, ISMST classifies all the general indications as follows.

- Approved standard indications by ISMST (indications are exactly reported as described by the guidelines)
  - Chronic tendinopathies
    - Plantar fasciitis with or without heel spur
    - Achilles tendinopathy
    - Radial epicondylopathy (tennis elbow)
    - Rotator cuff diseases with or without calcification
    - Patella tendinopathy
    - Greater trochanteric pain syndrome
  - Impaired bone healing function
    - Delayed bone healing
    - Stress fractures
    - Early stage of avascular bone necrosis (native X-ray without pathology)
    - Early stage osteochondritis dissecans post-skeletal maturity
  - Urology
    - lithotripsy (extracorporeal and endocorporeal)
- Common empirically-tested clinical uses
  - Tendinopathy
    - Ulnar epicondylopathy
    - Adductor syndrome
    - *Pes anserinus* syndrome
    - Peroneal tendon syndrome
  - Muscular pathologies
    - Myofascial syndrome (fibromyalgia excluded)
    - Injury without discontinuity
  - Impaired wound healing
  - Burn injuries
  - Salivary stones
- Exceptional indications/expert indications
  - Spasticity
  - Early stage osteochondritis dissecans pre-skeletal maturity
  - Apophysitis (Osgood Schlatter disease)

- ○ La Peyronie's disease
- Uses under experimental conditions
  - ○ Myocardial ischemia (extracorporeal/endocorporeal)
  - ○ Peripheral nerve lesions
  - ○ Abacterial prostatitis
  - ○ Periodontal disease
  - ○ Osteoarthritis

According to the ISMST guidelines, while considering the results of ESWT, some important factors can have a positive influence:

- experience of the physician/SW therapist;
- possibility to use a proper device;
- correct therapeutic choice in the context of an integrated personalized program.

On the other hand, clinical results after ESW therapy can be negatively influenced:

- when exclusion criteria have not been respected or when there is not a general consensus about them;
- if there are some secondary orthopedic diseases;
- if there are some secondary not orthopedic diseases;
- according to the level of chronicity.

From a general point of view, ESWT can be classified in two main sections, accordingly to the type of tissue to be treated and consequently, to the different energy levels and number of impulses needed for the therapy. We distinguish the soft tissue treatments (such as those for tendons, muscles and skin) on one hand, while on the other hand, those for bone (mainly pseudoarthrosis/bone healing disturbances and bone vascular diseases, as osteonecrosis and bone marrow edema syndromes).

In the group of the soft tissues diseases for ESWT, tendinopathies play undoubtedly a predominant role in rotator cuff tendinopathies of the shoulder, lateral epicondylitis (or tennis elbow), medial epicondylitis (or golfer's elbow), plantar fasciitis (or heel spur), as well as Achilles tendinopathy and trochanteric syndromes [1, 3, 4, 8, 53].

It is useful to remember that the aim of this mechanotherapy on living tissues is not to make a pure mechanical (or "destructive") effect, but rather determine some positive biological pathways. Calcification can disappear in some cases (more evident for shoulder, for example), due to dissolution (that is a biological action), not for direct fragmentation or disruption of the calcium deposits. A similar mechanism can be advocated for explaining the regenerative potential of SW in bone healing disturbances: osteoregeneration capacity is not due to micro-fractures induced by SW, but rather to a direct stimulation of bone cells, local stem cells and endothelial precursors, thus improving callus maturation and new bone formation as well [1, 3, 4, 8, 53].

The effectiveness of ESWT in the treatment of chronic tendinopathy is reported in many clinical trials have evaluated the efficacy in the treatment of rotator cuff syndrome, epicondylitis, plantar fasciitis, and other tendinopathies.

Although ESWT has been reported to be effective in some trials, in some other ones, it was not more effective than placebo.

The multiple variables associated with this therapy (besides the possible heterogeneity of the disease), such as the type of SW source, amount of energy delivered, method of focusing the shock waves, frequency and timing of delivery, and whether or not anesthetics are used, make it difficult to compare some different clinical trials [89].

Since from a biological point of view, (especially *in vitro* and animal experiments) nowadays there seem to be many valid and incontrovertible scientific evidences of a direct action of SW on tendon structures and cells, a statement of Rompe and Maffulli seems gaining more and more value. In 2007, Rompe and Maffulli [90] concluded that (cit.) «with current studies heterogeneous in terms of the duration of the disorder, type, frequency and total dose of SWT, period of time between SWT, type of management and control group, timing of follow-up and outcomes assessed, a pooled meta-analysis of SWT for lateral elbow tendinopathy was considered inappropriate. In a qualitative systematic per-study analysis identifying common and diverging details of 10 randomized-controlled trials, evidence was found for effectiveness of shock wave treatment for tennis elbow under well-defined, restrictive conditions only».

It could be stated that some different parameters could influence the results, in designing clinical studies, due to their high variability and heterogeneity, especially among different individuals.

Very recently again, Dingemanse *et al:* wrote that to draw more definite conclusions, high-quality randomized controlled trials, examining different intensities, are needed, as well as studies with long-term follow-up results [91, 92].

Finally, it is possible to reasume some variables, responsible for affecting clinical results:

- disease duration
- different devices and different ESWT protocols, not always perfectly comparable (according to frequency and total dose of SW energy);
- type of treatment and control group;
- timing of follow-up;
- clinical evaluation scales

It seems that the reason of controversial results in literature regarding the success of ESWT in tendinopathies could not be a biological matter but rather a methodological one [93]. When considering, for example, well-designed randomized control trials for tennis elbow, there has been demonstrated evidence of the effectiveness of shock wave intervention [94].

This seems to be more proper nowadays, as, since that time, some other basic science studies were published, describing a positive influence of SW on tendon cells and metabolism, that can be added to the well-known anti-inflammatory effect, proving physiological vascularization at the tendon-bone junction [33, 93].

All the beneficial effects deriving on tenocytes and tendon metabolism after SW exposure can be summarized as follows [94 - 99]:

- the release of nitric oxide (NO) activates protein synthesis and increases the expression of TGF-β1 gene and the increased production of cell nuclear antigen (PCNA): these processes result in an increase in the number of tenocytes and collagen synthesis;
- decreased expression of several interleukins (ILs) and metalloproteinases (MMPs);
- possible influence on tendon healing and regeneration;
- increased expression of lubrycin;
- improvement in cell proliferation and vitality, while expressing some typical tendon markers and anti-inflammatory cytokines;
- enhanced functional activities of ruptured tendon-derived tenocytes *in vitro* (relatively to proliferation and migration), with possible influence on tendon healing *in vivo:*

Thanks to a physiological-like mechanism of ESWT emulating E.S.A.F. action (Endothelial Stimulating Angiogenetic Factor), a peptide that perforate the endothelial capillary membrane promoting neo-angiogenesis thanks to endothelial cells migration in the interstitial space [100]. This means that the anti-inflammatory response, observing after treatment, is due to the intense circulatory washout, in the target area, causing the removal of quinine and histamine-like molecules activities and substance P present in the inflammation reaction. Another biological explanation for the analgesic effect of ESWT is related to degeneration of the nerve fibers originating from the small neurons immune-reactive to ATF3 (Activating Transcription Factor 3), a protein linked to the activation of genes related to protein coding pro-inflammatory, which seems to derive a reduction in pain. Peripheral destruction of non-myelin fibers deputed to control of the release of the release of calcitonin gene-related peptide (CGRP) [101] and substance P determines the resolution of symptoms in the following weeks [102].

These basic science data suggest that in the field of tendinopathies, SW can be considered not only as a "palliative" therapy but rather a real curative treatment, able to relieve pain and inflammation at short-medium term follow-up but also to positively interfere with tendon structure and physiology (potential trophic effect at long term follow-up) [53]. The effects of ESWT studied in non-pathological tenocytes highlight the increase of growth and cell proliferation associated with the type I collagen deposition [103], on the pathological tenocytes is observed, in addition to the two already mentioned phenomena, the decrease in the expression of matrix metalloproteases and interleukins [104].

Studies available in scientific literature confirm that ESWT is a promoting tissue regeneration agent due to the increased turnover of collagen (restoring type I collagen) [105, 106], the increase of vascularization in myotendinous junction associated with a restore of physiological percent of elastin. In wound healing ESWT determine reduction of wound area and the increase of vascularization of the wound bed with a proliferation of granulation tissue [107, 108]. The pathogenesis process associated with degenerative tendon pathologies is related to the alteration of the mechanisms of adaptation to the mechanical and metabolic stress, with imbalance between the synthesis and degradation of collagen and extracellular matrix [109]. The remodeling phase is essential in response to repetitive micro trauma; this endogenous repair mechanism is performed by tenocytes that maintain homeostasis between the production and the degradation of collagen fibers and matrix. The remodeling is, also, related to the resistance of the tendon as a response to training, which represents a mechanical stress, thus prevents the partial or complete rupture. During the remodelling phase, it determines an increase in the mass tendon in cross section.

The remodeling phase adjustment occurs through the MMP expression [110]. Studies of tendon injuries in rats have shown the important role of MMPs in the synthesis of collagen modulation and conversion of type III collagen in type I collagen (MMP-9 and MMP-13) with extracellular matrix remodeling and healing (MMP-2, MMP-3 and MMP-14) [111].

With regard to chronic wounds, the mechanism linked to the non-healing, is associated to an alteration of the inflammatory state [112]. Physiologically phase of inflammation is related to the release of growth factors and cytokines from platelets, polymorph nuclear leukocytes, macrophages and other inflammatory cells that induce vasodilation, angiogenesis with activation of fibroblasts and tenocytes, collagen proliferation. A pathological extension of inflammation slows down the healing process[113].

Nitric oxide is a radical with a short half-life but with many biological actions, in fact possesses a bactericidal action, can induce programmed cell death of inflammatory cells, is the most potent inducer of vasodilatation and neo-angiogenesis [114, 115] favoring thus healing. The synthesis of NO takes place from the L-arginine by the enzyme NO synthase (NOS). It is observed that the levels of NOS have a peak during the week following a damage tendon and they are stable up to the 14th day. Furthermore, the inhibition of NOS production determines not only a delayed healing but also an alteration of the tendinous section with less resistance and risk of rupture [107,108]. There are three NOS isoforms encoded by different genes: endothelial NOS (eNOS or type 3), neuronal NOS (nNOS or type 1), inducible NOS (iNOS or type 2) is not normally expressed but is induced by endotoxins and inflammatory mediators (lipopolysaccharide, cytokines) [117].

The levels of neuronal NOS (nNOS or type 1) coincides with the formation of small nerve fibers in animal models of tendon injury between 2 and 6 weeks [118]. These nerve fibers are the expression of the reparative phenomenon; they provide neuropeptides that act as second messengers in the complex of the tendon healing process [118]. Involved in this phenomenon are substance P and CGRP molecules released in the inflammatory stage and which cause vasodilatation and extravasation of proteins [119, 120]. ESWT Determines peripheral destruction of non-myelinic fibers deputed to control of the release of substance P determines the resolution of symptoms in the Following weeks; in some experimental protocols after 4-6 weeks from the treatment there was a significant reduction in pain symptomatology [121].

Berta *et al:*, [122] showed that, the ESWT applied at low-to medium-energy, on healthy fibroblasts in suspension, increase fibroblastic growth rate, enhance gene expression for TGF-β1 and type I and III collagen, the main factors involved in the process of repair and cell proliferation according to earlier work by Wang *et al:*, [123, 124] and Martini *et al:*, [125].

Number of pulses influences proliferation of fibroblasts, as well as the intensity of energy applied, in laboratory studies, they had a destructive dose-dependent effect on cells in suspension, as they had a stimulating effect on dose-dependent cell proliferation. The increase in the rate of proliferation is observed in the treated cells and the greatest increase is observed from the 6th to the 12th day. The authors conclude that the parameters which should be used to stimulate the reparative processes of the tendon are 0,22 mJ/mm^2 with 1,000 pulses with a piezoelectric device, in order to obtain a proliferative stimulus for fibroblasts. In addition, the expression of TGF-β1 mRNA of fibroblasts is greater at 9 days compared to 6 days, in particular the expression of the mRNA for the type I and III collagen in a different way, at day 6 for collagen type I and 9 days for type III collagen [126]. The fibroblast growth times are in agreement with those reported in the literature for TGF-β1 and collagen types I and III demonstrating the important role of collagen in reparative differentiation processes.

Other studies investigate the effect of ESWT on biochemical and biomechanical properties of Achilles tendons. They evaluated a single session of ESWT at 0.16 mJ/mm^2 density at different number of pulses demonstrating that a low number of pulses (200) leads to an improvement of biomechanical and biochemical characteristics after 12 sessions, while high numbers of pulses (between 500 and 1000) have inhibitory effects. After 6 weeks, tenocytes express high levels of PCNA (Proliferating Cell Nuclear Antigen) expression of a reactivation of the cell cycle so of mitosis. Furthermore, it is observed an increased expression of TGF-β1, which is associated with the aggregation of the hypertrophied cells and new tendon tissue, and IGF-1 for all the reparative period [99].

Tsai *et al:*, [127] confirm the stimulating effect of ESWT on the tendon cell proliferation, in rats after tendon injury. The proliferative effect, according to this author, appears to be greater in degenerative tendon rather than in inflammatory phases where the reactive component prevails [128]. This is supported by other data in the literature [129, 130]. The comparability of approaches is not homogeneous because not all studies have applied the use of ESWT according to degenerative or inflammatory characteristics of tendinopathy.

Overall, in literature, positive results are reported for tendinitis of the rotator cuff, jumper's knee, Achilles tendinopathy, plantar fasciitis (from 60 to 91%), and lateral epicondylitis (more than 60%); only 27% for the medial epicondylitis [1 - 3]. Other tendinopathies can be treated with ESWT as trochanteric pain syndrome [131], chronic proximal hamstring tendinopathy [132] and medial tibial stress syndrome [133, 134].

Comparison of some alternative therapeutic procedures with SW would underline the efficacy of this mechanotherapy and mechanostrasduction. Ozturan *et al:* compared the short-, medium-, and long-term effects of corticosteroid injection, autologous blood injection, and ESWT for lateral epicondylitis. Corticosteroid injection seemed to achieve a high success rate in the short-term follow-up, while autologous blood injection and ESWT resulted in better long-term results, especially considering the high recurrence percentage after corticosteroid injection. They describe a success rate of 50% of corticosteroid injection therapy, 83.3% of autologous blood injection and 89.9% of ESWT [135].

According to some other studies relatively to specific tendinopathies, not only ESWT revealed to be a noninvasive tool, useful for reducing the necessity of surgical interventions [136], but also a valid treatment option for all patients, when local steroid injection is ineffective or contraindicated [137].

CLINICAL APPLICATIONS

SW And Bone

Besides, tendinopathies, the second most representative clinical field where ESWT acts as vibratory mechanotherapy is among one of the bone healing disorders and bone vascular diseases.

First scientific evidence, of the efficacy of ESWT in improving osteogenesis in bone healing disturbances, was published in 1991 by Valchanov and Michailov, who reported positive results in 70 out of 82 patients affected by delayed or chronic bone nonunion at different sites [37]. This work can be considered a real milestone, as, until that time, the only therapeutic option for all these disturbances was surgery. Thereafter the therapeutic perspectives and scenario began to change: basic science studies and clinical trials were published in the following years, in order to explain the effects and mechanisms of action of ESWT in non-unions and delayed unions of bone fractures, reporting promising results with a success rate ranging from 50 to 85% [4, 5, 37, 138 - 140].

Another interesting field of SW application in bone healing disturbances is represented by stress fractures. Due to an altered biomechanical environment (repeated strains and overload), eventually sustained by an abnormal anatomical conformation (especially in the foot), there is an imbalance in local bone turnover, with a prevailing resorption phase, that, as a final results, if not properly and early treated, can result in a real fracture besides persisting and sometimes worsening pain,. ESWT application, in association with some other prescriptions (mainly rest and not weight-bearing), turns out to be a good strategy for accelerating bone healing and pain relief, thus allowing a more rapid return to sport and daily activities [141].

From a general point of view, bone can be considered a tissue where mechano-biological pathways are better expressed in their different forms: this in partly due to its mechanosensitivity and its complexity at the tissutal and physiologic level. Basic researches, in fact, would demonstrate that mechanical stimulation can act on the bone at different levels: surely SW action is exerted on bone, periosteal cells and their precursors, bone microvessels, and in the cross-talk between osteoblasts and osteoclasts as well [61, 142, 143].

Low-risk stress fractures in athletes usually can successfully be treated conservatively, but up to one third of them may not respond, and develope high-risk stress fractures. Surgical treatment may be the final solution, but it is in any case an invasive procedure, with potential complications. ESWT has been proposed for the treatment of stress fractures, since 1999, with interesting results, without complications. After many years and studies confirming this efficacy, it has been recently recommended that SW should be the primary standard of care in low risk patients with stress fracture and poor response to conventional treatments [141].

From a general point of view, all the following effects have been described in bone after SW exposure:

• osteogenic cells differentiation from mesenchymal precursors [62];
• direct stimulation of osteoblasts/periosteal cells [125, 144 - 148];
• orthotopic bone regeneration through stimulation of the periosteum [60];
• reduction of osteoclasts activity, through inhibition of pro-osteoclastogenic factors [61].
• accelerated migration of osteoblasts [149];
• early expression of angiogenesis-related growth factors, endothelial NOS, VEGF [143].

SW and Muscle Disorders

Spasticity: As anticipated, since the original description presented by Lohse-Busch, in 1997 [20], SW can be considered a valid therapeutic tool also in the field of spasticity and related syndromes, in children and adults, both for upper and lower limbs, although further standardization of treatment protocols (including treatment intervals and intensities) needs to be established and long-term follow-up studies are needed [21].

Interestingly, as mechanotherapies, both focal and radial SW seem to be effective in reducing spastic signs and symptoms of different origins, although the mechanisms of action are still under study and described only as hypothesis, as, all instrumental studies, until now, indeed did not reveal particular alterations or variations in peripheral neurophysiologic activities [150].

For example, it has been described that ESWT enhances the effect of botulinum toxin type A than better than electrical stimulation, probably by modulating rheology of the muscle and neurotransmission at the neuromuscular junction [151]. Furthermore, it has been postulated that the application of SW on muscles induced a transient dysfunction of nerve conduction at the neuromuscular junctions, but surely further studies have to be performed, in order to confirm and study this possible mechanism in more details [152].

More recently, some authors began and proposed some experimental studies in humans, based on SW transcranial stimulation, that is directed to the central nervous system, thus obtaining interesting preliminary results. Moreover, focused SW transcranial stimulations were able to stimulate vigilance in patients with unresponsive wakefulness syndrome. In addition, in this case, the precise neurophysiological effects remain to be verified by a study on clinical results. Although surely with promising perspectives, these applications have to be considered as experimental ones, thus requiring further confirmations and controlled studies [153].

Besides its effectiveness in spasticity until now, relatively few studies have been published in literature regarding SW treatment for muscle disturbances.

Myofascial pain syndrome: Some authors reported beneficial effects by applying SW also in myofascial pain syndromes and fibromyalgia, even if the exact mechanisms of action are still under study.

Some hypotheses have already been proposed in any case, as for example, a different concentration of pain related substances, enhanced angiogenesis and perfusion in ischemic tissues [154]. Moreover, mechanical stimulation of SW can be useful, according to many authors, in diagnosing and treating myofascial pain syndrome [155].

Gleitz *et al:*, [156] described in details which can be the non-invasive procedures employed in myofascial pain syndrome. In this case, combination of focal and radial SW seems to be a good strategy as medical intervention. In details, focal SW can be used for diagnosis, by evoking pain referral, immediately followed by therapy that can be carried out by radial SW.

Moreover, Moghtaderi *et al:*, in treating some cases of myofascial pain related to plantar fasciitis, concluded that by combining ESWT, both for plantar fasciitis and gastrocnemius-soleus trigger points, it is possible to obtain better results [157]. Preliminary results are surely very encouraging, but further studies and a standardization of the treatment protocol are needed as well, for optimizing therapy and results.

Myositis ossificans: Myositis ossificans, as a sequela of a direct trauma or secondary to repeated micro-injuries, can be considered a fairly common complication in sport activity. This pathologic condition is critical from the therapeutic point of view, as, in clinical practice, common "physical therapies" lack evidence. On the other hand, surgical removal, as an invasive and demolitive procedure, has to be considered the last resource, because it is frequently associated with a significative functional impairment. Relatively few articles have been published in literature about the treatment of post-traumatic myositis ossificans, and fewer about ESWT effects [158, 159].

From a general point of view, although further studies and researches are needed, preliminary experiences seem to suggest that SWs represent an interesting therapeutic tool for improving and partially restoring muscle functions and extensibility. Moreover, clinical positive results, in this disorder, can be even more evident, by associating ESWT to classical rehabilitation procedures, also by considering that this vibratory mechanotherapy is safe, economic and has no side effects; in other words, a good alternative to surgery [160].

Another revolutionary and recent field of application for ESWT is represented by regenerative medicine, especially in wound care management, where this mechanotherapy can be applied, together with some other therapeutic tools that represent a standard of care. As already described for the mechanisms of action, SW can induce tissue regeneration, in virtue of their angiogenetic potential and stem cells stimulation. Through a series of experimental and clinical studies, besides *in vitro* researches, it has been possible to enlarge its field of action to wide categories of regenerative disturbances; for example, wounds of different origin and ulcers that do not heal, as well as painful scars, diabetic ulcers, burns and some other similar disturbances [14 - 16, 18, 19].

Always recently, aiming to the angiogenic effect and trophic stimulation exerted by SW, we assisted to a growing interest and diffusion of this therapy in some andrological fields, namely *induratio penis plastica* (La Peyronie's disease) and erectile dysfunctions. From this point of view, nowadays, we can consider rapid experimental phase, already being involved in clinical practice [22 - 28].

Moreover, as anticipated, already since many years, many scientists all over the world, both in animals and in humans, as well as *in vitro*, are studying possible applications in cardiology, in order to regenerate ischaemic myocardium. This shows new interesting perspectives, in limiting hypoxic damage soon after noxious and increasing myocardial performance in the follow-up, as well as improving heart contraction in chronic insufficiency [29 - 32].

CONFLICT OF INTEREST

The author (editor) declares no conflict of interest, financial or otherwise.

ACKNOWLEDGEMENTS

Declared none.

REFERENCES

[1]   Notarnicola A, Moretti B. The biological effects of extracorporeal shock wave therapy (eswt) on tendon tissue. Muscles Ligaments Tendons J 2012; 2(1): 33-7.
[PMID: 23738271]

[2]   Romeo P, Lavanga V, Pagani D, Sansone V. Extracorporeal shock wave therapy in musculoskeletal disorders: a review. Med Princ Pract 2014; 23(1): 7-13.
[http://dx.doi.org/10.1159/000355472] [PMID: 24217134]

[3]   Wang CJ. Extracorporeal shockwave therapy in musculoskeletal disorders. J Orthop Surg 2012; 7: 11.
[http://dx.doi.org/10.1186/1749-799X-7-11] [PMID: 22433113]

[4]   Schaden W, Fischer A, Sailler A. Extracorporeal shock wave therapy of nonunion or delayed osseous union. Clin Orthop Relat Res 2001; (387): 90-4.
[http://dx.doi.org/10.1097/00003086-200106000-00012] [PMID: 11400900]

[5]   Cacchio A, Giordano L, Colafarina O, *et al.* Extracorporeal shock-wave therapy compared with surgery for hypertrophic long-bone nonunions. J Bone Joint Surg Am 2009; 91(11): 2589-97.
[http://dx.doi.org/10.2106/JBJS.H.00841] [PMID: 19884432]

[6]   Furia JP, Rompe JD, Cacchio A, Maffulli N. Shock wave therapy as a treatment of nonunions, avascular necrosis, and delayed healing of stress fractures. Foot Ankle Clin 2010; 15(4): 651-62.
[http://dx.doi.org/10.1016/j.fcl.2010.07.002] [PMID: 21056863]

[7]   Furia JP, Juliano PJ, Wade AM, Schaden W, Mittermayr R. Shock wave therapy compared with intramedullary screw fixation for nonunion of proximal fifth metatarsal metaphyseal-diaphyseal fractures. J Bone Joint Surg Am 2010; 92(4): 846-54.
[http://dx.doi.org/10.2106/JBJS.I.00653] [PMID: 20360507]

[8]   Ioppolo F, Rompe JD, Furia JP, Cacchio A. Clinical application of shock wave therapy (SWT) in musculoskeletal disorders. Eur J Phys Rehabil Med 2014; 50(2): 217-30.
[PMID: 24667365]

[9]   Wang CJ, Wang FS, Huang CC, Yang KD, Weng LH, Huang HY. Treatment for osteonecrosis of the femoral head: comparison of extracorporeal shock waves with core decompression and bone-grafting. J Bone Joint Surg Am 2005; 87(11): 2380-7.
[PMID: 16264111]

[10]   Alves EM, Angrisani AT, Santiago MB. The use of extracorporeal shock waves in the treatment of osteonecrosis of the femoral head: a systematic review. Clin Rheumatol 2009; 28(11): 1247-51.
[http://dx.doi.org/10.1007/s10067-009-1231-y] [PMID: 19609482]

[11]   DAgostino C, Romeo P, Amelio E, Sansone V. Effectiveness of ESWT in the treatment of Kienböcks disease. Ultrasound Med Biol 2011; 37(9): 1452-6.
[http://dx.doi.org/10.1016/j.ultrasmedbio.2011.06.003] [PMID: 21767905]

[12]   Vulpiani MC, Vetrano M, Trischitta D, *et al.* Extracorporeal shock wave therapy in early osteonecrosis of the femoral head: prospective clinical study with long-term follow-up. Arch Orthop Trauma Surg 2012; 132(4): 499-508.
[http://dx.doi.org/10.1007/s00402-011-1444-9] [PMID: 22228278]

[13]   dAgostino C, Romeo P, Lavanga V, Pisani S, Sansone V. Effectiveness of extracorporeal shock wave therapy in bone marrow edema syndrome of the hip. Rheumatol Int 2014; 34(11): 1513-8.
[http://dx.doi.org/10.1007/s00296-014-2991-5] [PMID: 24658812]

[14]   Saggini R, Figus A, Troccola A, Cocco V, Saggini A, Scuderi N. Extracorporeal shock wave therapy for management of chronic ulcers in the lower extremities. Ultrasound Med Biol 2008; 34(8): 1261-71.
[http://dx.doi.org/10.1016/j.ultrasmedbio.2008.01.010] [PMID: 18394777]

[15]   Arnó A, García O, Hernán I, Sancho J, Acosta A, Barret JP. Extracorporeal shock waves, a new non-surgical method to treat severe burns. Burns 2010; 36(6): 844-9.
[http://dx.doi.org/10.1016/j.burns.2009.11.012] [PMID: 20071091]

[16]   Qureshi AA, Ross KM, Ogawa R, Orgill DP. Shock wave therapy in wound healing. Plast Reconstr Surg 2011; 128(6): 721e-7e.
[http://dx.doi.org/10.1097/PRS.0b013e318230c7d1] [PMID: 21841528]

[17]   Romeo P, dAgostino MC, Lazzerini A, Sansone VC. Extracorporeal shock wave therapy in pillar pain after carpal tunnel release: a preliminary study. Ultrasound Med Biol 2011; 37(10): 1603-8.
[http://dx.doi.org/10.1016/j.ultrasmedbio.2011.07.002] [PMID: 21856074]

[18]   Fioramonti P, Cigna E, Onesti MG, Fino P, Fallico N, Scuderi N. Extracorporeal shock wave therapy for the management of burn scars. Dermatol Surg 2012; 38(5): 778-82.
[http://dx.doi.org/10.1111/j.1524-4725.2012.02355.x] [PMID: 22335776]

[19]   Mittermayr R, Antonic V, Hartinger J, *et al.* Extracorporeal shock wave therapy (ESWT) for wound healing: technology, mechanisms, and clinical efficacy. Wound Repair Regen 2012; 20(4): 456-65.
[PMID: 22642362]

[20]   Lohse-Busch H, Kraemer M, Reime U. A pilot investigation into the effects of extracorporeal shock waves on muscular dysfunction in children with spastic movement disorders. Schmerz 1997; 11(2): 108-12.
[http://dx.doi.org/10.1007/s004820050071] [PMID: 12799827]

[21]   Lee JY, Kim SN, Lee IS, Jung H, Lee KS, Koh SE. Effects of extracorporeal shock wave therapy on spasticity in patients after brain injury: A meta-analysis. J Phys Ther Sci 2014; 26(10): 1641-7.
[http://dx.doi.org/10.1589/jpts.26.1641] [PMID: 25364134]

[22]   Chung E, Cartmill R. Evaluation of clinical efficacy, safety and patient satisfaction rate after low-intensity extracorporeal shockwave therapy for the treatment of male erectile dysfunction: an Australian first open-label single-arm prospective clinical trial. BJU Int 2015; 115 (Suppl. 5): 46-9.
[http://dx.doi.org/10.1111/bju.13035] [PMID: 25828173]

[23]   Bechara A, Casabé A, De Bonis W, Nazar J. [Effectiveness of low-intensity extracorporeal shock wave therapy on patients with Erectile Dysfunction (ED) who have failed to respond to PDE5i therapy. A pilot study]. Arch Esp Urol 2015; 68(2): 152-60.
[PMID: 25774822]

[24]   Abu-Ghanem Y, Kitrey ND, Gruenwald I, Appel B, Vardi Y. Penile low-intensity shock wave therapy: a promising novel modality for erectile dysfunction. Korean J Urol 2014; 55(5): 295-9.
[http://dx.doi.org/10.4111/kju.2014.55.5.295] [PMID: 24868332]

[25]   Lei H, Liu J, Li H, *et al.* Low-intensity shock wave therapy and its application to erectile dysfunction. World J Mens Health 2013; 31(3): 208-14.
[http://dx.doi.org/10.5534/wjmh.2013.31.3.208] [PMID: 24459653]

[26] Gruenwald I, Appel B, Kitrey ND, Vardi Y. Shockwave treatment of erectile dysfunction. Ther Adv Urol 2013; 5(2): 95-9.
[http://dx.doi.org/10.1177/1756287212470696] [PMID: 23554844]

[27] Paulis G, Brancato T. Inflammatory mechanisms and oxidative stress in Peyronies disease: therapeutic rationale and related emerging treatment strategies. Inflamm Allergy Drug Targets 2012; 11(1): 48-57.
[http://dx.doi.org/10.2174/187152812798889321] [PMID: 22309083]

[28] Gruenwald I, Appel B, Vardi Y. Low-intensity extracorporeal shock wave therapy a novel effective treatment for erectile dysfunction in severe ED patients who respond poorly to PDE5 inhibitor therapy. J Sex Med 2012; 9(1): 259-64.
[http://dx.doi.org/10.1111/j.1743-6109.2011.02498.x] [PMID: 22008059]

[29] Holfeld J, Tepeköylü C, Blunder S, et al. Low energy shock wave therapy induces angiogenesis in acute hind-limb ischemia via VEGF receptor 2 phosphorylation. PLoS One 2014; 9(8): e103982.
[http://dx.doi.org/10.1371/journal.pone.0103982] [PMID: 25093816]

[30] Tepeköylü C, Lobenwein D, Blunder S, et al. Alteration of inflammatory response by shock wave therapy leads to reduced calcification of decellularized aortic xenografts in mice. Eur J Cardiothorac Surg 2015; 47(3): e80-90.
[http://dx.doi.org/10.1093/ejcts/ezu428] [PMID: 25422292]

[31] Ito K, Fukumoto Y, Shimokawa H. Extracorporeal shock wave therapy for ischemic cardiovascular disorders. Am J Cardiovasc Drugs 2011; 11(5): 295-302.
[http://dx.doi.org/10.2165/11592760-000000000-00000] [PMID: 21846155]

[32] Ito K, Fukumoto Y, Shimokawa H. Extracorporeal shock wave therapy as a new and non-invasive angiogenic strategy. Tohoku J Exp Med 2009; 219(1): 1-9.
[http://dx.doi.org/10.1620/tjem.219.1] [PMID: 19713678]

[33] Haupt G. Shock waves in orthopedics. Urologe A 1997; 36(3): 233-8.
[http://dx.doi.org/10.1007/s001200050096] [PMID: 9265344]

[34] Rompe JD, Furia J, Maffulli N. Eccentric loading versus eccentric loading plus shock-wave treatment for midportion Achilles tendinopathy: a randomized controlled trial. Am J Sports Med 2009; 37(3): 463-70.
[http://dx.doi.org/10.1177/0363546508326983] [PMID: 19088057]

[35] Al-Abbad H, Simon JV. The effectiveness of extracorporeal shock wave therapy on chronic Achilles tendinopathy: a systematic review. Foot Ankle Int 2013; 34(1): 33-41.
[http://dx.doi.org/10.1177/1071100712464354] [PMID: 23386759]

[36] Shrivastava SK, Kailash . Shock wave treatment in medicine. J Biosci 2005; 30(2): 269-75.
[http://dx.doi.org/10.1007/BF02703708] [PMID: 15933416]

[37] Valchanou VD, Michailov P. High energy shock waves in the treatment of delayed and nonunion of fractures. Int Orthop 1991; 15(3): 181-4.
[http://dx.doi.org/10.1007/BF00192289] [PMID: 1743828]

[38] Huang C, Holfeld J, Schaden W, Orgill D, Ogawa R. Mechanotherapy: revisiting physical therapy and recruiting mechanobiology for a new era in medicine. Trends Mol Med 2013; 19(9): 555-64.
[http://dx.doi.org/10.1016/j.molmed.2013.05.005] [PMID: 23790684]

[39] Ueberle F. Shock wave technology. In: Siebert W, Buch M, Eds. Extracorporeal shock waves in orthopaedics. Berlin: Springer 1997; pp. 59-87.

[40] Wess O, Ueberle F, Dührssen RN, et al. Working group technical developments – consensus report. In: Chaussy C, Eisenberger F, Jocham D, Wilbert D, Eds. High Energy Shock Waves in Medicine. Stuttgart: Thieme 1997; pp. 59-71.

[41]   Gerdesmeyer L, Henne M, Göbel M, Diehl P. Physical principles and generation of shockwaves. Extracorporeal shock wave therapy: Clinical results, technologies, basics. Towson: Data Trace Publishing Company 2006; pp. 11-20.

[42]   Speed C. A systematic review of shockwave therapies in soft tissue conditions: focusing on the evidence. Br J Sports Med 2014; 48(21): 1538-42.
[http://dx.doi.org/10.1136/bjsports-2012-091961] [PMID: 23918444]

[43]   Gerdesmeyer L, Maier M, Haake M, Schmitz C. Physical-technical principles of extracorporeal shockwave therapy (ESWT). Orthopade 2002; 31(7): 610-7.
[http://dx.doi.org/10.1007/s00132-002-0319-8] [PMID: 12219657]

[44]   Ogden JA, Tóth-Kischkat A, Schultheiss R. Principles of shock wave therapy. Clin Orthop Relat Res 2001; (387): 8-17.
[http://dx.doi.org/10.1097/00003086-200106000-00003] [PMID: 11400898]

[45]   Bosco V, Buselli P. Proprietà fisiche delle onde d'urto. In: Moretti B, Amelio E, Notarnicola A, Eds. Le onde d'urto nella pratica medica. Bari: WIP Edizioni 2010; pp. 19-39.

[46]   Wang CJ, Yang KD, Wang FS, Hsu CC, Chen HH. Shock wave treatment shows dose-dependent enhancement of bone mass and bone strength after fracture of the femur. Bone 2004; 34(1): 225-30.
[http://dx.doi.org/10.1016/j.bone.2003.08.005] [PMID: 14751581]

[47]   Moretti B, Notarnicola A. Le onde radiali. In: Moretti B, Amelio E, Notarnicola A, Eds. Le onde d'urto nella pratica medica. Bari: WIP Edizioni 2010; pp. 15-7.

[48]   Melegati G, Tornese D, Bandi M, Rubini M. Comparison of two ultrasonographic localization techniques for the treatment of lateral epicondylitis with extracorporeal shock wave therapy: a randomized study. Clin Rehabil 2004; 18(4): 366-70.
[http://dx.doi.org/10.1191/0269215504cr762oa] [PMID: 15180119]

[49]   Pettrone FA, McCall BR. Extracorporeal shock wave therapy without local anesthesia for chronic lateral epicondylitis. J Bone Joint Surg Am 2005; 87(6): 1297-304.
[PMID: 15930540]

[50]   Wang CJ, Chen HS. Shock wave therapy for patients with lateral epicondylitis of the elbow: a one- to two-year follow-up study. Am J Sports Med 2002; 30(3): 422-5.
[PMID: 12016085]

[51]   Furia JP. Safety and efficacy of extracorporeal shock wave therapy for chronic lateral epicondylitis. Am J Orthop 2005; 34(1): 13-9.
[PMID: 15707134]

[52]   Ko JY, Chen HS, Chen LM. Treatment of lateral epicondylitis of the elbow with shock waves. Clin Orthop Relat Res 2001; (387): 60-7.
[http://dx.doi.org/10.1097/00003086-200106000-00008] [PMID: 11400895]

[53]   D'Agostino MC, Amelio E, Frairia R. Evoluzione delle onde d'urto – Apporto scientifico dell'Italia. Meccanismi d'azione della terapia. In: Moretti B, Amelio E, Notarnicola A, Eds. Le onde d'urto nella pratica medica. Bari: WIP Edizioni 2010; pp. 41-84.

[54]   Tara S, Miyamoto M, Takagi G, *et al.* Low-energy extracorporeal shock wave therapy improves microcirculation blood flow of ischemic limbs in patients with peripheral arterial disease: pilot study. J Nippon Med Sch 2014; 81(1): 19-27.
[http://dx.doi.org/10.1272/jnms.81.19] [PMID: 24614391]

[55]   Tepeköylü C, Wang FS, Kozaryn R, *et al.* Shock wave treatment induces angiogenesis and mobilizes endogenous CD31/CD34-positive endothelial cells in a hindlimb ischemia model: implications for angiogenesis and vasculogenesis. J Thorac Cardiovasc Surg 2013; 146(4): 971-8.
[http://dx.doi.org/10.1016/j.jtcvs.2013.01.017] [PMID: 23395097]

[56]   Visco V, Vulpiani MC, Torrisi MR, Ferretti A, Pavan A, Vetrano M. Experimental studies on the

biological effects of extracorporeal shock wave therapy on tendon models. A review of the literature. Muscles Ligaments Tendons J 2014; 4(3): 357-61.
[PMID: 25489555]

[57]   Sansone V, D Agostino MC, Bonora C, Sizzano F, De Girolamo L, Romeo P. Early angiogenic response to shock waves in a three-dimensional model of human microvascular endothelial cell culture (HMEC-1). J Biol Regul Homeost Agents 2012; 26(1): 29-37.
[PMID: 22475095]

[58]   Suhr F, Delhasse Y, Bungartz G, Schmidt A, Pfannkuche K, Bloch W. Cell biological effects of mechanical stimulations generated by focused extracorporeal shock wave applications on cultured human bone marrow stromal cells. Stem Cell Res (Amst) 2013; 11(2): 951-64.
[http://dx.doi.org/10.1016/j.scr.2013.05.010] [PMID: 23880536]

[59]   Raabe O, Shell K, Goessl A, *et al.* Effect of extracorporeal shock wave on proliferation and differentiation of equine adipose tissue-derived mesenchymal stem cells *in vitro:* Am J Stem Cells 2013; 2(1): 62-73.
[PMID: 23671817]

[60]   Kearney CJ, Hsu HP, Spector M. The use of extracorporeal shock wave-stimulated periosteal cells for orthotopic bone generation. Tissue Eng Part A 2012; 18(13-14): 1500-8.
[http://dx.doi.org/10.1089/ten.tea.2011.0573] [PMID: 22519654]

[61]   Tamma R, dellEndice S, Notarnicola A, *et al.* Extracorporeal shock waves stimulate osteoblast activities. Ultrasound Med Biol 2009; 35(12): 2093-100.
[http://dx.doi.org/10.1016/j.ultrasmedbio.2009.05.022] [PMID: 19679388]

[62]   Hausdorf J, Sievers B, Schmitt-Sody M, Jansson V, Maier M, Mayer-Wagner S. Stimulation of bone growth factor synthesis in human osteoblasts and fibroblasts after extracorporeal shock wave application. Arch Orthop Trauma Surg 2011; 131(3): 303-9.
[http://dx.doi.org/10.1007/s00402-010-1166-4] [PMID: 20730589]

[63]   Wang FS, Yang KD, Chen RF, Wang CJ, Sheen-Chen SM. Extracorporeal shock wave promotes growth and differentiation of bone-marrow stromal cells towards osteoprogenitors associated with induction of TGF-β1. J Bone Joint Surg Br 2002; 84(3): 457-61.
[http://dx.doi.org/10.1302/0301-620X.84B3.11609] [PMID: 12002511]

[64]   Ciampa AR, de Prati AC, Amelio E, *et al.* Nitric oxide mediates anti-inflammatory action of extracorporeal shock waves. FEBS Lett 2005; 579(30): 6839-45.
[http://dx.doi.org/10.1016/j.febslet.2005.11.023] [PMID: 16325181]

[65]   Gotte G, Amelio E, Russo S, Marlinghaus E, Musci G, Suzuki H. Short-time non-enzymatic nitric oxide synthesis from L-arginine and hydrogen peroxide induced by shock waves treatment. FEBS Lett 2002; 520(1-3): 153-5.
[http://dx.doi.org/10.1016/S0014-5793(02)02807-7] [PMID: 12044888]

[66]   Davis TA, Stojadinovic A, Anam K, *et al.* Extracorporeal shock wave therapy suppresses the early proinflammatory immune response to a severe cutaneous burn injury. Int Wound J 2009; 6(1): 11-21.
[http://dx.doi.org/10.1111/j.1742-481X.2008.00540.x] [PMID: 19291111]

[67]   Fischer S, Mueller W, Schulte M, *et al.* Multiple extracorporeal shock wave therapy degrades capsular fibrosis after insertion of silicone implants. Ultrasound Med Biol 2015; 41(3): 781-9.
[http://dx.doi.org/10.1016/j.ultrasmedbio.2014.10.018] [PMID: 25619782]

[68]   Heine N, Prantl L, Eisenmann-Klein M. Extracorporeal shock wave treatment of capsular fibrosis after mammary augmentation - Preliminary results. J Cosmet Laser Ther 2013; 15(6): 330-3.
[http://dx.doi.org/10.3109/14764172.2012.738915] [PMID: 23384126]

[69]   Holfeld J, Tepeköylü C, Kozaryn R, *et al.* Shockwave therapy differentially stimulates endothelial cells: implications on the control of inflammation *via* toll-Like receptor 3. Inflammation 2014; 37(1): 65-70.
[http://dx.doi.org/10.1007/s10753-013-9712-1] [PMID: 23948864]

[70]   Alunni G, Marra S, Meynet I, *et al.* The beneficial effect of extracorporeal shockwave myocardial revascularization in patients with refractory angina. Cardiovasc Revasc Med 2015; 16(1): 6-11.
[http://dx.doi.org/10.1016/j.carrev.2014.10.011] [PMID: 25555620]

[71]   Gennari M, Gambini E, Bassetti B, Capogrossi M, Pompilio G. Emerging treatment options for refractory angina pectoris: ranolazine, shock wave treatment, and cell-based therapies. Rev Cardiovasc Med 2014; 15(1): 31-7.
[PMID: 24762464]

[72]   Mariotto S, de Prati AC, Cavalieri E, Amelio E, Marlinghaus E, Suzuki H. Extracorporeal shock wave therapy in inflammatory diseases: molecular mechanism that triggers anti-inflammatory action. Curr Med Chem 2009; 16(19): 2366-72.
[http://dx.doi.org/10.2174/092986709788682119] [PMID: 19601786]

[73]   Kuo YR, Wang CT, Wang FS, Yang KD, Chiang YC, Wang CJ. Extracorporeal shock wave treatment modulates skin fibroblast recruitment and leukocyte infiltration for enhancing extended skin-flap survival. Wound Repair Regen 2009; 17(1): 80-7.
[http://dx.doi.org/10.1111/j.1524-475X.2008.00444.x] [PMID: 19152654]

[74]   Shao PL, Chiu CC, Yuen CM, *et al.* Shock wave therapy effectively attenuates inflammation in rat carotid artery following endothelial denudation by balloon catheter. Cardiology 2010; 115(2): 130-44.
[http://dx.doi.org/10.1159/000262331] [PMID: 19955748]

[75]   Sukubo NG, Tibalt E, Respizzi S, Locati M, D'Agostino MC. Effect of shock waves on macrophages: A possible role in tissue regeneration and remodeling. Int J Surg 2015; 24(Pt B): 124-30.
[http://dx.doi.org/10.1016/j.ijsu.2015.07.719]

[76]   Vulpiani MC, Vetrano M, Savoia V, Di Pangrazio E, Trischitta D, Ferretti A. Jumpers knee treatment with extracorporeal shock wave therapy: a long-term follow-up observational study. J Sports Med Phys Fitness 2007; 47(3): 323-8.
[PMID: 17641600]

[77]   Vulpiani MC, Trischitta D, Trovato P, Vetrano M, Ferretti A. Extracorporeal shockwave therapy (ESWT) in Achilles tendinopathy. A long-term follow-up observational study. J Sports Med Phys Fitness 2009; 49(2): 171-6.
[PMID: 19528895]

[78]   Saggini R, Di Stefano A, Galati V, *et al.* Long-term effectiveness of combined mechanotransduction treatment in jumper's knee. Eur J Inflamm 2012; 10(3): 483-90.
[http://dx.doi.org/10.1177/1721727X1201000324]

[79]   Saggini R, Cavezza T, Di Pancrazio L, *et al.* Treatment of lesions of the rotator cuff. J Biol Regul Homeost Agents 2010; 24(4): 453-9.
[PMID: 21122285]

[80]   Saggini R, Fioramonti P, Bellomo RG, *et al.* Chronic ulcers: treatment with unfocused extracorporeal shock waves. Eur J Inflamm 2013; 11(2): 499-509.
[http://dx.doi.org/10.1177/1721727X1301100219]

[81]   Wang CJ, Ko JY, Chou WY, *et al.* Shockwave therapy improves anterior cruciate ligament reconstruction. J Surg Res 2014; 188(1): 110-8.
[http://dx.doi.org/10.1016/j.jss.2014.01.050] [PMID: 24560350]

[82]   Saggini R, Saggini A, Spagnoli AM, *et al.* Extracorporeal shock wave therapy: An emerging treatment modality for retracting scars of the hands. Ultrasound Med Biol 2016; 42(1): 185-95.
[http://dx.doi.org/10.1016/j.ultrasmedbio.2015.07.028] [PMID: 26454624]

[83]   Battery L, Maffulli N. Inflammation in overuse tendon injuries. Sports Med Arthrosc Rev 2011; 19(3): 213-7.
[http://dx.doi.org/10.1097/JSA.0b013e31820e6a92] [PMID: 21822104]

[84]   Saggini R, Carmignano SM, Buoso S, Pestelli G. La meccanotrasduzione e il dolore. In: Saggini R,

Buoso S, Pestelli G, Eds. Dolore e Riabilitazione. Torino: Edizioni. Minerva Med 2014; pp. 85-91.

[85]   Richardson JD, Vasko MR. Cellular mechanisms of neurogenic inflammation. J Pharmacol Exp Ther 2002; 302(3): 839-45.
[http://dx.doi.org/10.1124/jpet.102.032797] [PMID: 12183638]

[86]   Schepsis AA, Leach RE, Gorzyca J. Plantar fasciitis. Etiology, treatment, surgical results, and review of the literature. Clin Orthop Relat Res 1991; (266): 185-96.
[PMID: 2019049]

[87]   Roetert EP, Brody H, Dillman CJ, Groppel JL, Schultheis JM. The biomechanics of tennis elbow. An integrated approach. Clin Sports Med 1995; 14(1): 47-57.
[PMID: 7712557]

[88]   Uchio Y, Ochi M, Ryoke K, Sakai Y, Ito Y, Kuwata S. Expression of neuropeptides and cytokines at the extensor carpi radialis brevis muscle origin. J Shoulder Elbow Surg 2002; 11(6): 570-5.
[http://dx.doi.org/10.1067/mse.2002.126769] [PMID: 12469081]

[89]   Sems A, Dimeff R, Iannotti JP. Extracorporeal shock wave therapy in the treatment of chronic tendinopathies. J Am Acad Orthop Surg 2006; 14(4): 195-204.
[http://dx.doi.org/10.5435/00124635-200604000-00001] [PMID: 16585361]

[90]   Rompe JD, Maffulli N. Repetitive shock wave therapy for lateral elbow tendinopathy (tennis elbow): a systematic and qualitative analysis. Br Med Bull 2007; 83: 355-78.
[http://dx.doi.org/10.1093/bmb/ldm019] [PMID: 17626054]

[91]   Dingemanse R, Randsdorp M, Koes BW, Huisstede BM. Evidence for the effectiveness of electrophysical modalities for treatment of medial and lateral epicondylitis: a systematic review. Br J Sports Med 2014; 48(12): 957-65.
[http://dx.doi.org/10.1136/bjsports-2012-091513] [PMID: 23335238]

[92]   Rompe JD, Theis C, Maffulli N. Shock wave treatment for tennis elbow. Orthopade 2005; 34(6): 567-70.
[http://dx.doi.org/10.1007/s00132-005-0805-x] [PMID: 15886855]

[93]   Wang CJ. An overview of shock wave therapy in musculoskeletal disorders. Chang Gung Med J 2003; 26(4): 220-32.
[PMID: 12846521]

[94]   de Girolamo L, Stanco D, Galliera E, *et al.* Soft-focused extracorporeal shock waves increase the expression of tendon-specific markers and the release of anti-inflammatory cytokines in an adherent culture model of primary human tendon cells. Ultrasound Med Biol 2014; 40(6): 1204-15.
[http://dx.doi.org/10.1016/j.ultrasmedbio.2013.12.003] [PMID: 24631378]

[95]   Leone L, Vetrano M, Ranieri D, *et al.* Extracorporeal Shock Wave Treatment (ESWT) improves *in vitro* functional activities of ruptured human tendon-derived tenocytes. PLoS One 2012; 7(11): e49759.
[http://dx.doi.org/10.1371/journal.pone.0049759] [PMID: 23189160]

[96]   Vetrano M, dAlessandro F, Torrisi MR, Ferretti A, Vulpiani MC, Visco V. Extracorporeal shock wave therapy promotes cell proliferation and collagen synthesis of primary cultured human tenocytes. Knee Surg Sports Traumatol Arthrosc 2011; 19(12): 2159-68.
[http://dx.doi.org/10.1007/s00167-011-1534-9] [PMID: 21617986]

[97]   Han SH, Lee JW, Guyton GP, Parks BG, Courneya JP, Schon LC. J.Leonard Goldner Award 2008. Effect of extracorporeal shock wave therapy on cultured tenocytes. Foot Ankle Int 2009; 30(2): 93-8.
[PMID: 19254500]

[98]   Chao YH, Tsuang YH, Sun JS, *et al.* Effects of shock waves on tenocyte proliferation and extracellular matrix metabolism. Ultrasound Med Biol 2008; 34(5): 841-52.
[http://dx.doi.org/10.1016/j.ultrasmedbio.2007.11.002] [PMID: 18222032]

[99]   Chen YJ, Wang CJ, Yang KD, *et al.* Extracorporeal shock waves promote healing of collagenase-

induced Achilles tendinitis and increase TGF-beta1 and IGF-I expression. J Orthop Res 2004; 22(4): 854-61.
[http://dx.doi.org/10.1016/j.orthres.2003.10.013] [PMID: 15183445]

[100] Bjordal JM, Lopes-Martins RA, Joensen J, *et al.* A systematic review with procedural assessments and meta-analysis of low level laser therapy in lateral elbow tendinopathy (tennis elbow). BMC Musculoskelet Disord 2008; 9(9): 75.
[http://dx.doi.org/10.1186/1471-2474-9-75] [PMID: 18510742]

[101] Emanet SK, Altan LI, Yurtkuran M. Investigation of the effect of GaAs laser therapy on lateral epicondylitis. Photomed Laser Surg 2010; 28(3): 397-403.
[http://dx.doi.org/10.1089/pho.2009.2555] [PMID: 19877824]

[102] Hu J, Qu J, Xu D, Zhang T, Qin L, Lu H. Combined application of low-intensity pulsed ultrasound and functional electrical stimulation accelerates bone-tendon junction healing in a rabbit model. J Orthop Res 2014; 32(2): 204-9.
[http://dx.doi.org/10.1002/jor.22505] [PMID: 24136665]

[103] Vetrano M, dAlessandro F, Torrisi MR, Ferretti A, Vulpiani MC, Visco V. Extracorporeal shock wave therapy promotes cell proliferation and collagen synthesis of primary cultured human tenocytes. Knee Surg Sports Traumatol Arthrosc 2011; 19(12): 2159-68.
[http://dx.doi.org/10.1007/s00167-011-1534-9] [PMID: 21617986]

[104] Han SH, Lee JW, Guyton GP, Parks BG, Courneya JP, Schon LC. J.Leonard Goldner Award 2008. Effect of extracorporeal shock wave therapy on cultured tenocytes. Foot Ankle Int 2009; 30(2): 93-8.
[PMID: 19254500]

[105] Bosch G, Lin YL, van Schie HT, van De Lest CH, Barneveld A, van Weeren PR. Effect of extracorporeal shock wave therapy on the biochemical composition and metabolic activity of tenocytes in normal tendinous structures in ponies. Equine Vet J 2007; 39(3): 226-31.
[http://dx.doi.org/10.2746/042516407X180408] [PMID: 17520973]

[106] Bosch G, de Mos M, van Binsbergen R, van Schie HT, van de Lest CH, van Weeren PR. The effect of focused extracorporeal shock wave therapy on collagen matrix and gene expression in normal tendons and ligaments. Equine Vet J 2009; 41(4): 335-41.
[http://dx.doi.org/10.2746/042516409X370766] [PMID: 19562893]

[107] Ito Y, Ito K, Shiroto T, *et al.* Cardiac shock wave therapy ameliorates left ventricular remodeling after myocardial ischemia-reperfusion injury in pigs *in vivo:* Coron Artery Dis 2010; 21(5): 304-11.
[http://dx.doi.org/10.1097/MCA.0b013e32833aec62] [PMID: 20617568]

[108] Kuo YR, Wang CT, Wang FS, Chiang YC, Wang CJ. Extracorporeal shock-wave therapy enhanced wound healing via increasing topical blood perfusion and tissue regeneration in a rat model of STZ-induced diabetes. Wound Repair Regen 2009; 17(4): 522-30.
[http://dx.doi.org/10.1111/j.1524-475X.2009.00504.x] [PMID: 19614917]

[109] Leadbetter WB. Cell-matrix response in tendon injury. Clin Sports Med 1992; 11(3): 533-78.
[PMID: 1638640]

[110] Riley GP, Curry V, DeGroot J, *et al.* Matrix metalloproteinase activities and their relationship with collagen remodelling in tendon pathology. Matrix Biol 2002; 21(2): 185-95.
[http://dx.doi.org/10.1016/S0945-053X(01)00196-2] [PMID: 11852234]

[111] Oshiro W, Lou J, Xing X, Tu Y, Manske PR. Flexor tendon healing in the rat: a histologic and gene expression study. J Hand Surg Am 2003; 28(5): 814-23.
[http://dx.doi.org/10.1016/S0363-5023(03)00366-6] [PMID: 14507513]

[112] Evans CH. Cytokines and the role they play in the healing of ligaments and tendons. Sports Med 1999; 28(2): 71-6.
[http://dx.doi.org/10.2165/00007256-199928020-00001] [PMID: 10492026]

[113] Molloy T, Wang Y, Murrell G. The roles of growth factors in tendon and ligament healing. Sports

Med 2003; 33(5): 381-94.
[http://dx.doi.org/10.2165/00007256-200333050-00004] [PMID: 12696985]

[114]   Evans TJ, Buttery LD, Carpenter A, Springall DR, Polak JM, Cohen J. Cytokine-treated human neutrophils contain inducible nitric oxide synthase that produces nitration of ingested bacteria. Proc Natl Acad Sci USA 1996; 93(18): 9553-8.
[http://dx.doi.org/10.1073/pnas.93.18.9553] [PMID: 8790368]

[115]   Ziche M, Morbidelli L, Masini E, *et al.* Nitric oxide mediates angiogenesis *in vivo* and endothelial cell growth and migration in vitro promoted by substance P. J Clin Invest 1994; 94(5): 2036-44.
[http://dx.doi.org/10.1172/JCI117557] [PMID: 7525653]

[116]   Murrell GA, Szabo C, Hannafin JA, *et al.* Modulation of tendon healing by nitric oxide. Inflamm Res 1997; 46(1): 19-27.
[http://dx.doi.org/10.1007/s000110050027] [PMID: 9117513]

[117]   Lin JH, Wang MX, Wei A, Zhu W, Diwan AD, Murrell GA. Temporal expression of nitric oxide synthase isoforms in healing Achilles tendon. J Orthop Res 2001; 19(1): 136-42.
[http://dx.doi.org/10.1016/S0736-0266(00)00019-X] [PMID: 11332610]

[118]   Ackermann PW. Peptidergic innervation of periarticular tissue (Thesis). Stockholm: Karolinska Institutet 2001. Thesis Institutionen för kirurgisk vetenskap / Department of Surgical Science https://openarchive.ki.se/xmlui/handle/10616/38953

[119]   Nakamura-Craig M, Smith TW. Substance P and peripheral inflammatory hyperalgesia. Pain 1989; 38(1): 91-8.
[http://dx.doi.org/10.1016/0304-3959(89)90078-X] [PMID: 2476709]

[120]   Brain SD, Williams TJ, Tippins JR, Morris HR, MacIntyre I. Calcitonin gene-related peptide is a potent vasodilator. Nature 1985; 313(5997): 54-6.
[http://dx.doi.org/10.1038/313054a0] [PMID: 3917554]

[121]   Vasko MR, Campbell WB, Waite KJ. Prostaglandin E2 enhances bradykinin-stimulated release of neuropeptides from rat sensory neurons in culture. J Neurosci 1994; 14(8): 4987-97.
[PMID: 7519258]

[122]   Berta L, Fazzari A, Ficco AM, Enrica PM, Catalano MG, Frairia R. Extracorporeal shock waves enhance normal fibroblast proliferation in vitro and activate mRNA expression for TGF-β1 and for collagen types I and III. Acta Orthop 2009; 80(5): 612-7.
[http://dx.doi.org/10.3109/17453670903316793] [PMID: 19916698]

[123]   Wang FS, Wang CJ, Huang HJ, Chung H, Chen RF, Yang KD. Physical shock wave mediates membrane hyperpolarization and Ras activation for osteogenesis in human bone marrow stromal cells. Biochem Biophys Res Commun 2001; 287(3): 648-55.
[http://dx.doi.org/10.1006/bbrc.2001.5654] [PMID: 11563844]

[124]   Wang FS, Yang KD, Chen RF, Wang CJ, Sheen-Chen SM. Extracorporeal shock wave promotes growth and differentiation of bone-marrow stromal cells towards osteoprogenitors associated with induction of TGF-β1. J Bone Joint Surg Br 2002; 84(3): 457-61.
[http://dx.doi.org/10.1302/0301-620X.84B3.11609] [PMID: 12002511]

[125]   Martini L, Fini M, Giavaresi G, *et al.* Primary osteoblasts response to shock wave therapy using different parameters. Artif Cells Blood Substit Immobil Biotechnol 2003; 31(4): 449-66.
[http://dx.doi.org/10.1081/BIO-120025415] [PMID: 14672419]

[126]   Chao YH, Tsuang YH, Sun JS, *et al.* Effects of shock waves on tenocyte proliferation and extracellular matrix metabolism. Ultrasound Med Biol 2008; 34(5): 841-52.
[http://dx.doi.org/10.1016/j.ultrasmedbio.2007.11.002] [PMID: 18222032]

[127]   Tsai WC, Hsu CC, Tang FT, Chou SW, Chen YJ, Pang JH. Ultrasound stimulation of tendon cell proliferation and upregulation of proliferating cell nuclear antigen. J Orthop Res 2005; 23(4): 970-6.
[http://dx.doi.org/10.1016/j.orthres.2004.11.013] [PMID: 16023014]

[128] Andres BM, Murrell GA. Treatment of tendinopathy: what works, what does not, and what is on the horizon. Clin Orthop Relat Res 2008; 466(7): 1539-54.
[http://dx.doi.org/10.1007/s11999-008-0260-1] [PMID: 18446422]

[129] Maier M, Schmitz C. Shock wave therapy: what really matters. Ultrasound Med Biol 2008; 34(11): 1868-9.
[http://dx.doi.org/10.1016/j.ultrasmedbio.2008.03.016] [PMID: 18471951]

[130] Peers K. Extracorporeal shock wave therapy in chronic Achilles and patellar tendinopathy. Leuven: Leuven University Press 2003.

[131] Furia JP, Rompe JD, Maffulli N. Low-energy extracorporeal shock wave therapy as a treatment for greater trochanteric pain syndrome. Am J Sports Med 2009; 37(9): 1806-13.
[http://dx.doi.org/10.1177/0363546509333014] [PMID: 19439756]

[132] Cacchio A, Rompe JD, Furia JP, Susi P, Santilli V, De Paulis F. Shockwave therapy for the treatment of chronic proximal hamstring tendinopathy in professional athletes. Am J Sports Med 2011; 39(1): 146-53.
[http://dx.doi.org/10.1177/0363546510379324] [PMID: 20855554]

[133] Rompe JD, Cacchio A, Furia JP, Maffulli N. Low-energy extracorporeal shock wave therapy as a treatment for medial tibial stress syndrome. Am J Sports Med 2010; 38(1): 125-32.
[http://dx.doi.org/10.1177/0363546509343804] [PMID: 19776340]

[134] Winters M, Eskes M, Weir A, Moen MH, Backx FJ, Bakker EW. Treatment of medial tibial stress syndrome: a systematic review. Sports Med 2013; 43(12): 1315-33.
[http://dx.doi.org/10.1007/s40279-013-0087-0] [PMID: 23979968]

[135] Ozturan KE, Yucel I, Cakici H, Guven M, Sungur I. Autologous blood and corticosteroid injection and extracoporeal shock wave therapy in the treatment of lateral epicondylitis. Orthopedics 2010; 33(2): 84-91.
[http://dx.doi.org/10.3928/01477447-20100104-09] [PMID: 20192142]

[136] Radwan YA, ElSobhi G, Badawy WS, Reda A, Khalid S. Resistant tennis elbow: shock-wave therapy versus percutaneous tenotomy. Int Orthop 2008; 32(5): 671-7.
[http://dx.doi.org/10.1007/s00264-007-0379-9] [PMID: 17551726]

[137] Lee SS, Kang S, Park NK, *et al.* Effectiveness of initial extracorporeal shock wave therapy on the newly diagnosed lateral or medial epicondylitis. Ann Rehabil Med 2012; 36(5): 681-7.
[http://dx.doi.org/10.5535/arm.2012.36.5.681] [PMID: 23185733]

[138] Elster EA, Stojadinovic A, Forsberg J, Shawen S, Andersen RC, Schaden W. Extracorporeal shock wave therapy for nonunion of the tibia. J Orthop Trauma 2010; 24(3): 133-41.
[http://dx.doi.org/10.1097/BOT.0b013e3181b26470] [PMID: 20182248]

[139] Wang CJ, Chen HS, Chen CE, Yang KD. Treatment of nonunions of long bone fractures with shock waves. Clin Orthop Relat Res 2001; (387): 95-101.
[http://dx.doi.org/10.1097/00003086-200106000-00013] [PMID: 11400901]

[140] Rompe JD, Rosendahl T, Schöllner C, Theis C. High-energy extracorporeal shock wave treatment of nonunions. Clin Orthop Relat Res 2001; (387): 102-11.
[http://dx.doi.org/10.1097/00003086-200106000-00014] [PMID: 11400870]

[141] Leal C, D'Agostino C, Gomez-Garcia S, Fernandez A. Current concepts of shockwave therapy in stress fractures. Int J Surg 2015; 24(Pt B): 195-200.
[http://dx.doi.org/10.1016/j.ijsu.2015.07.723]

[142] Lai JP, Wang FS, Hung CM, Wang CJ, Huang CJ, Kuo YR. Extracorporeal shock wave accelerates consolidation in distraction osteogenesis of the rat mandible. J Trauma 2010; 69(5): 1252-8.
[http://dx.doi.org/10.1097/TA.0b013e3181cbc7ac] [PMID: 20404761]

[143] Ma HZ, Zeng BF, Li XL. Upregulation of VEGF in subchondral bone of necrotic femoral heads in

rabbits with use of extracorporeal shock waves. Calcif Tissue Int 2007; 81(2): 124-31.
[http://dx.doi.org/10.1007/s00223-007-9046-9] [PMID: 17629736]

[144]   Martini L, Giavaresi G, Fini M, *et al.* Effect of extracorporeal shock wave therapy on osteoblastlike cells. Clin Orthop Relat Res 2003; (413): 269-80.
[http://dx.doi.org/10.1097/01.blo.0000073344.50837.cd] [PMID: 12897619]

[145]   Martini L, Giavaresi G, Fini M, *et al.* Shock wave therapy as an innovative technology in skeletal disorders: study on transmembrane current in stimulated osteoblast-like cells. Int J Artif Organs 2005; 28(8): 841-7.
[PMID: 16211535]

[146]   Martini L, Giavaresi G, Fini M, Borsari V, Torricelli P, Giardino R. Early effects of extracorporeal shock wave treatment on osteoblast-like cells: a comparative study between electromagnetic and electrohydraulic devices. J Trauma 2006; 61(5): 1198-206.
[http://dx.doi.org/10.1097/01.ta.0000203575.96896.34] [PMID: 17099529]

[147]   Tam KF, Cheung WH, Lee KM, Qin L, Leung KS. Osteogenic effects of low-intensity pulsed ultrasound, extracorporeal shockwaves and their combination - an *in vitro* comparative study on human periosteal cells. Ultrasound Med Biol 2008; 34(12): 1957-65.
[http://dx.doi.org/10.1016/j.ultrasmedbio.2008.06.005] [PMID: 18771844]

[148]   Wang FS, Wang CJ, Huang HJ, Chung H, Chen RF, Yang KD. Physical shock wave mediates membrane hyperpolarization and Ras activation for osteogenesis in human bone marrow stromal cells. Biochem Biophys Res Commun 2001; 287(3): 648-55.
[http://dx.doi.org/10.1006/bbrc.2001.5654] [PMID: 11563844]

[149]   Xu JK, Chen HJ, Li XD, *et al.* Optimal intensity shock wave promotes the adhesion and migration of rat osteoblasts via integrin β1-mediated expression of phosphorylated focal adhesion kinase. J Biol Chem 2012; 287(31): 26200-12.
[http://dx.doi.org/10.1074/jbc.M112.349811] [PMID: 22654119]

[150]   Sohn MK, Cho KH, Kim YJ, Hwang SL. Spasticity and electrophysiologic changes after extracorporeal shock wave therapy on gastrocnemius. Ann Rehabil Med 2011; 35(5): 599-604.
[http://dx.doi.org/10.5535/arm.2011.35.5.599] [PMID: 22506181]

[151]   Santamato A, Notarnicola A, Panza F, *et al.* SBOTE study: extracorporeal shock wave therapy versus electrical stimulation after botulinum toxin type a injection for post-stroke spasticity-a prospective randomized trial. Ultrasound Med Biol 2013; 39(2): 283-91.
[http://dx.doi.org/10.1016/j.ultrasmedbio.2012.09.019] [PMID: 23245824]

[152]   Kenmoku T, Ochiai N, Ohtori S, *et al.* Degeneration and recovery of the neuromuscular junction after application of extracorporeal shock wave therapy. J Orthop Res 2012; 30(10): 1660-5.
[http://dx.doi.org/10.1002/jor.22111] [PMID: 22457214]

[153]   Lohse-Busch H, Reime U, Falland R. Symptomatic treatment of unresponsive wakefulness syndrome with transcranially focused extracorporeal shock waves. NeuroRehabilitation 2014; 35(2): 235-44.
[PMID: 24990026]

[154]   Ji HM, Kim HJ, Han SJ. Extracorporeal shock wave therapy in myofascial pain syndrome of upper trapezius. Ann Rehabil Med 2012; 36(5): 675-80.
[http://dx.doi.org/10.5535/arm.2012.36.5.675] [PMID: 23185732]

[155]   Jeon JH, Jung YJ, Lee JY, *et al.* The effect of extracorporeal shock wave therapy on myofascial pain syndrome. Ann Rehabil Med 2012; 36(5): 665-74.
[http://dx.doi.org/10.5535/arm.2012.36.5.665] [PMID: 23185731]

[156]   Gleitz M, Hornig K. Trigger points - Diagnosis and treatment concepts with special reference to extracorporeal shockwaves. Orthopade 2012; 41(2): 113-25.
[http://dx.doi.org/10.1007/s00132-011-1860-0] [PMID: 22349369]

[157]   Moghtaderi A, Khosrawi S, Dehghan F. Extracorporeal shock wave therapy of gastroc-soleus trigger

points in patients with plantar fasciitis: a randomized, placebo-controlled trial. Adv Biomed Res 2014; 3: 99.
[http://dx.doi.org/10.4103/2277-9175.129369] [PMID: 24800188]

[158] Buselli P, Coco V, Notarnicola A, *et al.* Shock waves in the treatment of post-traumatic myositis ossificans. Ultrasound Med Biol 2010; 36(3): 397-409.
[http://dx.doi.org/10.1016/j.ultrasmedbio.2009.11.007] [PMID: 20133043]

[159] Miller AE, Davis BA, Beckley OA. Bilateral and recurrent myositis ossificans in an athlete: a case report and review of treatment options. Arch Phys Med Rehabil 2006; 87(2): 286-90.
[http://dx.doi.org/10.1016/j.apmr.2005.09.002] [PMID: 16442986]

[160] Torrance DA, Degraauw C. Treatment of post-traumatic myositis ossificans of the anterior thigh with extracorporeal shock wave therapy. J Can Chiropr Assoc 2011; 55(4): 240-6.
[PMID: 22131560]

CHAPTER 5

The Electromagnetic Vibration: Physical Principles and Biomolecular Effects

Livio Giuliani[1,2,*], **Elisabetta Giuliani**[1], **Manuela Lucarelli**[1,3] and **Raoul Saggini**[4]

[1] *International Commission for Electromagnetic Safety (ICEMS), Venice, Italy*

[2] *University of Tuscia, Viterbo*

[3] *Istituto Nazionale per l'Assicurazione contro gli Infortuni sul Lavoro e le malattie professionali (INAIL), Rome, Italy*

[4] *Physical and Rehabilitation Medicine, Department of Medical Oral and Biotechnological Sciences, School of Specialty in Physical and Rehabilitation Medicine, "Gabriele d'Annunzio" University, Chieti-Pescara, Italy; National Coordinator of Schools of Specialty in Physical and Rehabilitation Medicine*

Abstract: Life on Earth has evolved in a sea of natural electromagnetic fields. Electromagnetic waves show a biological interaction with living matter, even when they are so weak (as in the case of the so-called long radio waves, which have frequencies lower than 80 kHz) to have non-thermal effects, which seem to be both negative and positive, depending on the frequency and on the coupling with the geomagnetic field.

Many studies report that exposure to man-made electromagnetic fields affects cellular and systemic function and metabolism, with risk for malignancy and pharmacological effects. Hence, the employment of low-frequency electromagnetic fields – especially pulsed electromagnetic fields – seems to be promising, having potential applications in biomedical engineering, biotechnology, biology, oncology, and regenerative medicine.

Keywords: Blackman-Liboff-Zhadin effect, Electromagnetic fields, coherent domains, extremely low frequency, microbiological spectroscopy, pulsed electromagnetic fields, regenerative medicine, thermal and non-thermal effects, tumor-specific frequencies.

INTRODUCTION

Life on earth has evolved in a sea of natural electromagnetic fields (EMF). Like other waveforms, electromagnetic waves also are physically characterized based

---

* **Corresponding authors Manuela Lucarelli:** International Commission for Electromagnetic Safety (ICEMS), Venice, Italy; Tel: +393334059595; E-mail: giuliani.livio@gmail.com

on wavelength (λ) and frequency (v), that are related through the following relationship:

$$\lambda \cdot v = c \qquad \textbf{(1)}$$

Where c is the speed of light (299,792.458 km/s).

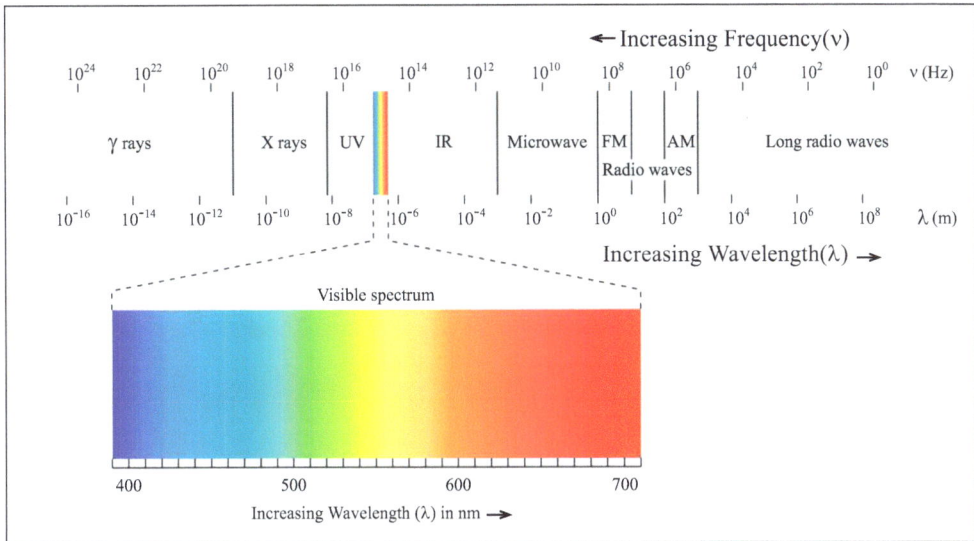

Fig. (1). The electromagnetic spectrum.

The electromagnetic spectrum is very wide and includes phenomena so different such as gamma rays, X-rays, ultraviolet, visible light, infrared, microwave, and radio waves. Gamma rays and X-rays and the more energetic ultraviolet are able to ionize molecules, because their photons transfer an energy to molecules so high to cause the escape of one or more electrons. The other frequencies, of light included, are not so energetic, and cannot ionize molecule in empty space, therefore, they are called non-ionizing radiations (NIR). All waves with frequencies lower than 80 kHz are generically referred as "long radio waves". Properly, this name has to be referred to waves with frequency higher than 3 kHz, employed to communicate by air, while frequencies under such threshold are only used for marine radio-communication between ships and submarines or between submarines. Thus their use cannot only be referred as long radio waves. In the range of frequency under 3 kHz, different bands can be distinguished: the Very Low Frequency (VLF) between 3-30 kHz, the Ultra Low Frequency (ULF) between 300-3000 Hz, the Super Low frequency (SLF) between 30-300 Hz, and Extremely Low Frequency (ELF) below 30 Hz.

THERMAL AND NON-THERMAL EFFECTS OF ELECTROMAGNETIC VIBRATIONS

Electromagnetic vibrations show a biological interaction with living matter, even when they are so weak (as in the case of long radio waves) to be considered non-thermal waves, *i.e.* when they are unable to induce a transfer of thermal energy to the living matter. The expression "non-thermal", referred to waves or to electric or magnetic or electromagnetic fields, is significant only with reference to the nature of the target that is exposed to the wave or the field [1].

Even if NIR are not able to ionize matter in empty space (and then in air, since the speed of light does not change significantly from empty space to air), their intensity can be so high that they become able to transfer thermic energy to living matter inducing several thermal biological effect. The best known thermal effects are burns, sunstrokes, and other shocks due to short term exposures; other possible effects are due to the thermal interaction of electromagnetic fields with animals and humans.

In May 2011, the International Agency for Research on Cancer (IARC) of the World Health Organization (WHO) classified the microwaves of wireless telephony as a «possibly carcinogen» (group 2B of the scale of carcinogenicity) [2]. As proposed in the draft of the WHO EMF Project, discussed in the WHO Conference on the precautionary principle in Luxembourg (25-26 February 2003), the possible carcinogenic effect of microwaves on humans should be due to the circumstance that portable devices can generate power in the same order of the limit established in Europe for the exposure of head (2 W/kg) [3], thus in the same order of the thermal threshold established for human exposures, set at 4 W/kg. The thermal threshold is the specific power of the incident wave able to induce an increase of the basal temperature equal to 0.5°C within 12 minutes. Power is the time derivative of energy, thus the amount above is the specific energy rate that is actually absorbed by the exposed human target; such amount is named Specific Absorption Rate (SAR). The thermal threshold is referred to a male with 70 kg weight and 175 cm highness (this standard was established in 1953 by the American Conference of Governmental Industrial Hygienists, based on studies about United States Navy sailors exposed to radar). Above the thermal threshold, the incident wave or field is able to induce an increase of basal temperature as 0.5°C or more; under the threshold it is not able to induce any durable increase of temperature, since after 6 minutes the homeostasis of human body compensate for the thermal absorption, reaching the basal temperature. Furthermore, the power of 4 W has to be the average of the absorbed energy for unit of time and of mass of the whole body of the target, *i.e.* of the exposed man. For the standard man, as above, the absorption of 280 W (J/s) is required to achieve the thermal threshold;

and such amount has to be continuously absorbed for 12 minutes (*i.e.* 720 seconds), summing on 201.6 kW.

The power of an incident wave or field is not completely absorbed by the target. It depends on several factors, as the thickness and conductivity of the skin and of the underling layers, under the dependence of the conductivity and of the resistivity of human muscle [4] (Fig. **2**).

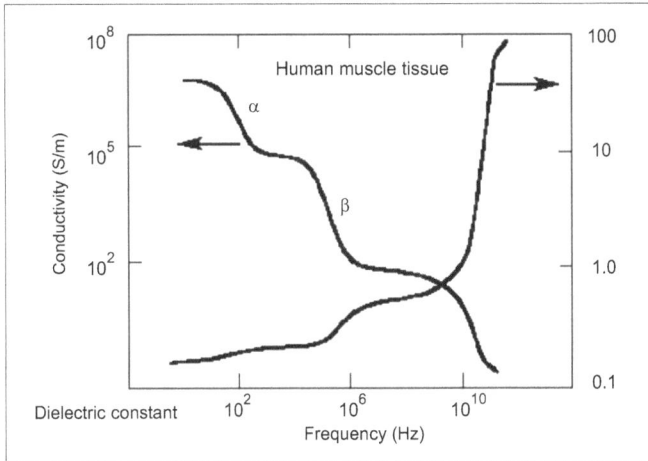

Fig. (2). The dielectric constant and conductivity of typical biological tissue as functions of frequency. From: Schwan HP. Biophysical principles of interactions and forces. In: Grandolfo M, Michaelson SM, Rindi A, Eds. Biological effects and dosimetry of static and ELF electromagnetic fields. New York, London: Plenum Press 1958; pp. 243-71.

The variation of normalized SAR with frequency and related absorption characteristics in living organisms is illustrated in Fig. (**3**).

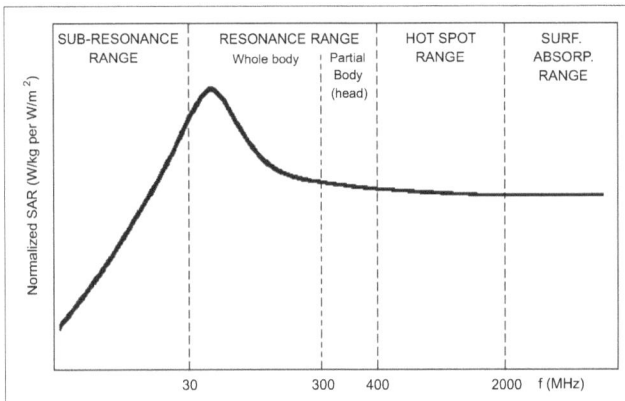

Fig. (3). Variation of normalized SAR with frequency and related absorption characteristics in living organisms. From: http://www.inchem.org/documents/ehc/ehc/ehc137.htm.

From (1) it can be calculated the peak of resonance of the standard man, who works as an antenna whose height, $h = 175$ cm, tunes a radio wave with length equal to its double:

$$v = c / \lambda = c / (2 \cdot h) = 299{,}792.458 \cdot 10^5 \text{ cm} \cdot \text{s}^{-1} / (2 \cdot 175 \text{ cm}) = 85{,}655 \text{ kHz} = 85.655 \text{ MHz}$$
(2)

The human body is a good conductor and its conductivity increases as the frequency of the incident radio wave: the conductivity of human tissues roughly is one thousand times higher with reference to the frequency of a radio wave at 85,655 MHz (a frequency employed by broadcast at frequency modulation) than with the frequency of an electromagnetic vibration, in the SHF band (Fig. **2**). Thus, the absorption of the rate of energy (*i.e.* the electromagnetic power) is higher, for the standard man, in the frequency modulation band than in the SHF/ELF band, due to both factors: resonance and conductivity of tissue.

Also the size of the target, mainly with reference to the length of the incident wave, plays a relevant role, due to the physical phenomenon of resonance: that is why an antenna is able to magnify the reception (or the emission) of an electromagnetic wave when its length is half of the length of the incident electromagnetic wave. For a child or a newborn the peak of resonance increases inversely to the size (Fig. **4**); this explain of the increased risk of children and newborns with respect to adult men for exposures to powerful radio waves in the band of microwaves [5 - 7].

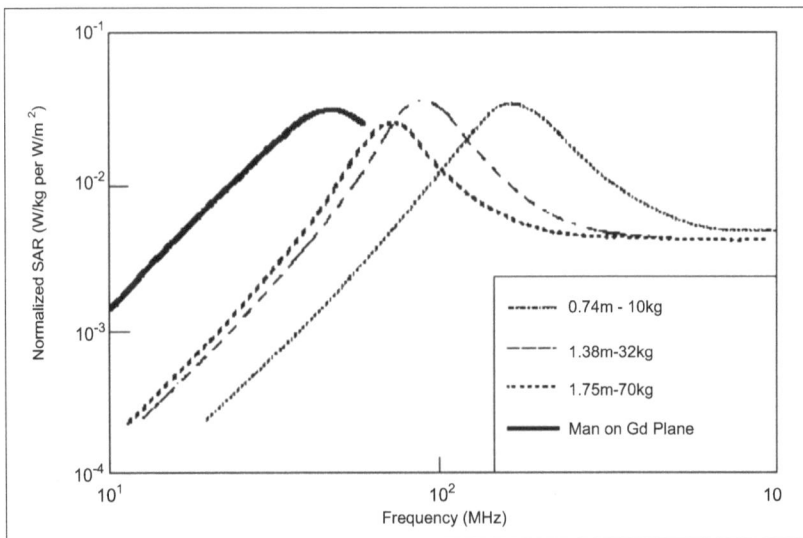

Fig. (4). Specific absorption rate for humans, according to size. From: http://www.inchem.org/ documents/ ehc/ehc/ehc137.htm.

In different organisms, the frequency of the peak of SAR shifts toward higher or lower frequencies depending respectively on the smaller or larger size of the organism.

Nonetheless, if the considered organism is a vertebrate animal the size is not the only factor influencing the absorption, the conductivity have to be considered too: for example, a jellyfish has so much water in the body to be quite different from an adult man as regards the two parameters (Fig. **5**).

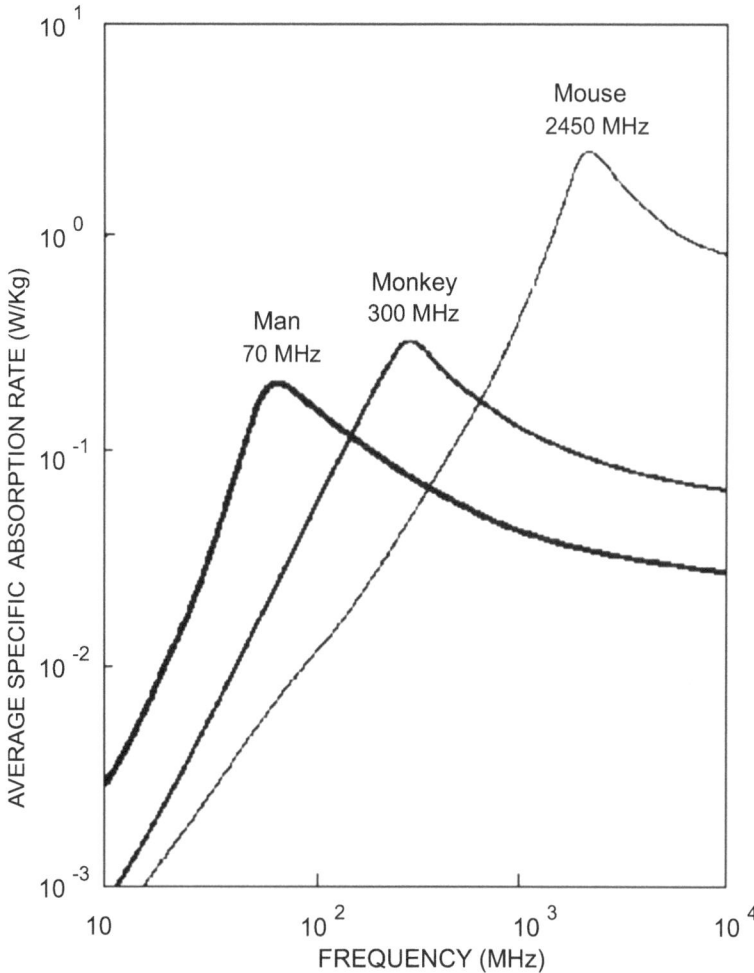

Fig. (5). Average SAR for three different species exposed to 10 W/m² with the E vector parallel to the long axis of the body. From: Durney CH, Johnson CC, Barber PW, *et al*. Radiofrequency radiation dosimetry handbook. 2nd ed. Texas, Brooks Air Force Base, USAF School of Aerospace Medicine 1978 (Report SAM-TR-78-22).

The SAR also depends on exposure conditions, that can be altered considerably by the presence of objects, the degree of perturbation depending on their size, shape, orientation in the field, and electrical properties (Fig. **6**).

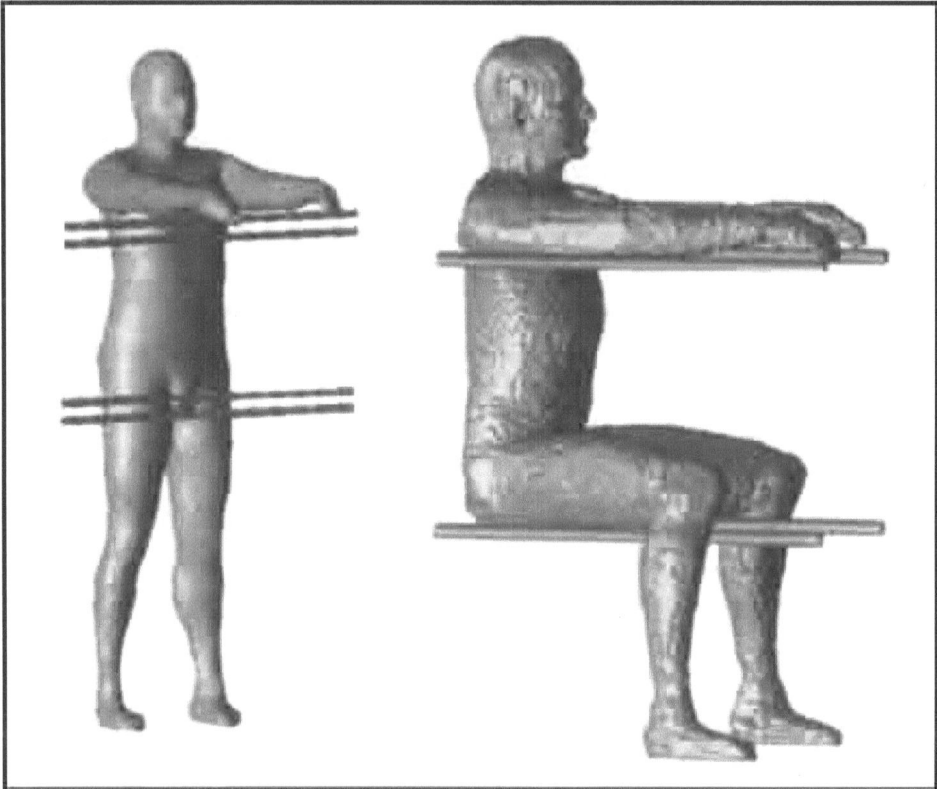

Fig. (6). Body positions in two exposure scenarios. From: Stuchly MA, Dawson TW. Interaction of low frequency electric and magnetic fields with the human body. Proc IEEE 2000; 88(5): 643-64.

Thermal effects are often associated with high frequencies of NIR, radio waves and microwaves, whereas non-thermal effects are mostly associated with long radio waves EMF.

While the thermal interaction has often adverse effects for human health (we recall the possible carcinogenic effect due to industrial frequencies, as classified on June 2001 by the IARC in the class 2B of the list of carcinogens [8]), the non-thermal interaction seems to have both adverse and positive effects, depending on the frequency and on the coupling with the geomagnetic field. Many studies report that exposure to man-made radiofrequency EMF affects cellular and systemic function and metabolism, with risk for malignancy and pharmacological effects (Fig. **7**).

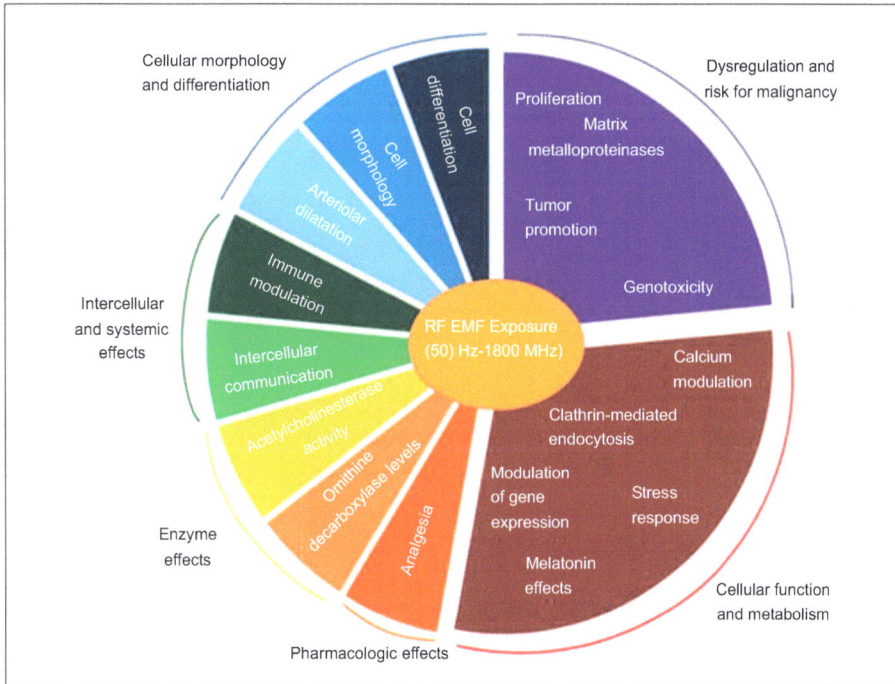

Fig. (7). Reported biological effects of radiofrequency EMF exposure. From: Zimmerman JW, Jimenez H, Pennison MJ, *et al*. Targeted treatment of cancer with radiofrequency electromagnetic fields amplitude-modulated at tumor-specific frequencies. Chin J Cancer 2013; 32(11): 573-81.

Nevertheless, the use of high-energy ionizing radiation is very common in medicine for both the diagnosis (as with radiography and computed tomography) and treatment (for example, radiotherapy) of diseases. On the other hand, the employment of low-intensity radiofrequency EMF seems to be promising, having potential applications in biomedical engineering, biotechnology, biology, and medicine, as illustrated in Fig. (**8**).

THE BLACKMAN-LIBOFF-ZHADIN EFFECT AND BIOLOGICAL IMPLICATIONS

Many currently marketed devices have no scientific rationale behind their design, but use empiric protocols. Recent achievements in bioelectromagnetics provided a conceptual frame for the evolution of such devices suitable for several purposes in therapy, based on non-thermal effects of the interaction between electromagnetic fields and living matter, the so-called Blackman-Liboff-Zhadin effect, whose pioneers were Blackman, Liboff, and Zhadin.

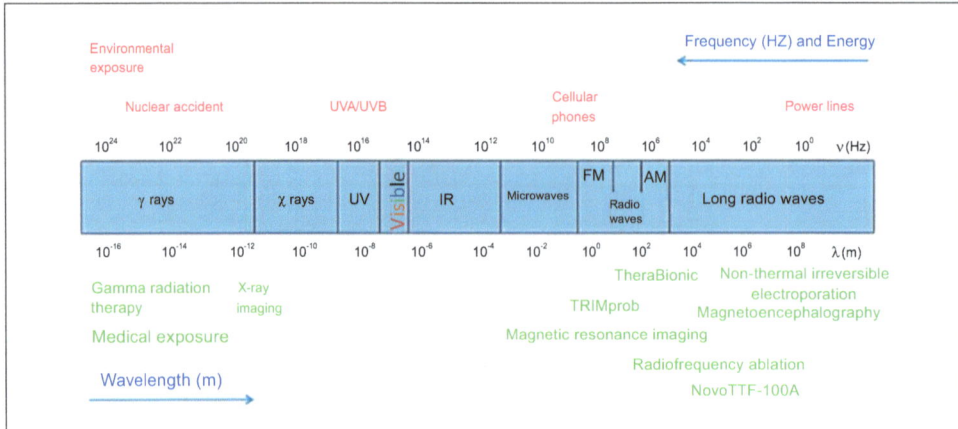

Fig. (8). The electromagnetic spectrum is depicted in blue. Environmental exposures with known or possible negative consequences are shown in red. Exposures received as part of medical diagnosis or treatment are shown in green. From: Zimmerman JW, Jimenez H, Pennison MJ, *et al*. Targeted treatment of cancer with radiofrequency electromagnetic fields amplitude-modulated at tumor-specific frequencies. Chin J Cancer 2013; 32(11): 573-81.

Since the mid 1970s, Bawin and Adey showed that weak sinusoidal electric fields modify the calcium efflux from freshly isolated chick and cat cerebral tissues bathed in Ringer's solution at 36°C [9 - 11]. In the early 1980s, Blackman *et al.* showed that an increased efflux of calcium ion is observed in brain tissue exposed to long radio waves *in vitro* [12 - 20].

In 1985, Liboff discovered that cyclotron resonance drives calcium ion motions in water solutions within electrolytic cells. Calcium ion current peaks were detected when an external alternating current (AC) EMF was applied, being tuned with the charge to mass ratio of calcium and with the intensity of local static direct current (DC) EMF. The amplitude of the AC-EMF should be lower than the amplitude of the DC-EMF (ordinary the geomagnetic field) [21].

In the early 1990s, Liboff's model was recalled by Zhadin [22], who proved that when change the DC-EMF also the AC-EMF is proportionally shifted in order to get the effect, and vice versa. Moreover, the effect could be extended to many ions and zwitterions, as well as nucleic acids. In the latter case, the amplitude of the AC-EMF should be three orders of magnitude lower than the one of the DC-EMF [23, 24].

Criticism was opposed by Adair, who observed that weak AC-EMF could not be the source of currents of ions in water (the medium of a cytoplasm), since the generated Lorentz force was not enough to overcome the kT threshold *i.e.* the

Brownian force, which resulted to be able to destroy any arising ion current due to the Lorentz force [25]. Such criticism was based on a classical gas-like model of water.

Preparata related the effect to a quantum property of water: besides the usually known liquid state, a fraction of water (at 0°C the percentages are 50% and 50%; at 30°C they are 40% coherent, 60% incoherent [26]) is in coherent state, *i.e.* there are clusters (or more correctly "coherent domains") of water molecules that oscillate in phase solvated in single molecules bulk water. They are systems able to store energy from environment, because of the shell of quasi-free electrons of excited water molecules (that are always 13% of all the molecules of clusters); furthermore, water coherent domains are able to capture solvated ions forming mixed domains. This coherent fraction is able to provide energy to ion currents arising from an aqueous solution under the influence of electric or magnetic fields or of the chemical potential due to other ion currents. Thus, when AC-EMF – tuned with the cyclotron frequency of ions – is applied, clusters release ions, providing them their own energy [27 - 33].

In 2006, Zhadin and Giuliani argued that coherent domains are also able to protonate the captured zwitterions and to release the so-formed ions when the suitable cyclotron frequency is applied [34].

In 2008, a group of Italian researchers from CNR and ISPESL with Zhadin observed that the Blackman-Liboff-Zhadin effect could be reproduced in a vessel filled of water instead of an electrolytic cell [35]. In the following year, the same group with Del Giudice showed that the water floating bridge can transport copper ions inside [36]. In 2015, the group showed that water can be protonated when it is exposed to the cyclotron frequency of hydrates of $H O^+$ [37].

NEW THERAPEUTIC INSIGHTS

There have been many attempts to develop a theoretical explanation of the phenomena of electromagnetic field interactions with biological systems. None of the reported efforts has been entirely successful in accounting for the observed experimental results, in particular with respect to the reports of interactions between ELF magnetic fields and biological systems at ion cyclotron resonance frequencies [38].

Nowadays, the main areas of research in bioelectromagnetics focuses on widely separated areas of biology and medicine:

• nucleic acid electromagnetic signaling;
• electromagnetic diagnosis and interference with spectra of bacteria and their

films, viruses, and cancer cells and their growth (introducing the new electromagnetic oncology);
- trans-membrane and cytoplasm ion currents modulation;
- induction or promotion of stem cell differentiation and regenerative medicine;
- heart attacks and congestive heart failure treatment;
- treatment and rehabilitation of pain conditions, and musculoskeletal, neurological, urological and gynecological diseases;
- electromagnetically driven drug delivery and endogenous nanoparticles transport and targeting.

Discoveries by Montagnier, Goodman and Blank show that biological processes at cellular level are driven by electromagnetic fields. In 2009, Montagnier detected electromagnetic signals of viral and bacterial DNA in water solutions [39, 41]. In 2011, Blank and Goodman provided a general theory of DNA signaling: DNA is a fractal antenna in electromagnetic fields [42 - 44]. The discovery of DNA signals coming from bacteria and viruses opens to a new technology – the microbiological spectroscopy – that could lead on the one hand to a new physical way for diagnosis of infections and the creation of a database of spectra of pathogenic bacteria and viruses (making the diagnosis of infections simpler and faster), on the other hand to the development of devices able to deliver electromagnetic signals that could interfere with signals coming from bacteria or viruses (thus inactivating their pathogenicity, as demonstrated against biofilm-related infections caused by cystic fibrosis pathogens [45]), hence ensuring a significant progress in microbiology and clinic of infective diseases.

The influx and the efflux of any ion through the cell membrane at every time is not electrically zero. Thus, at every time, there is an electric charge at the extremities of the body, that is variable in time. If an electric signal (electric probe) is sent to the extremities it is possible to measure the impedance of the signal. This point is usually exploited by the clinic bioelectrical impedance analysis or impedancemetry. Since the Blackman-Liboff-Zhadin effect associates an external ELF electromagnetic field to so-induced ion motion across the cell membranes, this could have potential diagnostic and therapeutic implications [46]. Indeed, a device able to provide the suitable signal depending on the detected impedance at the extremities of the body can be driven by such feedback in order to select suitable frequencies to be delivered to patients; that is the way of working, in principle, of the so-called "Talpo's machine" [30, 47, 48].

Using biofeedback devices and techniques, Barbault *et al.* discovered that the growth of human tumors is sensitive to specific modulation of a small number of frequencies (above 1,000 Hz), irrespective of their sex, age, or ethnic status [49] (Table **1**).

Table 1. Frequencies identified in 163 patients with cancer.

Tumor type	Number of patients	Number of frequency detection sessions	Number of frequencies	Tumor-specific frequencies Nb and (%)	Frequencies common to two or more tumor types
Brain tumors	8	22	57	41 (71.9)	16
Hematologic malignancies	7	13	56	44 (78.6)	12
Colorectal cancer	19	40	99	67 (67.7)	32
Hepatocellular carcinoma	46	63	170	144 (84.7)	26
Pancreatic cancer	6	44	162	125 (77.2)	37
Ovarian cancer	10	66	278	219 (78.8)	59
Breast cancer	32	93	188	141 (75.0)	47
Prostate cancer	17	80	187	150 (80.2)	37
Lung cancer	6	17	80	57 (71.3)	23
Renal cell cancer	2	3	36	33 (91.7)	3
Thyroid cancer	1	14	112	89 (79.5)	23
Neuroendocrine tumor	5	5	30	17 (56.7)	13
Bladder cancer	2	4	31	25 (80.6)	6
Leiomyosarcoma	1	2	36	31 (86.1)	5
Thymoma	1	1	2	0 N/A	2
Total	163	467	1524	1183 (77.6)	341

From: Barbault A, Costa FP, Bottger B, *et al.* Amplitude-modulated electromagnetic fields for the treatment of cancer: discovery of tumor-specific frequencies and assessment of a novel therapeutic approach. J Exp Clin Cancer Res 2009; 28(1): 51.

Conversely, examination of healthy individuals without a diagnosis of cancer did not reveal any biofeedback responses to the frequencies identified in patients with a diagnosis of cancer [46]. Tumor-specific modulation frequencies block the growth of cancer cells, modify gene expression, and disrupt the mitotic spindle (Fig. **9**).

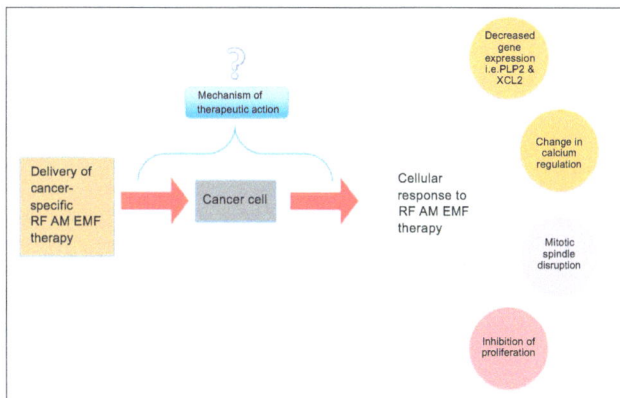

Fig. (9).   Cancer-specific treatment and responses. Theoretical flowchart representing the published biological responses to amplitude-modulated radiofrequency EMF therapy that may in part explain the antitumor effect. From: Zimmerman JW, Jimenez H, Pennison MJ, *et al.* Targeted treatment of cancer with radiofrequency electromagnetic fields amplitude-modulated at tumor-specific frequencies. Chin J Cancer 2013; 32(11): 573-81.

In 2009, Novikov with Fesenko showed that Ehrlich tumor cells (transplantable cells derived from breast carcinoma in mice, that grow in solid and ascitic form), are no more able to develop ascites when previously treated with a suitable DC/AC-EMF combination [50, 51].

In 2011, Costa *et al.* assessed the safety and effectiveness of the three-daily 60-minute intrabuccal administration of very low levels of amplitude-modulated radiofrequency EMF at HCC-specific frequencies in 41 patients with advanced HCC and limited therapeutic options (Fig. **10**) [52].

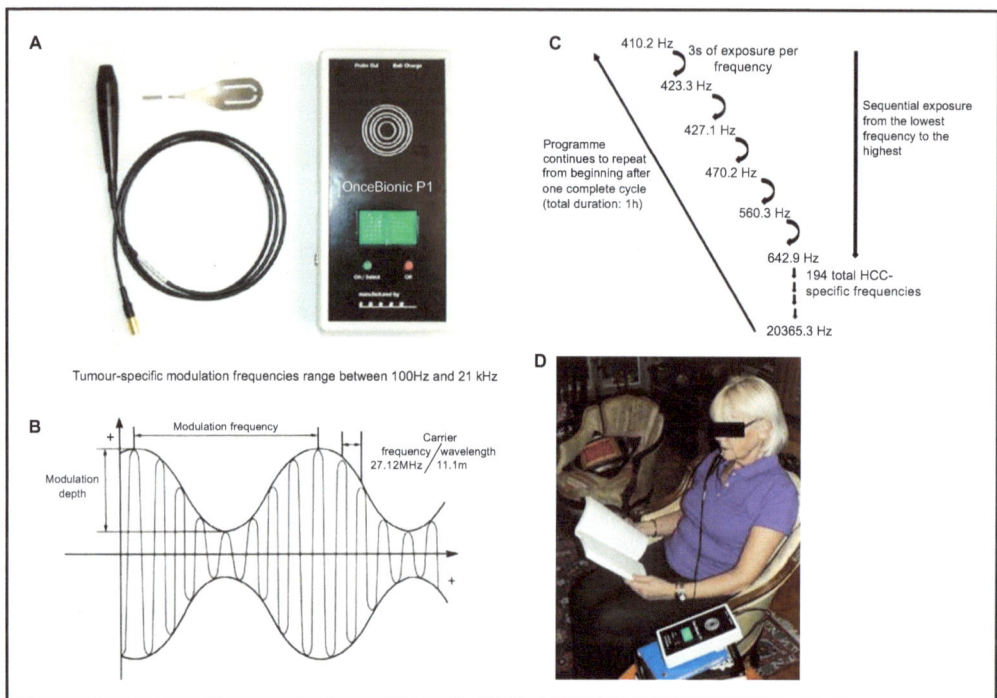

Fig. (10). Delivery of HCC-specific modulation frequencies. (A) The generator of amplitude-modulated EMF is a battery-driven radiofrequency EMF generator connected to a spoon-shaped mouthpiece. (B) Schematic description of amplitude-modulated EMF. The carrier frequency (27.12 MHz) is sinusoidally modulated at specific frequencies. (C) Patient receiving treatment with AM EMF. (D) HCC treatment programme consisting of sequential emission of 194 modulation frequencies for 60 min. From: Costa FP, de Oliveira AC, Meirelles R, *et al.* Treatment of advanced hepatocellular carcinoma with very low levels of amplitude-modulated electromagnetic fields. Br J Cancer 2011; 105(5): 640-8.

The following year, Zimmerman *et al.* showed that the growth of HCC and breast cancer cells was significantly decreased by HCC-specific and breast cancer-specific modulation frequencies, respectively (importantly, the same frequencies did not affect proliferation of nonmalignant hepatocytes or breast epithelial cells);

furthermore, inhibition of HCC cell proliferation was associated with downregulation of expression of specific genes (XCL2 and PLP2) and disruption of the mitotic spindle through specific modulation frequencies [53]. As Blackman notices, an elucidation of induced genomic pathway modifications, the responsiveness of cells different stages of transformation, the definition of the duration and the species-specificity of the observed inhibition effects need to be clarified [54].

In the same year, the Food and Drug Administration approved a non-invasive electromagnetic device (Optune/NovoTTF-100A System) that delivers low-intensity, intermediate-frequency, alternating electric fields – referred to as Tumor Treating Fields (TTF) – for treatment of glioma and glioblastoma in combination with or as an alternative to radiotherapy [55].

Regulating ion flux through the cell membrane can regulate osmotic gradient across intracellular and extracellular districts, restoring the osmotic equilibrium, where altered. Moreover, acting on metallic ions that constitute contained in some enzymes, specific ELF devices could interfere with certain chemical reactions, including cytochrome-catalyzed reactions that involve transient radical pairs and production of free radicals (such as reactive oxygen or nitric oxide) [56 - 60].

Thus, such devices can be employed tools of some help in pathological conditions as edemas and inflammatory disorders [61].

The first clinical employments of pulsed EMF date back to the mid 1970s, and were applications on longstanding non-union of fractures [62 - 82], failed arthrodesis [83, 84], avascular necrosis of the hip in adults [85, 86], and Legg-Calvé-Perthes's disease in children [87].

In the following decade, a number of studies were conducted based on first qualitative evidence that pulsed EMF might regenerate cartilage tissue through promoting cell proliferation and increasing glycosaminoglycan synthesis, having potential application in osteoarthritis [88 - 92]. Further evidence for the effectiveness of the so-called "magnetic resonance therapy" was given by *in vitro* studies on chondrocytes, osteoblasts, fibroblasts, and keratinocytes [93 - 98]. These last evidences lead to the ultimate frontier of EMF: the employment in regenerative medicine, with implications from wound healing [99 - 105] to cardiology [106, 107] and from peripheral nerve regeneration [108 - 117] to neurodegenerative disorders [118 - 122].

CONCLUDING REMARKS

Over a span of a few years, our point of view has moved from organs to tissues, to cells, and most recently to the physical and chemical reactions that are the actual basis of all the biological processes and hence of all living systems. In prospect, bioelectromagnetism is emerging as a separate biological discipline, having developed experimental approaches embracing new technologies in a search for ultimate order in living systems. Future research on submolecular signaling pathways may answer challenging question as structural deformations after application of mechanical loads, conformational modifications during receptor-ligand binding, or possible electromagnetic signals associated with enzyme action.

CONFLICT OF INTEREST

The author (editor) declares no conflict of interest, financial or otherwise.

ACKNOWLEDGEMENTS

Declared none.

REFERENCES

[1]   Giuliani L. Why investigate the non thermal mechanisms and effects of electromagnetic fields on living systems? An introduction. In: Giuliani L, Soffritti M, Eds. Non-thermal mechanisms and effects of interaction between electromagnetic fields and living matter. Eu J Oncology 2010; 5: ix-xi.

[2]   IARC classifies radiofrequency electromagnetic fields as possibly carcinogenic to humans (press release n° 208). Lyon, France, 31 May 2011. http://www.iarc.fr/ en/ media-centre/pr/2011/ pdfs/pr208_E.pdf.

[3]   Council Recommendation. 1999/519/EC of 12 July 1999 on the limitation of exposure of the general public to electromagnetic fields (0 Hz to 300 GHz). Official Journal of the European Communities 1999.

[4]   IPCS INCHEM. Environmental health criteria 137.. http://www.inchem.org/ documents/ehc/ ehc/ ehc137.htm.

[5]   Hyland GJ. Physics and biology of mobile telephony. Lancet 2000; 356(9244): 1833-6. [http://dx.doi.org/10.1016/S0140-6736(00)03243-8] [PMID: 11117927]

[6]   Kheifets L, Repacholi M, Saunders R, van Deventer E. The sensitivity of children to electromagnetic fields. Pediatrics 2005; 116(2): e303-13. [http://dx.doi.org/10.1542/peds.2004-2541] [PMID: 16061584]

[7]   Han Y-Y, Ghandi OP, DeSalles A, Heberman RB, Davis DL. Comparative assessment of models of electromagnetic absorption of the head for children and adults indicates the needs for policy changes. In: Giuliani L, Soffritti M, Eds. Non-thermal mechanisms and effects of interaction between electromagnetic fields and living matter. Eu J Oncology 2010; 5: 301-18.

[8]   IARC Monographs on the Evaluation of Carcinogenic Risks to Humans. Non-Ionizing Radiation, Part 1: Static and Extremely Low-Frequency (ELF) Electric and Magnetic Fields. Lyon, France, 19-26 June 2001. 2002; 80: 338. http://monographs.iarc.fr/ENG/Monographs/vol80/mono80.pdf.

[9]   Bawin SM, Kaczmarek LK, Adey WR. Effects of modulated VHF fields on the central nervous system. Ann N Y Acad Sci 1975; 247: 74-81. [http://dx.doi.org/10.1111/j.1749-6632.1975.tb35984.x] [PMID: 1054258]

[10] Bawin SM, Adey WR. Sensitivity of calcium binding in cerebral tissue to weak environmental electric fields oscillating at low frequency. Proc Natl Acad Sci USA 1976; 73(6): 1999-2003.

[http://dx.doi.org/10.1073/pnas.73.6.1999] [PMID: 1064869]

[11]   Bawin SM, Adey WR, Sabbot IM. Ionic factors in release of $^{45}Ca^{2+}$ from chicken cerebral tissue by electromagnetic fields. Proc Natl Acad Sci USA 1978; 75(12): 6314-8.
[http://dx.doi.org/10.1073/pnas.75.12.6314] [PMID: 282648]

[12]   Blackman CF, Elder JA, Weil CM, Benane SG, Eichinger DC, House DE. Induction of calcium-ion efflux from brain tissue by radio-frequency radiation: Effects of modulation frequency and field strength. Radio Sci 1979; 14(63): 93-8.
[http://dx.doi.org/10.1029/RS014i06Sp00093]

[13]   Blackman CF, Benane SG, Elder JA, House DE, Lampe JA, Faulk JM. Induction of calcium-ion efflux from brain tissue by radiofrequency radiation: effect of sample number and modulation frequency on the power-density window. Bioelectromagnetics 1980; 1(1): 35-43.
[http://dx.doi.org/10.1002/bem.2250010104] [PMID: 7284014]

[14]   Joines WT, Blackman CF. Power density, field intensity, and carrier frequency determinants of RF-energy-induced calcium-ion efflux from brain tissue. Bioelectromagnetics 1980; 1(3): 271-5.
[http://dx.doi.org/10.1002/bem.2250010303] [PMID: 7284025]

[15]   Blackman CF, Benane SG, Joines WT, Hollis MA, House DE. Calcium-ion efflux from brain tissue: power-density versus internal field-intensity dependencies at 50-MHz RF radiation. Bioelectromagnetics 1980; 1(3): 277-83.
[http://dx.doi.org/10.1002/bem.2250010304] [PMID: 7284026]

[16]   Joines WT, Blackman CF, Hollis MA. Broadening of the RF power-density window for calcium-ion efflux from brain tissue. IEEE Trans Biomed Eng 1981; 28(8): 568-73.
[http://dx.doi.org/10.1109/TBME.1981.324829] [PMID: 7262896]

[17]   Blackman CF, Joines WT, Elder JA. Calcium-ion efflux in brain tissue by radiofrequency radiation. In: Illinger KH, Ed. Biological Effects of Nonionizing Radiation. Washington: American Chemical Society 1981; pp. 299-314.
[http://dx.doi.org/10.1021/bk-1981-0157.ch017]

[18]   Blackman CF, Benane SG, Kinney LS, Joines WT, House DE. Effects of ELF fields on calcium-ion efflux from brain tissue *in vitro*. Radiat Res 1982; 92(3): 510-20.
[http://dx.doi.org/10.2307/3575923] [PMID: 7178417]

[19]   Blackman CF, Benane SG, Rabinowitz JR, House DE, Joines WT. A role for the magnetic field in the radiation-induced efflux of calcium ions from brain tissue *in vitro*. Bioelectromagnetics 1985; 6(4): 327-37.
[http://dx.doi.org/10.1002/bem.2250060402] [PMID: 3836676]

[20]   Blackman CF, Benane SG, House DE, Joines WT. Effects of ELF (1120 Hz) and modulated (50 Hz) RF fields on the efflux of calcium ions from brain tissue *in vitro*. Bioelectromagnetics 1985; 6(1): 1-11.
[http://dx.doi.org/10.1002/bem.2250060102] [PMID: 3977964]

[21]   Liboff AR. Geomagnetic cyclotron resonance in living cells. J Biol Phys 1985; 13(4): 99-102.
[http://dx.doi.org/10.1007/BF01878387]

[22]   Zhadin MN, Fesenko EE. Ionic cyclotron resonance in biomolecules. Biomed Sci 1990; 1(3): 245-50.
[PMID: 2103827]

[23]   Novikov VV, Zhadin MN. Combined action of weak static and alternating low frequency magnetic fields on ionic currents in aqueous amino-acid solutions. Biofizika 1994; 39: 45-9.

[24]   Zhadin MN, Novikov VV, Barnes FS, Pergola NF. Combined action of static and alternating magnetic fields on ionic current in aqueous glutamic acid solution. Bioelectromagnetics 1998; 19(1): 41-5.
[http://dx.doi.org/10.1002/(SICI)1521-186X(1998)19:1<41::AID-BEM4>3.0.CO;2-4]   [PMID: 9453705]

[25]   Adair RK. Constraints on biological effects of weak extremely-low-frequency electromagnetic fields.

Phys Rev A 1991; 43(2): 1039-48.
[http://dx.doi.org/10.1103/PhysRevA.43.1039] [PMID: 9905119]

[26] Arani R, Bono I, Del Giudice E, Preparata G. QED coherence and the thermodynamic of water. Int J Mod Phys B 1995; 9(15): 1813-41.
[http://dx.doi.org/10.1142/S0217979295000744]

[27] Preparata G, Vitiello G, Vitiello G. Water as a free electric dipole laser. Phys Rev Lett 1988; 61(9): 1085-8.
[http://dx.doi.org/10.1103/PhysRevLett.61.1085] [PMID: 10039515]

[28] Preparata G. QED Coherence in Matter. Singapore: World Scientific 1995.
[http://dx.doi.org/10.1142/2738]

[29] Buzzacchi M, Del Giudice E, Preparata G. Coherence of the glassy state. Int J Mod Phys B 2002; 16(25): 3771-86.
[http://dx.doi.org/10.1142/S0217979202012116]

[30] Del Giudice E, Fleischmann M, Preparata G, Talpo G. On the unreasonable effects of ELF magnetic fields upon a system of ions. Bioelectromagnetics 2002; 23(7): 522-30.
[http://dx.doi.org/10.1002/bem.10046] [PMID: 12224056]

[31] Del Giudice E, Tedeschi A. Water and autocatalysis in living matter. Electromagn Biol Med 2009; 28(1): 46-52.
[http://dx.doi.org/10.1080/15368370802708728] [PMID: 19337894]

[32] Yinnon CA, Yinnon TA. Domains in aqueous solutions: theory and experimental evidence. Mod Phys B 2009; 23(16): 1959-73.
[http://dx.doi.org/10.1142/S0217984909020138]

[33] Marchettini N, Del Giudice E, Voeikov V, Tiezzi E. Water: a medium where dissipative structures are produced by a coherent dynamics. J Theor Biol 2010; 265(4): 511-6.
[http://dx.doi.org/10.1016/j.jtbi.2010.05.021] [PMID: 20493195]

[34] Zhadin M, Giuliani L. Some problems in modern bioelectromagnetics. Electromagn Biol Med 2006; 25(4): 227-43.
[http://dx.doi.org/10.1080/15368370601066195] [PMID: 17178583]

[35] Giuliani L, Grimaldi S, Lisi A, DEmilia E, Bobkova N, Zhadin M. Action of combined magnetic fields on aqueous solution of glutamic acid: the further development of investigations. Biomagn Res Technol 2008; 6: 1.
[http://dx.doi.org/10.1186/1477-044X-6-1] [PMID: 18218145]

[36] Giuliani L, D'Emilia E, Lisi A, Grimaldi S, Foletti A, Del Giudice E. The Floating Water Bridge Under Strong Electric Potential. Neural Network World 2009; 19(4): 393-8.

[37] DEmilia E, Giuliani L, Lisi A, *et al.* Lorentz force in water: evidence that hydronium cyclotron resonance enhances polymorphism. Electromagn Biol Med 2015; 34(4): 370-5.
[http://dx.doi.org/10.3109/15368378.2014.937873] [PMID: 25020009]

[38] McLeod BR, Liboff AR, Smith SD. Electromagnetic gating in ion channels. J Theor Biol 1992; 158(1): 15-31.
[http://dx.doi.org/10.1016/S0022-5193(05)80646-0] [PMID: 1282185]

[39] Montagnier L, Aïssa J, Ferris S, Montagnier JL, Lavallée C. Electromagnetic signals are produced by aqueous nanostructures derived from bacterial DNA sequences. Interdiscip Sci 2009; 1(2): 81-90.
[http://dx.doi.org/10.1007/s12539-009-0036-7] [PMID: 20640822]

[40] Montagnier L, Aïssa J, Lavallée C, Mbamy M, Varon J, Chenal H. Electromagnetic detection of HIV DNA in the blood of AIDS patients treated by antiretroviral therapy. Interdiscip Sci 2009; 1(4): 245-53.
[http://dx.doi.org/10.1007/s12539-009-0059-0] [PMID: 20640802]

[41]   Montagnier L, Del Giudice E, Aïssa J, *et al.* Transduction of DNA information through water and electromagnetic waves. Electromagn Biol Med 2015; 34(2): 106-12.
[http://dx.doi.org/10.3109/15368378.2015.1036072] [PMID: 26098521]

[42]   Goodman R, Blank M. Insights into electromagnetic interaction mechanisms. J Cell Physiol 2002; 192(1): 16-22.
[http://dx.doi.org/10.1002/jcp.10098] [PMID: 12115732]

[43]   Blank M, Goodman R. Initial interactions in electromagnetic field-induced biosynthesis. J Cell Physiol 2004; 199(3): 359-63.
[http://dx.doi.org/10.1002/jcp.20004] [PMID: 15095282]

[44]   Blank M, Goodman R. A mechanism for stimulation of biosynthesis by electromagnetic fields: charge transfer in DNA and base pair separation. J Cell Physiol 2008; 214(1): 20-6.
[http://dx.doi.org/10.1002/jcp.21198] [PMID: 17620313]

[45]   Di Bonaventura G, Pompilio A, Crocetta V, *et al.* Exposure to extremely low-frequency magnetic field affects biofilm formation by cystic fibrosis pathogens. Future Microbiol 2014; 9(12): 1303-17.
[http://dx.doi.org/10.2217/fmb.14.96] [PMID: 25517897]

[46]   Zimmerman JW, Jimenez H, Pennison MJ, *et al.* Targeted treatment of cancer with radiofrequency electromagnetic fields amplitude-modulated at tumor-specific frequencies. Chin J Cancer 2013; 32(11): 573-81.
[http://dx.doi.org/10.5732/cjc.013.10177] [PMID: 24206915]

[47]   Comisso N, Del Giudice E, De Ninno A, *et al.* Dynamics of the ion cyclotron resonance effect on amino acids adsorbed at the interfaces. Bioelectromagnetics 2006; 27(1): 16-25.
[http://dx.doi.org/10.1002/bem.20171] [PMID: 16283642]

[48]   Gerardi G, De Ninno A, Prosdocimi M, *et al.* Effects of electromagnetic fields of low frequency and low intensity on rat metabolism. Biomagn Res Technol 2008; 6: 3.
[http://dx.doi.org/10.1186/1477-044X-6-3] [PMID: 18380892]

[49]   Barbault A, Costa FP, Bottger B, *et al.* Amplitude-modulated electromagnetic fields for the treatment of cancer: discovery of tumor-specific frequencies and assessment of a novel therapeutic approach. J Exp Clin Cancer Res 2009; 28(1): 51.
[http://dx.doi.org/10.1186/1756-9966-28-51] [PMID: 19366446]

[50]   Novikov VV, Novikov GV, Fesenko EE. Effect of weak combined static and extremely low-frequency alternating magnetic fields on tumor growth in mice inoculated with the Ehrlich ascites carcinoma. Bioelectromagnetics 2009; 30(5): 343-51.
[http://dx.doi.org/10.1002/bem.20487] [PMID: 19267367]

[51]   Novikov GV, Novikov VV, Fesenko EE. [Effect of weak combined static and low-frequency alternating magnetic fields on the Ehrlich ascites carcinoma in mice]. Biofizika 2009; 54(6): 1120-7.
[PMID: 20067194]

[52]   Costa FP, de Oliveira AC, Meirelles R, *et al.* Treatment of advanced hepatocellular carcinoma with very low levels of amplitude-modulated electromagnetic fields. Br J Cancer 2011; 105(5): 640-8.
[http://dx.doi.org/10.1038/bjc.2011.292] [PMID: 21829195]

[53]   Zimmerman JW, Pennison MJ, Brezovich I, *et al.* Cancer cell proliferation is inhibited by specific modulation frequencies. Br J Cancer 2012; 106(2): 307-13.
[http://dx.doi.org/10.1038/bjc.2011.523] [PMID: 22134506]

[54]   Blackman CF. Treating cancer with amplitude-modulated electromagnetic fields: a potential paradigm shift, again? Br J Cancer 2012; 106(2): 241-2.
[http://dx.doi.org/10.1038/bjc.2011.576] [PMID: 22251967]

[55]   Stupp R, Wong ET, Kanner AA, *et al.* NovoTTF-100A versus physicians choice chemotherapy in recurrent glioblastoma: a randomised phase III trial of a novel treatment modality. Eur J Cancer 2012; 48(14): 2192-202.

[http://dx.doi.org/10.1016/j.ejca.2012.04.011] [PMID: 22608262]

[56]   Adey WR. Collective properties of cell membranes. In: Norden B, Ramel C, Eds. Interaction Mechanisms of Low-Level Electromagnetic Fields in Living Systems. Oxford: University Press 1992; pp. 47-77.

[57]   Grundler W, Kaiser F, Keilmann F, Walleczek J. Mechanisms of electromagnetic interaction with cellular systems. Naturwissenschaften 1992; 79(12): 551-9.
[http://dx.doi.org/10.1007/BF01131411] [PMID: 1480219]

[58]   Adey WR. Biological effects of electromagnetic fields. J Cell Biochem 1993; 51(4): 410-6.
[http://dx.doi.org/10.1002/jcb.2400510405] [PMID: 8388394]

[59]   Patruno A, Amerio P, Pesce M, *et al.* Extremely low frequency electromagnetic fields modulate expression of inducible nitric oxide synthase, endothelial nitric oxide synthase and cyclooxygenase-2 in the human keratinocyte cell line HaCat: potential therapeutic effects in wound healing. Br J Dermatol 2010; 162(2): 258-66.
[http://dx.doi.org/10.1111/j.1365-2133.2009.09527.x] [PMID: 19799606]

[60]   Patruno A, Tabrez S, Amerio P, *et al.* Kinetic study on the effects of extremely low frequency electromagnetic field on catalase, cytochrome P450 and inducible nitric oxide synthase in human HaCaT and THP-1 cell lines. CNS Neurol Disord Drug Targets 2011; 10(8): 936-44.
[http://dx.doi.org/10.2174/187152711799219325] [PMID: 22229327]

[61]   Selvam R, Ganesan K, Narayana Raju KV, Gangadharan AC, Manohar BM, Puvanakrishnan R. Low frequency and low intensity pulsed electromagnetic field exerts its antiinflammatory effect through restoration of plasma membrane calcium ATPase activity. Life Sci 2007; 80(26): 2403-10.
[http://dx.doi.org/10.1016/j.lfs.2007.03.019] [PMID: 17537462]

[62]   Bassett CA, Pawluk RJ, Pilla AA. Augmentation of bone repair by inductively coupled electromagnetic fields. Science 1974; 184(4136): 575-7.
[http://dx.doi.org/10.1126/science.184.4136.575] [PMID: 4821958]

[63]   Bassett CA, Pilla AA, Pawluk RJ. A non-operative salvage of surgically-resistant pseudarthroses and non-unions by pulsing electromagnetic fields. A preliminary report. Clin Orthop Relat Res 1977; (124): 128-43.
[PMID: 598067]

[64]   Heckman JD, Ingram AJ, Loyd RD, Luck JV Jr, Mayer PW. Nonunion treatment with pulsed electromagnetic fields. Clin Orthop Relat Res 1981; (161): 58-66.
[PMID: 6975692]

[65]   Barker AT, Dixon RA, Sharrard WJ, Sutcliffe ML. Pulsed magnetic field therapy for tibial non-union. Interim results of a double-blind trial. Lancet 1984; 1(8384): 994-6.
[http://dx.doi.org/10.1016/S0140-6736(84)92329-8] [PMID: 6143970]

[66]   de Haas WG, Beaupré A, Cameron H, English E. The Canadian experience with pulsed magnetic fields in the treatment of ununited tibial fractures. Clin Orthop Relat Res 1986; (208): 55-8.
[PMID: 3720140]

[67]   Meskens MW, Stuyck JA, Mulier JC. Treatment of delayed union and nonunion of the tibia by pulsed electromagnetic fields. A retrospective follow-up. Bull Hosp Jt Dis Orthop Inst 1988; 48(2): 170-5.
[PMID: 2854484]

[68]   Bassett CA. Fundamental and practical aspects of therapeutic uses of pulsed electromagnetic fields (PEMFs). Crit Rev Biomed Eng 1989; 17(5): 451-529.
[PMID: 2686932]

[69]   Meskens MW, Stuyck JA, Feys H, Mulier JC. Treatment of nonunion using pulsed electromagnetic fields: a retrospective follow-up study. Acta Orthop Belg 1990; 56(2): 483-8.

[PMID. 2239195]

[70]   Sharrard WJ. A double-blind trial of pulsed electromagnetic fields for delayed union of tibial fractures. J Bone Joint Surg Br 1990; 72(3): 347-55.
[PMID: 2187877]

[71]   Adams BD, Frykman GK, Taleisnik J. Treatment of scaphoid nonunion with casting and pulsed electromagnetic fields: a study continuation. J Hand Surg Am 1992; 17(5): 910-4.
[http://dx.doi.org/10.1016/0363-5023(92)90467-4] [PMID: 1401805]

[72]   Deibert MC, Mcleod BR, Smith SD, Liboff AR. Ion resonance electromagnetic field stimulation of fracture healing in rabbits with a fibular ostectomy. J Orthop Res 1994; 12(6): 878-85.
[http://dx.doi.org/10.1002/jor.1100120616] [PMID: 7983563]

[73]   Ryaby JT. Clinical effects of electromagnetic and electric fields on fracture healing. Clin Orthop Relat Res 1998; (355): (Suppl.)S205-15.
[http://dx.doi.org/10.1097/00003086-199810001-00021] [PMID: 9917640]

[74]   Chao EY, Inoue N. Biophysical stimulation of bone fracture repair, regeneration and remodelling. Eur Cell Mater 2003; 6: 72-84.
[http://dx.doi.org/10.22203/eCM.v006a07] [PMID: 14722904]

[75]   Aaron RK, Ciombor DM, Simon BJ. Treatment of nonunions with electric and electromagnetic fields. Clin Orthop Relat Res 2004; (419): 21-9.
[http://dx.doi.org/10.1097/00003086-200402000-00005] [PMID: 15021127]

[76]   Punt BJ, den Hoed PT, Fontijne WP. Pulsed electromagnetic fields in the treatment of nonunion. Eur J Orthop Surg Traumatol 2008; 18(2): 127-33.
[http://dx.doi.org/10.1007/s00590-007-0271-8]

[77]   Griffin XL, Warner F, Costa M. The role of electromagnetic stimulation in the management of established non-union of long bone fractures: what is the evidence? Injury 2008; 39(4): 419-29.
[http://dx.doi.org/10.1016/j.injury.2007.12.014] [PMID: 18321512]

[78]   Mollon B, da Silva V, Busse JW, Einhorn TA, Bhandari M. Electrical stimulation for long-bone fracture-healing: a meta-analysis of randomized controlled trials. J Bone Joint Surg Am 2008; 90(11): 2322-30.
[http://dx.doi.org/10.2106/JBJS.H.00111] [PMID: 18978400]

[79]   Griffin XL, Costa ML, Parsons N, Smith N. Electromagnetic field stimulation for treating delayed union or non-union of long bone fractures in adults. Cochrane Database Syst Rev 2011; 4(4): CD008471.
[PMID: 21491410]

[80]   Adie S, Harris IA, Naylor JM, *et al.* Pulsed electromagnetic field stimulation for acute tibial shaft fractures: a multicenter, double-blind, randomized trial. J Bone Joint Surg Am 2011; 93(17): 1569-76.
[http://dx.doi.org/10.2106/JBJS.J.00869] [PMID: 21915570]

[81]   Assiotis A, Sachinis NP, Chalidis BE. Pulsed electromagnetic fields for the treatment of tibial delayed unions and nonunions. A prospective clinical study and review of the literature. J Orthop Surg 2012; 7: 24.
[http://dx.doi.org/10.1186/1749-799X-7-24] [PMID: 22681718]

[82]   Shi HF, Xiong J, Chen YX, *et al.* Early application of pulsed electromagnetic field in the treatment of postoperative delayed union of long-bone fractures: a prospective randomized controlled study. BMC Musculoskelet Disord 2013; 14: 35.
[http://dx.doi.org/10.1186/1471-2474-14-35] [PMID: 23331333]

[83]   Bassett CA, Mitchell SN, Gaston SR. Pulsing electromagnetic field treatment in ununited fractures and failed arthrodeses. JAMA 1982; 247(5): 623-8.
[http://dx.doi.org/10.1001/jama.1982.03320300027017] [PMID: 7054564]

[84]   Bassett CA. The development and application of pulsed electromagnetic fields (PEMFs) for ununited

fractures and arthrodeses. Clin Plast Surg 1985; 12(2): 259-77.
[PMID: 3886262]

[85] Bassett CA, Schink-Ascani M, Lewis SM. Effects of pulsed electromagnetic fields on Steinberg ratings of femoral head osteonecrosis. Clin Orthop Relat Res 1989; (246): 172-85.
[PMID: 2670386]

[86] Aaron RK, Lennox D, Bunce GE, Ebert T. The conservative treatment of osteonecrosis of the femoral head. A comparison of core decompression and pulsing electromagnetic fields. Clin Orthop Relat Res 1989; (249): 209-18.
[PMID: 2582669]

[87] Harrison MH, Bassett CA. Use of pulsed electromagnetic fields in Perthes disease: report of a pilot study. J Pediatr Orthop 1984; 4(5): 579-84.
[http://dx.doi.org/10.1097/01241398-198409000-00010] [PMID: 6490879]

[88] Trock DH, Bollet AJ, Dyer RH Jr, Fielding LP, Miner WK, Markoll R. A double-blind trial of the clinical effects of pulsed electromagnetic fields in osteoarthritis. J Rheumatol 1993; 20(3): 456-60.
[PMID: 8478852]

[89] Froböse I, Eckey U, Reiser M, *et al.* Evaluation of the effectiveness of MultiBioSignal-Therapy (MBST) 3D pulsing electro-magnetic fields on the regeneration of cartilage structures. Orthopädische Praxis 2000; 36: 510-5.

[90] Kullich W, Außerwinkler M. Functional improvement in finger joint osteoarthritis with therapeutic use of nuclear magnetic resonance. Orthopädische Praxis 2008; pp. 287-90.

[91] Levers A, Staat M, van Laack W. Analysis of the Long-Term Effect of the MBST® Nuclear Magnetic Resonance Therapy on Gonarthrosis. Orthopädische Praxis 2011; 47(11S): 536-43.

[92] Ryang We S, Koog YH, Jeong KI, Wi H. Effects of pulsed electromagnetic field on knee osteoarthritis: a systematic review. Rheumatology (Oxford) 2013; 52(5): 815-24.
[http://dx.doi.org/10.1093/rheumatology/kes063] [PMID: 22504115]

[93] Endo N. The effect of pulsing electromagnetic fields on differentiation and proliferation of rabbit costal chondrocytes in culture. J Niigata Med Soc 1987; 101: 367-81.

[94] Sakai A, Suzuki K, Nakamura T, Norimura T, Tsuchiya T. Effects of pulsing electromagnetic fields on cultured cartilage cells. Int Orthop 1991; 15(4): 341-6.
[http://dx.doi.org/10.1007/BF00186874] [PMID: 1809715]

[95] Temiz-Artmann A, Linder P, Kayser P, Digel I, Artmann GM, Lücker P. NMR in vitro effects on proliferation, apoptosis, and viability of human chondrocytes and osteoblasts. Methods Find Exp Clin Pharmacol 2005; 27(6): 391-4.
[http://dx.doi.org/10.1358/mf.2005.27.6.896831] [PMID: 16179956]

[96] Cricenti A, Generosi R, Luce M, *et al.* Low-frequency electromagnetic field effects on functional groups in human skin keratinocytes cells revealed by IR-SNOM. J Microsc 2008; 229(Pt 3): 551-4.
[http://dx.doi.org/10.1111/j.1365-2818.2008.01942.x] [PMID: 18331509]

[97] Vianale G, Reale M, Amerio P, Stefanachi M, Di Luzio S, Muraro R. Extremely low frequency electromagnetic field enhances human keratinocyte cell growth and decreases proinflammatory chemokine production. Br J Dermatol 2008; 158(6): 1189-96.
[http://dx.doi.org/10.1111/j.1365-2133.2008.08540.x] [PMID: 18410412]

[98] Zhang M, Li X, Bai L, *et al.* Effects of low frequency electromagnetic field on proliferation of human epidermal stem cells: An in vitro study. Bioelectromagnetics 2013; 34(1): 74-80.
[http://dx.doi.org/10.1002/bem.21747] [PMID: 22926783]

[99] Ottani V, De Pasquale V, Govoni P, Franchi M, Zaniol P, Ruggeri A. Effects of pulsed extremely-lo--frequency magnetic fields on skin wounds in the rat. Bioelectromagnetics 1988; 9(1): 53-62.
[http://dx.doi.org/10.1002/bem.2250090105] [PMID: 3345213]

[100] Callaghan MJ, Chang EI, Seiser N, *et al.* Pulsed electromagnetic fields accelerate normal and diabetic wound healing by increasing endogenous FGF-2 release. Plast Reconstr Surg 2008; 121(1): 130-41.
[http://dx.doi.org/10.1097/01.prs.0000293761.27219.84] [PMID: 18176216]

[101] Goudarzi I, Hajizadeh S, Salmani ME, Abrari K. Pulsed electromagnetic fields accelerate wound healing in the skin of diabetic rats. Bioelectromagnetics 2010; 31(4): 318-23.
[PMID: 20082338]

[102] Costin GE, Birlea SA, Norris DA. Trends in wound repair: cellular and molecular basis of regenerative therapy using electromagnetic fields. Curr Mol Med 2012; 12(1): 14-26.
[http://dx.doi.org/10.2174/156652412798376143] [PMID: 22082478]

[103] Cheing GL, Li X, Huang L, Kwan RL, Cheung KK. Pulsed electromagnetic fields (PEMF) promote early wound healing and myofibroblast proliferation in diabetic rats. Bioelectromagnetics 2014; 35(3): 161-9.
[http://dx.doi.org/10.1002/bem.21832] [PMID: 24395219]

[104] Cañedo-Dorantes L, Soenksen LR, García-Sánchez C, *et al.* Efficacy and safety evaluation of systemic extremely low frequency magnetic fields used in the healing of diabetic foot ulcersphase II data. Arch Med Res 2015; 46(6): 470-8.
[http://dx.doi.org/10.1016/j.arcmed.2015.07.002] [PMID: 26226416]

[105] Patruno A, Pesce M, Grilli A, *et al.* mTOR Activation by PI3K/Akt and ERK Signaling in Short ELF-EMF Exposed Human Keratinocytes. PLoS One 2015; 10(10): e0139644.
[http://dx.doi.org/10.1371/journal.pone.0139644] [PMID: 26431550]

[106] Lisi A, Ledda M, de Carlo F, *et al.* Ion cyclotron resonance as a tool in regenerative medicine. Electromagn Biol Med 2008; 27(2): 127-33.
[http://dx.doi.org/10.1080/15368370802072117] [PMID: 18568930]

[107] Gaetani R, Ledda M, Barile L, *et al.* Differentiation of human adult cardiac stem cells exposed to extremely low-frequency electromagnetic fields. Cardiovasc Res 2009; 82(3): 411-20.
[http://dx.doi.org/10.1093/cvr/cvp067] [PMID: 19228705]

[108] Wilson DH, Jagadeesh P. Experimental regeneration in peripheral nerves and the spinal cord in laboratory animals exposed to a pulsed electromagnetic field. Paraplegia 1976; 14(1): 12-20.
[http://dx.doi.org/10.1038/sc.1976.2] [PMID: 180476]

[109] Ito H, Bassett CA. Effect of weak, pulsing electromagnetic fields on neural regeneration in the rat. Clin Orthop Relat Res 1983; (181): 283-90.
[PMID: 6641063]

[110] Orgel MG, OBrien WJ, Murray HM. Pulsing electromagnetic field therapy in nerve regeneration: an experimental study in the cat. Plast Reconstr Surg 1984; 73(2): 173-83.
[http://dx.doi.org/10.1097/00006534-198402000-00001] [PMID: 6695016]

[111] Byers JM, Clark KF, Thompson GC. Effect of pulsed electromagnetic stimulation on facial nerve regeneration. Arch Otolaryngol Head Neck Surg 1998; 124(4): 383-9.
[http://dx.doi.org/10.1001/archotol.124.4.383] [PMID: 9559684]

[112] De Pedro JA, Pérez-Caballer AJ, Dominguez J, Collía F, Blanco J, Salvado M. Pulsed electromagnetic fields induce peripheral nerve regeneration and endplate enzymatic changes. Bioelectromagnetics 2005; 26(1): 20-7.
[http://dx.doi.org/10.1002/bem.20049] [PMID: 15605398]

[113] Güven M, Günay I, Ozgünen K, Zorludemir S. Effect of pulsed magnetic field on regenerating rat sciatic nerve: an in-vitro electrophysiologic study. Int J Neurosci 2005; 115(6): 881-92.
[http://dx.doi.org/10.1080/00207450590897950] [PMID: 16019581]

[114] Mert T, Gunay I, Gocmen C, Kaya M, Polat S. Regenerative effects of pulsed magnetic field on injured peripheral nerves. Altern Ther Health Med 2006; 12(5): 42-9.
[PMID: 17017754]

[115]   Gunay I, Mert T. Pulsed magnetic fields enhance the rate of recovery of damaged nerve excitability. Bioelectromagnetics 2011; 32(3): 200-8.
[http://dx.doi.org/10.1002/bem.20629] [PMID: 21365664]

[116]   Beck-Broichsitter BE, Lamia A, Geuna S, *et al.* Does pulsed magnetic field therapy influence nerve regeneration in the median nerve model of the rat? Biomed Res Int 2014; 2014: 401760.
[http://dx.doi.org/10.1155/2014/401760]

[117]   Geiger G, Mikus E, Dertinger H, Rick O. Low frequency magnetic field therapy in patients with cytostatic-induced polyneuropathy: a phase II pilot study. Bioelectromagnetics 2015; 36(3): 251-4.
[http://dx.doi.org/10.1002/bem.21897] [PMID: 25644670]

[118]   Sisken BF, Kanje M, Lundborg G, Kurtz W. Pulsed electromagnetic fields stimulate nerve regeneration *in vitro* and *in vivo*. Restor Neurol Neurosci 1990; 1(3): 303-9.
[PMID: 21551571]

[119]   Lisi A, Ciotti MT, Ledda M, *et al.* Exposure to 50 Hz electromagnetic radiation promote early maturation and differentiation in newborn rat cerebellar granule neurons. J Cell Physiol 2005; 204(2): 532-8.
[http://dx.doi.org/10.1002/jcp.20322] [PMID: 15754325]

[120]   Cho H, Seo YK, Yoon HH, *et al.* Neural stimulation on human bone marrow-derived mesenchymal stem cells by extremely low frequency electromagnetic fields. Biotechnol Prog 2012; 28(5): 1329-35.
[http://dx.doi.org/10.1002/btpr.1607] [PMID: 22848041]

[121]   Park JE, Seo YK, Yoon HH, Kim CW, Park JK, Jeon S. Electromagnetic fields induce neural differentiation of human bone marrow derived mesenchymal stem cells via ROS mediated EGFR activation. Neurochem Int 2013; 62(4): 418-24.
[http://dx.doi.org/10.1016/j.neuint.2013.02.002] [PMID: 23411410]

[122]   Choi YK, Lee DH, Seo YK, Jung H, Park JK, Cho H. Stimulation of neural differentiation in human bone marrow mesenchymal stem cells by extremely low-frequency electromagnetic fields incorporated with MNPs. Appl Biochem Biotechnol 2014; 174(4): 1233-45.
[http://dx.doi.org/10.1007/s12010-014-1091-z] [PMID: 25099373]

APPENDIX: Update on Therapeutic Applications of Vibrations

Scientific data illustrated in previous chapters and those collected by our personal experience allow us to summarize that each type of vibration has a proper applicability in terms of cost/benefit ratio. It is clear that using vibration therapy on the basis of scientific knowledge we can determine the tissue repair or modulate regeneration. The obtained results in rehabilitation essentially depends on type, extension and location of damaged tissue, type and set parameters of applied mechanical therapy, frequency and duration of treatment.

The best approach to bone damage varies depending on specific conditions:

- fresh fracture
  - 1st-line treatment: focused extracorporeal shock waves
  - 2nd-line treatment: pulsed electromagnetic fields
- delayed bone union, nonunion
  - 1st-line treatment: pulsed electromagnetic fields
  - 2nd-line treatment: focused extracorporeal shock waves

- pseudo arthrosis, osteonecrosis
  - 1st-line treatment: focused extracorporeal shock waves
  - 2nd-line treatment: medium- and low-intensity electromagnetic fields

The best approach to muscle tissue damage depends on the timing of the injury:

- acute muscle injury
  - 1st-line treatment: pulsed electromagnetic fields
  - 2nd-line treatment: low-frequency ultrasounds
  - 3rd-line treatment: *EndoSphères Therapy*®
- chronic muscle injury
  - 1st-line treatment: focused mechano-acoustic vibrations
  - 2nd-line treatment: low-frequency ultrasounds
  - 3rd-line treatment: focused or unfocused extracorporeal shock waves
  - 4th-line treatment: *EndoSphères Therapy*®

To modulate muscle activity it could be applied:

- to reduce muscle tone
  - 1st-line treatment: focused mechano-acoustic vibrations
- to enhance muscle tone
  - 1st-line treatment: focused mechano-acoustic vibrations
  - 2nd-line treatment: whole-body vibrations

The best approach to muscular fascia:

- 1st-line treatment: focused mechano-acoustic vibrations
- 2nd-line treatment: low-frequency ultrasounds
- 3rd-line treatment: *EndoSphères Therapy*®
- 4th-line treatment: unfocused extracorporeal shock waves

The best approach to tendon injury is:

- 1st-line treatment: focused or unfocused extracorporeal shock waves
- 2nd-line treatment: low-frequency ultrasounds

The best approach to acute and chronic skin lesions is low-frequency ultrasounds and unfocused extracorporeal shock waves, respectively (for more details, see below).

TREATMENT PROTOCOLS WITH FOCUSED MECHANO-ACOUSTIC SQUARE WAVEFORM VIBRATION

With regard to the focused mechano-acoustic vibration, some treatment protocols can be schematically summarized as follows (Tables **1**, **2**).

Table 1. Treatment protocols for the use of focal mechanical vibration.

Frequency	Target
30-50 Hz	Muscle relaxation
50 Hz	Delayed onset muscle soreness
80-100 Hz	Improvement of proprioception
100 Hz	Pyramidal spasticity
120 Hz	Muscle relaxation
100-120 Hz	Pain
200 Hz	Strengthening of slow muscle fibers
300 Hz	Strengthening of fast muscle fibers

Table 2. Treatment protocols for the use of focal mechanical vibration in different muscle conditions.

Muscle relaxation	50-120 Hz for 10 minutes (applied with an handpiece)	Treatment of tender points and fatigue
	120-200 Hz for 10 minutes (applied with an handpiece)	Treatment of trigger points and taut bands
Muscle strengthening in sport, upright position	200 Hz for 10 minutes 300 Hz for 10 minutes 120 Hz for 5 minutes (applied with segmental strips)	Strengthening of slow muscle fibers Strengthening of fast muscle fibers Deconditioning

(Table 2) contd.....

Muscle relaxation	50-120 Hz for 10 minutes (applied with an handpiece)	Treatment of tender points and fatigue
	120-200 Hz for 10 minutes (applied with an handpiece)	Treatment of trigger points and taut bands
Muscle strengthening and corticalization	200 Hz for 10 minutes 300 Hz for 10 minutes 120 Hz for 5 minutes (applied with segmental strips)	Working with squats through active work or isometric muscle contraction
Proprioceptive exercise in combination with *Synergy Mat* (Human Tecar® Unibell srl, Calco, Italy)	60-80-100-120-140-160-180-200-220-240-260-280-300 Hz, to increase every 2 minutes (applied with segmental strips)	Mono- and bipedal walking on unstable proprioceptive platforms

A disorder commonly responsible for many cases of chronic musculoskeletal pain is the myofascial pain syndrome, whose diagnosis is missed often. It can cause tenderness, tightness, stiffness, weakness (without atrophy), associated with hypersensitive areas called trigger points. Placed in taut muscle bands, trigger points cause referred pain in characteristic areas for specific muscles, restricted range of motion, and a visible or palpable local twitch response to local stimulation (Fig. **1**). The treatment of trigger points by a focal vibration system with a handpiece frequency of 120 Hz [1, 2] can be direct or start from the surrounding area and coming on it and the area of referred pain.

- *Direct treatment of trigger point*: it places the handpiece directly on the trigger point up to the relaxation of muscle.
- *Treatment of the taut band, of the trigger point, of the referred pain area*: it highlights the trigger point, the taut band and the referred pain area. It proceeds to treat taut band to 5cm in diameter area from the periphery and towards centripetal to the point of maximum tenderness, continuing the treatment area of referred pain.

Since following the application of a vibration stimulus, bone reacts changing its micro-architecture, at the same time, a balance training with focused mechano-acoustic vibration applied with segmental strips can reduce the likelihood of falling, and hence the risk of fall-related fractures (Fig. **2**), we adopt the following protocol to treat osteoporosis/osteopenia and prevent falls (Table **3**).

Integrated protocols involve the use of focal vibrations in combination with active exercises and systems that increase proprioceptive stimulation to determine the synergy between stimuli. For example, we work with *Synergy Viss*® (Synergy Viss Human Tecar® Unibell srl, Calco, Italy) to carry out eccentric exercises in upright position on Bosu ball, a half-spher--shaped unstable platform, composed of a hard and a rubber hemispherical platform (Fig. **3**).

Another type of integrated protocol used both in sports for functional recovery after muscle injury and in neurological diseases for the recovery of kinetic and kinematic characteristics of gait, as well as in developmental disorders and functional decline in the elders includes the use of *Synergy Viss*® (Synergy Viss Human Tecar® Unibell srl, Calco, Italy) with a proprioceptive system called *Synergy Mat*.

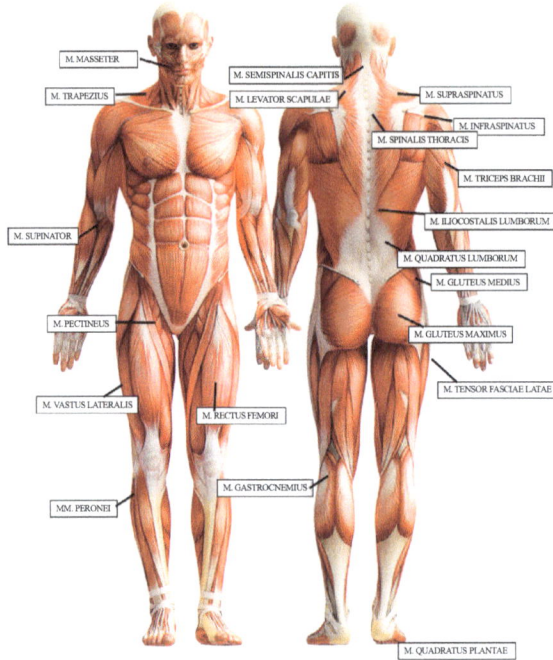

Fig. (1). Common trigger points.

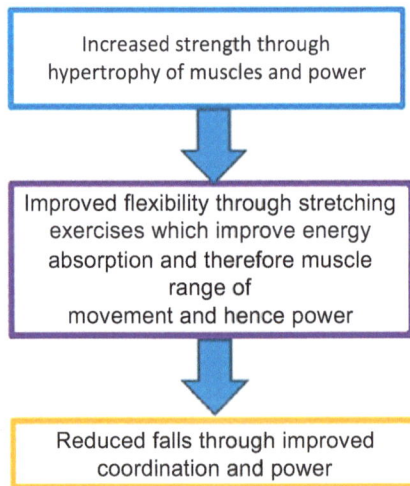

Fig. (2). Treatment goals.

Table 3. Treatment protocols for the use of focal mechanical vibration in osteoporosis/osteopenia and prevention of falls.

Sites of application	trapezius muscle (upper fibers) triceps brachii muscle latissimus dorsi muscle quadratus lumborum muscle rectus abdominis muscle	gluteus maximus muscle rectus femoris muscle biceps femoris muscle tibialis anterior muscle
Treatment parameters	*Wave frequency*: 200-300 Hz *Maximum wave pressure*: 500 mbar	
Duration and number of sessions	10 minutes per session, twice a week, for at least 6 months	

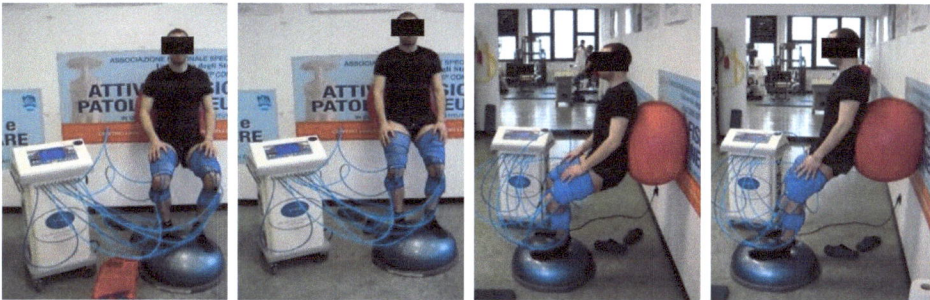

Fig. (3). *Synergy Viss* ® (Synergy Viss Human Tecar® Unibell srl, Calco, Italy) to carry out eccentric exercises in upright position on Bosu ball.

Synergy Mat (Human Tecar® Unibell srl, Calco, Italy) is the innovative response to these needs of training, rehabilitation and natural and harmonious reeducation of the body. Different surfaces give the possibility to work barefoot on routs instability with different levels, responding to the needs of personalized training and rehabilitation. Different densities correspond to different level of movement absorption, providing protection of the joints and increasing time the energy expenditure. The variety of interchangeable elements that composed the *Synergy Mat* set (mats and pillows) provides many combinations of routes adapted to the user specific needs (Fig. **4**).

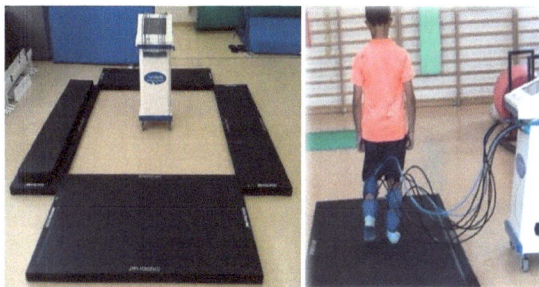

Fig. (4). Integrated protocol with *Synergy Viss® (Synergy Viss Human Tecar® Unibell srl, Calco, Italy)* and proprioceptive system- *Synergy Mat*.

TREATMENT PROTOCOLS WITH WHOLE-BODY VIBRATION

The following guidelines were developed over several years of clinical experience.

First of all the familiarization with the training whole-body vibration can be achieved in approximately 1 min with slow (5-12 Hz), subjectively comfortable frequency and middle amplitude of "swing" (where the subjective feeling of comfort is individual and varies significantly) (Table **4**, Fig. **5**).

Table 4. Guidelines for the use of whole-body vibration.

Stretching	*Frequency*: 10-18 Hz, subjectively comfortable "swing frequency" (varies with the individual's posture and hence resonance frequency). *Duration*: slowly attain the end position until a significant stretching can be felt; maintain this position for 10-30 s and then return to the starting position. Two or three repetitions. Repeat each exercise for 1 or 2 minutes.	Improvement of elasticity and joint range of motion. Stretching should be incorporated into the commencement of each training session so as to optimize the muscle elasticity.
Balance	*Frequency*: 5-12 Hz, the lower the frequency, the harder the exercise (varies with the individual client and posture). *Duration*: every exercise should be undertaken for 1 or 2 minutes, several repetitions of each exercise are possible, several times per day.	Improvement of stability.
Force	*Frequency*: 25-40 Hz (varies with the training device). *Duration*: To the point of fatigue of the musculature.	Improvement of muscle strength and muscle mass.

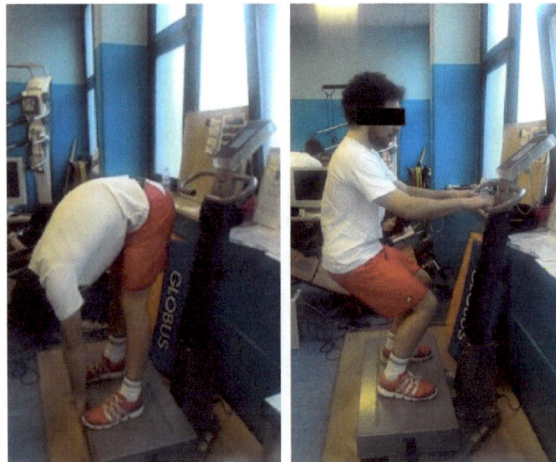

Fig. (5). Example of exercises on whole-body vibration platform.

Application of Whole-body Vibration Therapy in the Treatment of Osteoporosis/Osteopenia

Exercises on whole-body vibrating plates for osteoporosis/osteopenia should be conducted over a longer period (at least 6 months) and never conducted if the subject is experiencing pain. Strength training should be individually selected depending on the concept of progressive training. A training session should last 15-20 minutes, divided into series of 60 seconds with 60-second rest between each series. Within 6 months, two or three training sessions per week should be undertaken, with at least 1 rest day for recovery between training sessions (Table **5**).

Table 5.   Treatment sequence for the use of whole-body vibration in osteoporosis/osteopenia.

First session	*Frequency*: 5-12 Hz. *Duration*: 1-3 minutes.	Standing with slightly bent knees. If possible without holding on. The vibration can be directed to various body parts through changes in the center of gravity and slowly straightening the knees. Stretching exercises out of the stretching and balance series.
Protocols	*Frequency*: 15-30 Hz. *Duration*: 3-5 minutes for each exercise.	Exercises varying between the force and power series. Also some of the exercises from the balance series may be appropriate. 1 or 2 applications per series, without rest. 1-to-2-minute rest between the applications.
Relaxing	*Frequency*: 5-10 Hz. *Duration*: 1-2 minutes.	Relaxed, moving the body gently forwards and backwards with slightly bent knees while not holding on. The soles of the feet must stay fully on the vibration plate.

Application of Whole-body Vibration Therapy in Reducing the Likelihood of Falling

The duration of treatment in subjects who are at risk of falling varies between individuals. In order to maintain/sustain mobility and power the training in these individuals should become daily routine. Progression occurs with increasing strength of the client. Divide training into sets and repetitions. At least 48 hours rest between exercise sessions are required. Balance training can be carried out several times per day (Table **6**). Power training is attained through all series since power = force • velocity, which is a combination of coordination, balance and strength. Muscle power is essential to prevent falls. A reaction within milliseconds can reduce the risk of falling.

Application of Whole-body Vibration Therapy in Low Back Pain

The aim of the treatment is to improve the elasticity of paraspinal muscles, and hence the range of motion of the trunk (Table **7**).

Application of Whole-body Vibration Therapy in Weighted Dumbbell Training

Vibration dumbbell systems are less commonly used than the vibration platforms. Vibration dumbbells can be adjusted from 5 to 40 Hz with amplitude of approximately 2.0 mm. From the reflex-provoked muscle contraction arises an increase in strength and power, depending upon the training parameters. Improved inter- and intramuscular coordination occurs due to the nature of the cyclical and fast stimulation. The aim of the oscillatory dumbbells is improved strength of the shoulder and elbow muscles. In a sitting or standing position, grab the dumbbells with both hands with some light pre-tension. The starting position varies depending on pathology. If necessary, the elbow can be flexed and supported on a table (Table **8**).

Table 6. Treatment sequence for the use of whole-body vibration in prevention of falls.

Strength training	*Frequency*: 15-12 Hz. *Duration*: 3-5 minutes. *Amplitude*: medium to high, depending on comfort.	Starting position: exercises out of force and power series alternately. Sets of 10, 3 sets per exercise. 10-to-20-second rest between sets. 1-to-3-minute rest between the sets. Additional weights 70% of individual's maximal strength.
Stretching / balance exercises	*Frequency*: 15-30 Hz. *Duration*: 3-5 minutes for each exercise. *Amplitude*: low to medium.	Starting position: in standing, carry out exercises from balance and stretching series. The number of repetitions is individually tailored. Importantly, the whole body is gradually brought to an end-of-range stretching position. Balance: placing one foot alternately on the lowest position, slightly lift the other foot and hold at 5 Hz without support for 5-30 seconds.
Power training	*Frequency*: 18-30 Hz. *Duration*: 5-6 minutes. *Amplitude*: medium to high.	Carry out exercises without weights, concentrating on speed and changes in direction.

Table 7. Treatment sequence for the use of whole-body vibration in low back pain.

Stretching exercise	*Frequency*: 5-12 Hz. *Duration*: 3-10 minutes.	Standing, ideally not holding on. Bend the knees slightly. Direct vibration into the various body parts. Then bend the torso forwards, backwards, sideways and into rotation. Ideally, maintain the position at the end of range for 3-5 seconds.
Force and power training	*Frequency*: 15-30 Hz. *Duration*: 3-5 minutes for each exercise.	Exercises out of force and power series alternately. In principle exercise examples from balance-series could also be incorporated here.

(Table 7) contd.....

Post-training relaxation	*Frequency*: 5-10 Hz. *Duration*: 1-2 minutes.	Loose, with slightly bent knees and without holding on, move the whole body slightly. Importantly, the soles of the feet must remain completely on the vibration platform.

Table 8. Weighted dumbbell training.

First session	*Frequency*: 5-15 Hz. *Duration*: 1-2 minutes.	Starting position: individually selected. Arm movements: grab the dumbbells completely and move the arms in various directions. Similarly, move the neck and shoulders in various directions.
Strength training	*Frequency*: 18-40 Hz. *Duration*: 15-30 minutes, with 60-second rest each 120 seconds.	Position: weighted pulleys can also be used. The starting position is always individually attained through the examination process. Repetitions: from 2 to 10 repetitions with a 1-minute rest between repetitions. Sets: 2-5 sets with a 3-to-5-minute rest between sets.
Relaxing	*Frequency*: 5-10 Hz. *Duration*: 1-2 minutes.	Relaxed, moving the body gently forwards and backwards with slightly bent knees while not holding on. The soles of the feet must stay fully on the vibration plate.

TREATMENT PROTOCOLS WITH ULTRASOUNDS

Ultrasounds (US) can be delivered in continuous or pulsed mode. In the *continuous mode* the US wave has a constant amplitude, whereas in the *pulsed wave* the pressure amplitude is not constant and is zero for part of the time. In the latter mode, no acoustic energy is being emitted between pulses and the US propagates through the medium as small packages of acoustic energy. Pulsed waves can have any combination of "on"/"off" times. Thus, it is important to specify exactly the time regimen of the pulsed beam. The percentage of "on" time of US output is known as the "duty factor/cycle", which can be expressed as a percentage or as a ratio. Clearly, when output is continuous, the duty factor is 100%; the output must have an "off" time for it to be considered pulsed.

In literature, the use of US in the field of rehabilitation seems to play a minor role (Table **9**); in our experience, we use US as part of integrated protocols among others physical therapies.

Table 9. Summary of US clinical protocols.

Location and condition		Treatment parameters		
		frequency (MHz)	*duty cycle (%)*	*duration (minutes)*
Superficial muscle and/or tendon and/or ligament	subchronic injury	3.3	20	5-7
	chronic injury	3.3	100	5-7
	tissue scar or adhesion	3.3	100	5-7

(Table 9) contd.....

Location and condition		Treatment parameters		
		frequency (MHz)	duty cycle (%)	duration (minutes)
Deep muscle, tendon and/or ligament	subchronic injury	1	20	7-10
	chronic injury	1	100	7-10
	tissue scar or adhesion	1	100	7-10
Joint contracture and/or adhesive capsulitis	superficial joint	3.3	100	5-7
	deep joint	1	100	7-10

In recent years we experienced the use of continuous low-frequency US shock thermic LF Esasound (Table **10**) and of pulsed low-frequency US for the integrated treatment of soft tissue injuries with the following protocols (Table **11**).

Table 10. Therapeutic protocols with the use low-frequency US shock thermic (LF Esasound).

Condition	Treatment parameters		
	frequency (MHz)	duty cycle (%)	duration (minutes)
Low back pain	38	90-100	3-5
Myofascial pain	34	90-100	3-5
Muscular contracture	38	90-100	3-5
Muscular fibrosis	38	90-100	3-5
Edema	38	90-100	3-5
Lymphostasis	30	90-100	3-5
Localized fat deposit	38	90-100	3-5
Scar	30	90-100	3-5

Table 11. Therapeutic protocols with the use low-frequency US.

Condition	Treatment parameters		
	frequency (MHz)	duty cycle (%)	duration (minutes)
Low back pain	40	40-80	15
Myofascial pain	42	40-80	20
Muscular contracture	38	33-75	20 or 30
Muscular fibrosis	38	33-75	30

(Table 11) contd.....

Condition	Treatment parameters		
	frequency (MHz)	duty cycle (%)	duration (minutes)
Edema	42	40-80	15
Lymphostasis	15	50-80	20
Localized fat deposit	15	50-80	30
Scar	38	33-75	5

TREATMENT PROTOCOLS WITH EXTRACORPOREAL SHOCK WAVES

Extracorporeal Shock Waves (ESW) has been widely recognized in literature as a biological regulator on bone, ligament, tendon and muscle tissue. In musculo- skeletal disorders, ESW has been primarily used in the treatment of bone defects (delayed fracture healing, bone nonunion, avascular necrosis of femoral head) and tendinopathies (proximal plantar fasciopathy, lateral elbow tendinopathy, calcific tendinopathy of the shoulder, and patellar tendinopathy). Nowadays, ESW therapy represents a valid tool for a wide range of disorders, both in orthopedics and rehabilitative medicine (tendon pathologies, bone healing disturbances, vascular bone diseases), dermatology and vulnology (wound healing disturbances, ulcers, painful scars) and neurology (spastic hypertonia and related disturbances).

ESW can be generated by electrohydraulic, electromagnetic or piezoelectric methods. The focused shock waves concentrate acoustic energy in a well-defined point, or focal area. The physical parameters that influence treatment response are summarized in the following Table **12**.

Table 12. Therapeutic parameters of ESW therapy.

Treatment parameter	Description
Maximal positive pressure	The maximal positive pressure that is reached
Focal zone	A three-dimensional ellipsoid where the pressure is above a certain value
Energy flux density	The amount of energy per surface unit (expressed in mJ/mm^2)
Impulse frequency	The number of shock waves that is applied per second

The energy level is commonly categorized into three groups depending on the energy flux density [3] (Fig. **6**):

- low-energy ESW, with an energy flux density below 0.08 mJ/mm^2 ;
- medium-energy ESW, with an energy flux density from 0.08 to 0.28 mJ/mm^2;
- high-energy ESW, with an energy flux density from 0.28 to 0.60 mJ/mm^2.

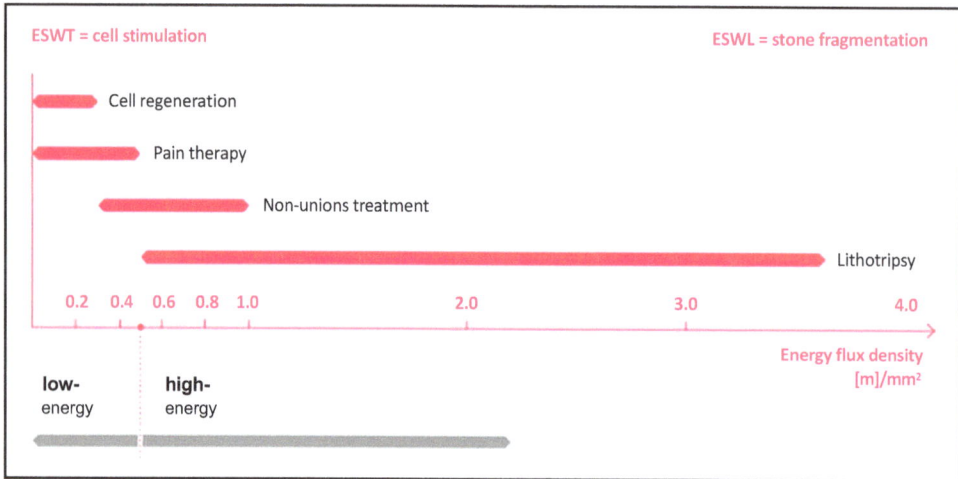

Fig. (6). Fields of application and relative energy levels of shock waves in medicine. ESWL, Extracorporeal Shock Waves Lithotripsy; ESWT, Extracorporeal Shock Waves Therapy.

ESW treatment protocols have not yet been standardized, with significant diversity between the studies in dosages, frequency of applications, density of energy and total energy applied. Other variations in technique include the treatment site and use of anaesthetic injections prior to shock wave application. The lack of standardized protocols in the use of shock waves comes from the variety of devices used, the parameters for the application, the application times that do not allow the comparison between the various studies. Our expertise in the use of shock waves is long lasting and it is the result of clinical practice and research [4 - 7].

From 1998, in our rehabilitation Center we utilize focused ESW generated by an electro-hydraulical source; from 2009 with *Orthogold 100®* (MTS Medical UG, Konstanz, Germany) (Fig. **7**).

Electrohydraulic systems incorporate an electrode, submerged in a water-filled housing composed of an ellipsoid and a patient interface. The electrohydraulic generator initiates the shock wave by an electrical spark produced between the tips of the electrode. Vaporization of the water molecules between the tips of the

electrode produce an explosion, thus creating a spherical shock wave. The wave is then reflected from the inside wall of a metal ellipsoid to create a focal point of shock wave energy in the target tissue. The size and shape of the ellipsoid control the focal size and the amount of energy within the target. Each operator aims to couple the generated pressure pulse to the tissue while minimizing energy loss, concentrating the shock waves so that they can be applied in sufficient quantity to stimulate a desired tissue response. For their clinical use, the head of the shock-wave generators are positioned over the area to be treated, which can be determined on the basis of previous diagnostic images or, if available on the device, by radiographic or US positioning systems. Once the position of the targeting site has been located, the treatment area is prepared with a coupling gel to minimize the loss of shock wave energy at the interface between the head of the device and the skin. The characteristics of the device are the following:

- applicator OE35
    therapeutic focus (-6dB): 0-79 mm
    energy flux density: 0.01- 0.16 mJ/mm^2
    focus energy (E total / -6 dB): 0.34-4.22 mJ
- applicator OE50
    therapeutic focus (- 6dB): 0-62 mm
    energy flux density: 0.03- 0.27 mJ/mm^2
    focus energy (E total / -6 dB): 0.3-6.15 mJ
- dimensions: 21.8 x 40 x 45.9 cm
- power supply: alternating current 100-240 V, 50- 60 Hz
- power input: 200 VA
- repetition rate: 0.5-8 Hz

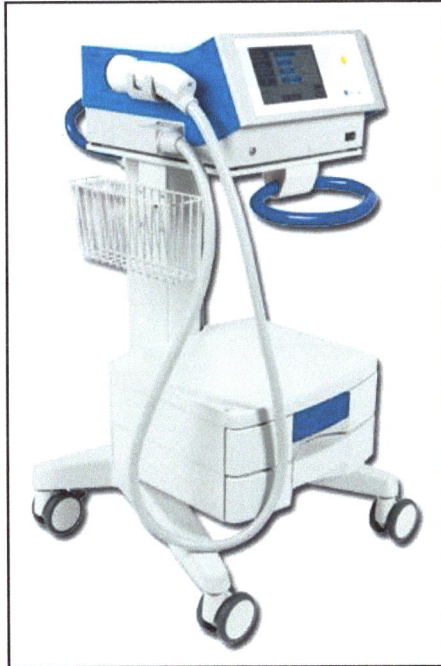

Fig. (7). *Orthogold 100*® (MTS Medical UG, Konstanz, Germany).

ESW in Bone Disorders

Several studies investigated the effects of ESW on acute fracture healing, delayed fracture healing, bone nonunion, and avascular necrosis. Experimental models demonstrate that ESW promotes bone healing through a biological response characterized by the upregulation of local expression of angiogenesis-related growth factors, endothelial nitric oxide synthase, and vascular endothelial growth factor, as well as bone growth factors and morphogenetic proteins. Table **13** summarizes our treatment protocols for bone diseases.

ESW in Tendinopathies

Though supported by clinical data, the validity, effectiveness and reliability of ESW in the treatment of tendinopathies do not always meet the criteria of evidence-based medicine. This is mainly due to an objective difficulty in comparing data from non-homogeneous studies, which have adopted various types of ESW generators, with differing energy parameters and treatment protocols. Nonetheless, the most frequent application of ESW is in the treatment of tendinopathies. Our treatment protocols for tendinopathies are summarized in Table **14**.

Table 13. Treatment protocols for bone diseases with *Orthogold 100*® (MTS Medical UG, Konstanz, Germany).

Condition	Energy flux density	Number of impulses per treatment	Repetition rate	Number of treatment sessions
Non-union, delayed union	0.10-0.17 mJ/mm^2	600-800	6 Hz	1 per week for 4-6 weeks
Stress fracture	0.12-0.19 mJ/mm^2	400 + 400	6 Hz	2 per week for 3-5 weeks
Avascular necrosis	0.14-0.21 mJ/mm^2	700-800	6 Hz	1 per week for 4-6 weeks
Bone marrow edema	0.10-0.21 mJ/mm^2	350 + 350	6 Hz	2 per week for 3-4 weeks

Table 14.   Treatment protocols for tendinopathies with *Orthogold 100*® (MTS Medical UG, Konstanz, Germany).

Condition	Energy flux density	Number of impulses per treatment	Repetition rate	Number of treatment sessions
Calcific tendinopathy of the shoulder	0.17-0.23 mJ/mm^2	600-700	6 Hz	1 per week for 3-5 weeks
Tendonitis of the rotator cuff	0.14-0.21 mJ/mm^2	600-800	6 Hz	1 per week for 3-4 weeks
Lateral epicondylitis	0.12-0.19 mJ/mm^2	600-700	6 Hz	1 per week for 3-4 weeks
Plantar fasciitis	0.15-0.21 mJ/mm^2	600-700	6 Hz	1 per week for 4-5 weeks

ESWT in Skin Pathologies

First investigations on the effect of ESW on wound healing were undertaken in 1986. However, systematic studies (experimental *in vitro* and *in vivo* studies and clinical trials) evaluating the efficacy of low-energy defocused ESW therapy on delayed healing or chronic wounds have only been performed in recent years. Nowadays, ESWT has become increasingly popular and it become accepted in scientific world. Successful application has been reported in the peer-reviewed literature for numerous medical indications. Despite this encouraging progress, the biomolecular mechanisms by which shock waves exert their positive clinical effects are yet to be completely understood. Advantages of ESW include: (1) non-invasiveness (avoidance of surgery); (2) low associated complication rates (*e.g.*, minimal petechial skin hemorrhage and hematoma); (3) efficacy for indications refractory to other standards of practice (*e.g.*, bone nonunion); (4) flat learning curve; and (5) cost-effectiveness.

Possible treatment of pathologic, retracting scars currently includes several options, such as intralesional corticosteroids, cryotherapy, dermabrasion, excision and scar revision surgery, laser therapy and radiation therapy; likewise, prophylactic strategies may include variable combinations of compression therapy, silicone gel and oral supplements such as flavonoids. Nonetheless, retractive scarring is characterized by a complex etiology related to both local and systemic factors, and the efficacy rate of available treatments is still far from satisfactory. As a consequence, treatment of pathologic scars often requires lengthy and expensive procedures, posing the need for clinical studies aimed at the development of novel therapeutic strategies for pathologic scarring. Saggini *et al.* support the role of ESW as an emerging option for the treatment of painful, retracting scars [8]; administration of ESW appears to result in significant improvements in scar clinical appearance, hand mobility and subjective pain.

In the cited studies chronic ulcer and retracting scars of skin were treated with unfocused ESWT probe with electrohydraulical ESW system *Dermagold 100*® (MTS Medical UG, Konstanz, Germany) (Fig. **8**).

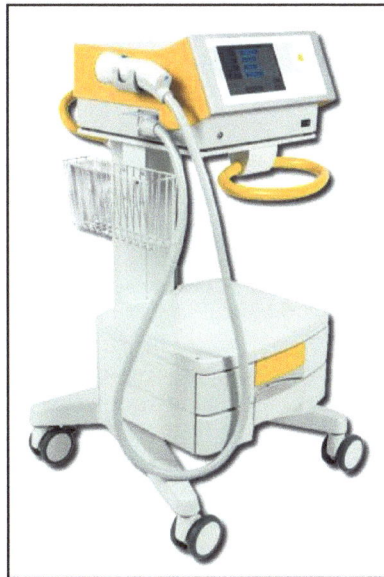

Fig. (8). *Dermagold 100*® (MTS Medical UG, Konstanz, Germany).

The characteristics of the device are the following:

- applicator OP155
- therapeutic Focus (-6dB): 0-82 mm
- energy flux density: 0.01-0.19 mJ/mm^2
- focus energy (E total / -6dB): 0.40- 3.88 mJ
- dimensions: 21.8 x 40 x 45.9 cm
- power supply: alternating current 100- 240 V, 50-60 Hz
- power input: 200 VA
- repetition rate: 0.5-8 Hz

Our treatment protocols for chronic ulcers of skin are summarized in Table **15**.

Table 15. Treatment protocols for chronic ulcers of the skin and retracting scars with *Dermagold 100*® (MTS Medical UG, Konstanz, Germany).

Condition	Energy flux density	Number of impulses per treatment	Repetition rate	Number of treatment sessions
Chronic ulcer	0.09-0.11 mJ/mm^2	300-500	4-6 Hz	2 per week for 5 weeks
Retracting scar	0.10-0.13 mJ/mm^2	500-600	4-6 Hz	2 per week for 4-5 weeks

CONFLICT OF INTEREST

The authors confirm that they have no conflict of interest to declare for this publication.

ACKNOWLEDGEMENTS

Declared none.

REFERENCES

[1]   Saggini R, Bellomo RG, Cancelli F, Iodice P. Treatment on myofascial pain syndromes: local acoustic vibration vs local lidocaine injection. J Musculoskel Pain. Haworth Medical Press Publ 2007; (Suppl. 13)15.

[2]   Saggini R, Iodice P, Galati V, Marri A, Bellomo RG. Treatment on myofascial pain syndromes: local selective acoustic vibration vs lidocaine injection. J Rehabil Med 2008; (Suppl. 47)94.

[3]   Rompe JD, Kirkpatrick CJ, Küllmer K, Schwitalle M, Krischek O. Dose-related effects of shock waves on rabbit tendo Achillis. A sonographic and histological study. J Bone Joint Surg Br 1998; 80(3): 546-52.
[http://dx.doi.org/10.1302/0301-620X.80B3.8434] [PMID: 9619954]

[4]   Romeo P, Lavanga V, Pagani D, Sansone V. Extracorporeal shock wave therapy in musculoskeletal disorders: a review. Med Princ Pract 2014; 23(1): 7-13.
[http://dx.doi.org/10.1159/000355472] [PMID: 24217134]

[5]   Ioppolo F, Rompe JD, Furia JP, Cacchio A. Clinical application of shock wave therapy (SWT) in musculoskeletal disorders. Eur J Phys Rehabil Med 2014; 50(2): 217-30.

[PMID: 24667365]

[6]   Saggini R, Di Stefano A, Saggini A, Bellomo RG. Clinical application of shock wave therapy in musculoskeletal disorders: part I. J Biol Regul Homeost Agents 2015; 29(3): 533-45.
        [PMID: 26403392]

[7]   Saggini R, Di Stefano A, Saggini A, Bellomo RG. Clinical application of shock wave therapy in musculoskeletal disorders: part II related to myofascial and nerve apparatus. J Biol Regul Homeost Agents 2015; 29(4): 771-85.
        [PMID: 26753637]

[8]   Saggini R, Saggini A, Spagnoli AM, *et al.* Extracorporeal Shock Wave Therapy: An Emerging Treatment Modality for Retracting Scars of the Hands. Ultrasound Med Biol 2016; 42(1): 185-95.
        [http://dx.doi.org/10.1016/j.ultrasmedbio.2015.07.028] [PMID: 26454624]

SUBJECT INDEX

A

Absorption characteristics 221
Absorption coefficients 99
Achilles tendinopathy 190, 195, 196, 201
Acoustic energy 102, 104, 115, 116, 249, 251
  small packages of 104, 249
Acoustic excitation frequency 112
Acoustic impedance 93, 94, 95, 97, 109, 151, 182
Acoustic pressures 113, 117
  applied 113
Acoustic streaming 106, 115
Acoustic waves 1, 4, 7, 14, 61, 62, 96, 116, 153, 181, 185
  so-modified 61, 62
Action of shock waves 186
Action potential (AP) 28, 50, 57, 141
Adipose tissue cavitation effect 147
Afferent fibers 36, 37, 58
Afferent neuron 28
Alpha motoneurons 37
Alternating current (AC) 226, 253, 256
Amplitude-modulated EMF 230
Angiogenesis 131, 143, 144, 187, 192, 200
Angle of incidence 97
Application 23, 48, 49, 54, 57, 58, 93, 100, 101, 117, 121, 122, 123, 124, 130, 132, 133, 136, 139, 142, 144, 145, 149, 150, 151, 154, 155, 180, 184, 186, 193, 205, 232, 243, 245, 247, 248, 252, 254, 255
  direct 123, 154
  frequent 254
Applications 66, 87, 107, 123, 145, 153, 155, 179, 181, 202, 218, 225, 231, 241
  aesthetic 87, 145
  clinical 155, 179, 181, 202
  potential 66, 218, 225, 231
  therapeutic 107, 123, 153, 241
Application times 122, 252
Audible sound frequencies 5
Avascular necrosis 231, 251, 253, 254
Average 102, 103, 127, 128
  spatial 102, 103, 127, 128
  temporal 102

B

Balance 24, 47, 57, 110, 121, 246, 247, 248
  homeostatic 24
Balance series 247
Bands, frequency modulation 222
Beam energy 94, 97
Beam nonuniformity ratio (BNR) 107, 108
Behaviour, elastic 3, 4
Biochemical substance 187
Biological media 94
Biopolymers 109, 116
Blackman 225, 226, 231
Blood flow 109, 110, 111
Blood vessels 26, 94, 95, 99, 123, 149
Body 20, 21, 24, 38, 40, 46, 52, 61, 64, 97, 98, 145, 149, 185, 187, 220, 223, 228, 245, 247, 248, 249
Body parts 33, 121, 247, 248
Body positions 35, 36, 224
Body surface 30, 32, 33, 121, 122, 185
Body tissues 21
Bone 4, 24, 38, 41, 42, 43, 44, 49, 50, 51, 52, 94, 95, 97, 99, 110, 125, 126, 129, 130, 131, 186, 187, 188, 190, 196, 202, 203, 243, 251
  biological effects of US on 129
Bone cells 188, 197
Bone diseases 179, 180, 253, 254
  treatment protocols for 253, 254
Bone disorders 186, 188, 253
Bone formation 127, 197
Bone growth 126, 127
Bone healing 128, 129, 194, 195, 253
  delayed 194, 195
Bone healing disturbances 180, 197, 202, 251
Bone mass 24, 52
Bone nonunion 251, 253, 255
Bones and skin 94, 190
Bone tissue 49, 50, 51, 99, 126
Bosu ball 243, 245
Bubble growth 113
Bubbles 113, 114, 117, 182
  single 114
Bulk module 20

www.ingramcontent.com/pod-product-compliance
Lightning Source LLC
Chambersburg PA
CBHW041725210326
41598CB00008B/785